Trauma Practice

# About the Authors

**Anna B. Baranowsky**, PhD, CPsych, is a registered clinical psychologist and the founder and director of Traumatology Institute (Canada). She was instrumental in developing training materials for the Traumatology Institute Training Curriculum (TITC). She is the developer of www.psychink.com, the e-learning site for TITC; the Trauma Recovery Program – self-guided online trauma informed care (http://www.whatisptsd.com/trauma-care-online); the 30-day video stabilization program (http://www.whatisptsd.com/find-calm/); and the WhatIs PTSD YouTube channel, filled with tips and tools for trauma recovery (https://youtube.com/whatisptsd). She is the clinical director of Bear Psychology in Toronto, Ontario Canada (https://annabaranowsky.com) with her talented team of clinicians and a remarkable and dedicated administrative team.

Dr. Baranowsky received her doctorate in clinical psychology from the University of Ottawa, Canada. Her accomplishments include the co-development of the Accelerated Recovery Program (ARP) for Compassion Fatigue, national and international presentations on the ARP, trauma assessment, treatment, and interventions. She has published in the area of posttraumatic stress disorder, secondary traumatization, compassion fatigue, the ARP, and therapeutic relationships (the silencing response). Dr. Baranowsky served on the Board of Directors of the Academy of Traumatology's Commission on Certification and Accreditation. She has been recognized by the American Academy of Experts in Traumatic Stress with Diplomate status and is a board-certified expert in traumatic stress.

Dr. Baranowsky dedicates a large portion of her clinical practice on the emotional well-being of trauma survivors. She has been trained in many cutting-edge trauma treatments now being recognized as highly effective in resolving the emotional aftermath of exposure to trauma and works with a wide range of trauma survivors, from airplane crash survivors to victims of violence as well as first responders at trauma scenes. Her dedication to the emotional recovery of survivors is demonstrated by her passion for training and supervising professionals working on skills development in the field of trauma informed care. For information contact: office@annabaranowsky.com

The Trauma Practice for Healthy Communities is a charitable organization that she launched in 2017. Since that time TPHC has provided thousands of direct client service hours using a trauma informed care model for those in need. This has been particularly crucial during the COVID-19 Pandemic in 2020–2021 where services have been provided virtually for those isolated, while struggling with post-traumatic stress. For details visit: https://traumapractice.org

**J. Eric Gentry**, PhD, LMHC, is an internationally recognized leader in the study and treatment of traumatic stress and compassion fatigue. His PhD is from Florida State University where he studied with Professor Charles Figley – a pioneer of these two fields. In 1997, he co-developed the Accelerated Recovery Program (ARP) for Compassion Fatigue – the world's only evidence-based treatment protocol for compassion fatigue. In 1998, he introduced the Certified Compassion Fatigue Specialist Training and Compassion Fatigue Prevention & Resiliency Training. These two trainings have demonstrated treatment effectiveness for the symptoms of compassion fatigue, and he published these effects in several journals. He has trained over 100,000 health professionals over the past 25 years.

Dr. Gentry was original faculty, curriculum designer, and Associate Director of the Traumatology Institute at Florida State University. In 2001, he became the co-director and moved this institute to the University of South Florida where it became the International Traumatology Institute. In 2010, he began the International Association of Trauma Professionals. He is currently the co-owner and vice president of the Arizona Trauma Institute/Trauma Institute International.

*Forward-Facing® Trauma Therapy: Healing the Moral Wound*, a landmark text for re-imaging trauma treatment, was published in 2016. *Forward-Facing® Professional Resilience* detailing the evidence-based practices for developing resilience and professional well-being was published in 2020. *Forward-Facing® Freedom: Healing the Past, Transforming the Present and a Future on Purpose* is the book that will introduce Forward-Facing® practices to the lay public was published in 2021. In 2005, Hogrefe and Huber published *Trauma Practice: Tools for Stabilization and Recovery* – a critically acclaimed text on the treatment of traumatic stress for which Dr. Gentry is a co-author. The Second Edition was released in 2010 and the Third Edition in 2015. *Professional Resilience: Helping Doesn't Have to Hurt*, a compassion workbook for the Professional Resilience and Optimization Workshop was published in 2017. *Transformative Care: A Trauma-Focused Approach to Caregiving* was published in 2018. He is the author of numerous chapters, papers, and peer-reviewed journal articles in the areas of traumatic stress and compassion fatigue. In 2021, He co-authored *Trauma Competency for the 21st Century: A Salutogenic Approach*. In 2022, Dr. Gentry co-authored *Forward-Facing for Educators: A Journey to Professional Resilience and Compassion Restoration* and published the Second Edition of *Forward-Facing Trauma Therapy: Healing the Moral Wound*.

Dr. Gentry is owner of Compassion Unlimited, LLC - a private coaching, training, and consulting practice - that he began in Tampa., FL in 2004 and is now in Phoenix, AZ.

In 2020, Dr. Gentry incorporated the Forward-Facing Institute, LLC. This institute provides training, consultation, and credentialing in all things Forward-Facing.

# Trauma Practice

A Cognitive Behavioral Somatic Therapy

4th edition

**Anna B. Baranowsky, PhD, CPsych**

**J. Eric Gentry, PhD, LMHC**

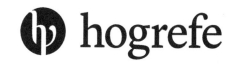

**Library of Congress of Congress Cataloging in Publication** information for the print version of this book is available via the Library of Congress Marc Database under the Library of Congress Control Number 2022949918

**Library and Archives Canada Cataloguing in Publication**

Title: Trauma practice : a cognitive behavioral somatic therapy / Anna B. Baranowsky, PhD, CPsych, J. Eric Gentry, PhD, LMHC.

Names: Baranowsky, Anna B., author. | Gentry, J. Eric, author.

Description: 4th edition. | Includes bibliographical references and index.

Identifiers: Canadiana (print) 20220470391 | Canadiana (ebook) 20220470456 | ISBN 9780889375925 (softcover) | ISBN 9781616765927 (PDF) | ISBN 9781613345924 (EPUB)

Subjects: LCSH: Post-traumatic stress disorder—Treatment. | LCSH: Psychic trauma—Treatment.

Classification: LCC RC552.P67 B37 2023 | DDC 616.85/2106—dc23

© 2023 by Hogrefe Publishing

www.hogrefe.com

The authors and publisher have made every effort to ensure that the information contained in this text is in accord with the current state of scientific knowledge, recommendations, and practice at the time of publication. In spite of this diligence, errors cannot be completely excluded. Also, due to changing regulations and continuing research, information may become outdated at any point. The authors and publisher disclaim any responsibility for any consequences which may follow from the use of information presented in this book.

Registered trademarks are not noted specifically as such in this publication. The use of descriptive names, registered names, and trademarks does not imply, even in the absence of a specific statement, that such names are exempt from the relevant protective laws and regulations and therefore free for general use.

Cover image: © Yuliia Khvyshchuk 14jan092017 – iStock.com

PUBLISHING OFFICES

USA:    Hogrefe Publishing Corporation, 44 Merrimac Street, Suite 207, Newburyport, MA 01950
        Phone (978) 255 3700; E-mail customersupport@hogrefe.com

EUROPE: Hogrefe Publishing GmbH, Merkelstr. 3, 37085 Göttingen, Germany
        Phone +49 551 99950 0, Fax +49 551 99950 111; E-mail publishing@hogrefe.com

SALES & DISTRIBUTION

USA:    Hogrefe Publishing, Customer Services Department,
        30 Amberwood Parkway, Ashland, OH 44805
        Phone (800) 228 3749, Fax (419) 281 6883; E-mail customersupport@hogrefe.com

UK:     Hogrefe Publishing, c/o Marston Book Services Ltd., 160 Eastern Ave.,
        Milton Park, Abingdon, OX14 4SB
        Phone +44 1235 465577, Fax +44 1235 465556; E-mail direct.orders@marston.co.uk

EUROPE: Hogrefe Publishing, Merkelstr. 3, 37085 Göttingen, Germany
        Phone +49 551 99950 0, Fax +49 551 99950 111; E-mail publishing@hogrefe.com

OTHER OFFICES

CANADA:       Hogrefe Publishing Corporation, 82 Laird Drive, East York, Ontario M4G 3V1

SWITZERLAND:  Hogrefe Publishing, Länggass-Strasse 76, 3012 Bern

Printed and bound in the USA

ISBN 978-0-88937-592-5 (print) • ISBN 978-1-61676-592-7 (PDF) • ISBN 978-1-61334-592-4 (EPUB)
http://doi.org/10.1027/00592-000

# Foreword

This book, *Trauma Practice: A Cognitive Behavioral Somatic Therapy (CBST)*, represents a new generation of resources for traumatologists – those who study or treat the traumatized. A good indication of this comes in the first few chapters of background and history, because by now the assessment and treatment of the traumatized are far from novel.

Today we know that traumatic stress treatments work. We know that learning how to attend gently to our inner fear response with acceptance and compassion combined with exposure to the conditioned (fear) stimulus are critical elements to resolution of traumatic stress symptoms or active ingredients. We also know that a person's ability to tolerate exposure to what they fear varies greatly and that it is counterproductive, if not a breach of professional standards of practice, to not offer gentle ways for individuals to reach a therapeutic threshold for such exposure.

We know today that iatrogenic effects of trauma therapy are real and that practitioners must be extraordinarily cautious when interviewing a patient, developing a treatment plan, and ensuring that there is sufficient safety as well as retraumatization containment strategies. Remission is expected and, therefore, relapse prevention training is a requirement.

We also know that the individual presentation and assessment of traumatized persons is not an exact science. Extraordinary events that would traumatize most people have little effect on some. Conversely, exposure to rather noxious stimuli can cause extraordinary traumatic stress reactions for others. Children tend to appear rather hardy springing back with less apparent negative effects. Their parents, on the other hand, have lingering symptoms. Although women present as more symptomatic, a desire to be seen as emotionally and psychologically well may be a more significant motivator in male than female patients. However, war-related PTSD is actually less frequently seen in women than men. This may be a factor related to women harnessing social support within a community setting during times of strain.

Clients with PTSD can pose unique clinical challenges to the practitioner. Most PTSD patients, for example, are dual diagnosed. It is rare to find clients with PTSD who do *not* have at least one additional diagnosis (i.e., panic disorder, somatic symptom disorder, depression, borderline personality disorder, addiction, etc). It is also important to recognize that a common comorbidity exists with addictions (drug dependency) and PTSD.

This important book both addresses what we know today at a theoretical level and, equally importantly, explains clinical methods in the context of treatment. More than the typical book about why and how the cognitive behavioral treatment approaches work, Baranowsky and Gentry offer a comprehensive guide for clinicians working with the traumatized. This book presents clear instructions to traumatologists – even the most experienced in working with the traumatized – to help the traumatized. The guidance is detailed. The authors direct practitioners to focus on symptoms of the body as well as on behavior and emotions associated with trauma. They also link their guidance to a tri-phasic treatment model that starts with establishing Safety, continues with Working through Trauma, and ends with Reconnection. This book is also an excellent resource for trainers, teachers, and educators of trauma practitioners, providing a how-to manual to address the challenges of clinical traumatology.

These authors represent the current and future generation of clinical traumatologists who are well-equipped to handle the extraordinary challenges of traumatized clients. We have come a long way in nearly thirty years, as illustrated by this useful book.

*Charles R. Figley, PhD*
*Florida State University Traumatology Institute*
*Tallahassee, November 2022*

# Acknowledgments

**Anna B. Baranowsky** – To my beloved parents who taught me love and life exist even after terrible losses. To my dear husband Chris, my compassionate warrior and companion in all life's joys. For Cassie, Jasper and Sukhi, who have enriched my every waking day. To Gold and the Golds, who are special in my heart; to Zahava, who showed me that love, strength, and intelligence live harmoniously together; to my dear Maj buddies; my incredibly talented team (Tamara, Betty Ann, Usha, Sandy, the BPPC, Ya'ara, and Jaime of the Trauma Practice Team). I am deeply fortunate to have found myself surrounded by incredible people. Without them I would be unable to dedicate my life to this work. In appreciation of Dr. Michael McCarrey, my ally and supervisor (University of Ottawa). To Marlene Mawhinney and B. K. S Iyengar, my yoga teachers of over 30 years, whose work has brought me the harmony and resiliency, which has enabled me to follow the call to trauma work.

I am grateful to Dr. Charles Figley for laying fertile ground at just the perfect time. To my friend and inspiration, Eric, who willingly joins me in challenging dialog and laughter. Mostly, to my clients, students, trainers, and friends over the years who have taught me more than they could imagine and helped me stay humble and continue to learn and grow... I am grateful.

**J. Eric Gentry** – Thanks go to the mentors in my life in order of their appearance: Charles "Charlie" Yeargan, PhD; Louis Tinnin, MD; Charles Figley, PhD; and Joseph Moore. Gratitude to N. A. and H. P. for keeping me alive long enough to write this work. Thanks to my support, in no particular order: Marjie, Jeffrey "Jim" Dietz, MD, Mike Dubi Mom, Bubbita, Augie, Rick O., Helen MaryJoan, PDR, Mason, Rosalina, TZap, Jennifer, Connor, Frank, Jim "Big Bro" Norman, Carlos & family, Eduardo & Maria, Jim Hussey, Joe Williams, Nacho & Lucy, ITI Site Directors, Sheryl Hakala, MD, Mason Hines & family, and my family. A special mention of gratitude for the creative and supportive relationship that I share with Anna – you are the BEST! I dedicate this text to all my clients and trainees – past, present, and future.

# Dedication

This text is dedicated to unsung heroes, the caregivers who maintain the courage and the stamina to bear witness to the stories and selves of trauma survivors, making healing a reality.

*See first that you yourself deserve to be a giver,*
*and an instrument of giving.*
*For in truth it is life that gives unto life –*
*while you, who deem yourself a giver,*
*are but a witness.*

Khalil Gibran

# Contents

# Introduction to Trauma Practice: A Cognitive Behavioral Somatic Therapy

*If you are perfect you don't need to learn anything
and if you don't need to learn anything, you wouldn't need to be a teacher.*

Stuart Wilde, *The Secrets of Life (1990)*

## The surprising act of arriving at 2023

After living through the unprecedented events of the COVID-19 pandemic, revelations of an encouraged white supremist mob, and the real cruelty to brown and black lives, my sense about the importance of human kindness, courage, and trauma-informed care has been reinforced. I could never imagine all of the complex layers of the last three years unfolding, but what I am aware of is the ongoing need for the use of the right tools, the ones that guide those in need toward their own growth and healing. After all, when you and I heal we are less likely to react from a place of fear and rigidity and more from a place of wisdom and kindness. At least that is what I have witnessed over the past 20 years of helping trauma survivors.

Since the last edition of *Trauma Practice* there has been awareness of post-trauma care. The public has become more educated on the need for specialized trauma-informed care and that clinicians need precise training in order to attend to trauma impact. It has been more than seven years since the authors collaborated together on *Trauma Practice*, yet independently we seem to have arrived at a similar place in terms of the meaning of our work, the new refinements in our field, and our sense of how to move the trauma practice approach forward. Although there are some differences in the use of language, the overall approach appreciates the need to face the ever-present moment and use it as the gift for growth while down-regulating the body to stay present and extinguish the past.

This is no regular revised edition but rather our 20-year anniversary edition! We are excited, grateful and humbled to announce our 21st year of offering *Trauma Practice* to you, our readers. We published the first edition of *Trauma Practice: Tools for Stabilization and Recovery* in 2001. Over twenty years later, this is our fourth publication of this book. We have heard from hundreds of you, kind folks, providing feedback about how much this book has assisted you in helping trauma survivors to recover from their painful history and begin to live lives of choice instead of continuing to live in fear and self-defense. It has been joyful for us to contribute to your growth as clinicians and to our field's growth in treating trauma survivors using gentler, more effective and accelerated methods of healing. We have matured along with you and we are excited to share our combined 60 years of experience with you in this, our 4th edition.

Since the publication of the previous edition of *Trauma Practice*, much has changed in the field of trauma treatment. The organic emergence of complex posttraumatic stress disorder (C-PTSD) as something distinctly different from PTSD, and the demand for more sophisticated clinicians and treatment strategies for these clients has been a powerful catalyst for the evolution of our field. The discovery that traditional evidence-based treatments, driven by narrative exposure and cognitive processing, were not sufficiently effective for clients with C-PTSD (and in some cases exacerbated symptoms) has led to an awakening among clinicians working with this population. Teaching somatic (in previous texts simply referred to as body) self-regulatory skills – which we have advocated in each previous edition of this book – has become a primary focus of early treatment when working with C-PTSD. As our clients develop competency with these skills of self-regulation and threat response interruption, we can then coach them to take these skills into their personal and professional lives to confront the plethora of perceived and real threats they encounter each day.

We have re-discovered the use of in vivo and imaginal exposure (Wolpe knew this in the 1950s) as a powerful mechanism for activating reciprocal inhibition that desensitizes and, ultimately, extinguishes intrusion and arousal caused by the trauma exposure (Criterion A in the DSM-5), including childhood attachment trauma. For us, the power and utility of in vivo and imaginal exposure paired with intentional self-regulation has become an essential triage for the treatment of *all* traumatic stress. We have discovered that teaching self-regulation skills early in treatment and then coaching our survivor clients to begin the process of confronting situations of perceived threat (instead of engaging the instinctual self-defense of avoidance in these contexts) provide a rapid relief of symptoms while simultaneously significantly augmenting well-being, a sense of accomplishment, and improved quality of life.

Thankfully, there has been an increased emphasis on addressing the somatic effects of trauma. For many, this somatic posttrauma impact metastasizes into instinctual procedural or "muscle" memory patterns of self-defense employed in situations where there is little or no danger (only perceived threat). In order to properly update this version of *Trauma Practice* we have begun to reference our approach as *Trauma Practice: A Cognitive Behavioral Somatic Therapy* (or CBST). In previous editions, where we have labeled the somatic response and related interventions as "body" interventions, in this edition we are now identifying them as "somatic-based" interventions. So, for this edition, interventions will include: cognitive, behavioral, somatic, and emotion-relational categories.

In addition to the emergence of C-PTSD as a catalyst for trauma treatment maturation over the past several years, there are many other phenomenon that have emerged that have also spurred us forward. The research by the Centers for Disease Control and Prevention (CDC) and Kaiser Permanente captured the original Adverse Childhood Experiences (ACE) data from 1995 to 1997. The reverberations and understandings of the ACE studies are now taking a more central role on reflections of lifetime trauma impact and posttrauma treatment. We have now witnessed that most of our clients have ACE scores above 5. This has led us to consider how much trauma contributes to the etiology of adult PTSD and other mental diseases and disorders. There are many clinicians that are discovering much of the distress experienced by our clients can be traced to an over-activation of their sympathetic nervous systems (SNS). We are also discovering that treating this over-active threat response with self-regulation is diminishing distress and enhancing quality of life with clients who have a trauma history but had actually been diagnosed with mood disorders or another psychiatric condition.

In 2017, we (along with Robert Rhoton, PsyD), published the article "Trauma Competency: An Active Ingredients Approach to Treating Posttraumatic Stress Disorder" in the *Journal of Counseling and Development*. In this article, we explored the integration of the "active ingredients/common factors" among *all* effective trauma treatment into a phased delivery that is fitted to the survivor's relational and processing style. This has been a focus of many researchers in the field of trauma treatment – looking for generic treatments that do not require adherence to treatment manuals and that are, instead, tailored to fit the individual needs of each client struggling with posttraumatic stress. In our article, we review several of the meta-analyses that have been conducted with evidence-based treatments for PTSD and have found four primary ingredients/factors embedded in each of these effective treatments. These are: (1) a good therapeutic relationship (using Miller's feedback informed treatment; Black et al., 2017; Duncan et al., 2010; Miller et al., 2015, 2020), (2) relaxation/self-regulation, (3) exposure (in vivo and imaginal), and (4) cognitive restructuring/psychoeducation. The intentional engagement and integration of these factors into a phased delivery with our clients, represents the nascent offering of a generic equivalent to evidence-based, manual-driven treatment. For sure, more research will be required before we can pronounce this delivery of the active ingredients/common factors as an evidence-based treatment, but we have found much success in our own application of these skills and principles with our clients.

The 2021 publication of *Trauma Competency for the 21st Century: A Salutogenic Active Ingredients Approach to Treatment* (Rhoton & Gentry, 2021) provides a deeper contemporary dive into these issues. In the first half of the book, the history and utilization of each of the four active ingredients/common factors is explored within current treatment models. In the second half, the salutogenic trauma treatment structure is presented as a semi-structured phased delivery for these factors. The four stages for delivery of treatment in the salutogenic trauma treatment structure are: (1) preparation and relationship-building, (2) psychoeducation and self-regulation (skills-building), (3) integration and desensitization, and (4) posttraumatic growth and resilience. *Trauma Compentency*, also addresses clinician preparation as the first and primary intervention for trauma treatment.

Inspired by the work on *Trauma Competency*, this edition of *Trauma Practice*, has been updated and augmented to include the discussion of the active ingredients/common factors from these recent developments.

In 1997, during our early collaborative efforts, we began to develop products and protocols for compassion fatigue treatment and professional resilience (i.e., accelerated recovery program for compassion fatigue) and are consensual with the a priori importance of clinician preparation as the bedrock of effective trauma treatment. Add to this the recent development of a body of research around "deliberate practice" as a primary means for augmenting treatment outcomes (Chow et al., 2015; Rousmaniere, 2016). Our instincts were later affirmed by the current researchers, (i.e., Miller et al., 2013, 2016, 2020) who, for the past decade, have identified the potency of individual therapist's preparation and on-going development as an important predictor of positive change in clients.

Individual therapist effects account for between 5–9 times more of the outcome variable than the difference between theory and techniques (Baldwin & Imel, 2013; Firth et al., 2019; Wampold & Imel, 2015). Embracing this contemporary research, we have addressed this important factor by adding a Phase 0 (or pre-phase) to the triphasic presentation of interventions in this book. In Phase 0, we focus upon the importance of trauma-specific training – beyond that of only developing expertise in any particular evidence-based model for treatment. We advocate that trauma clinicians develop expertise in also delivering the four active ingredients *inside* the models which they use. We also argue that a crucial clinician capacity is the ability to self-regulate the sympathetic nervous system so that they are able to remain ventral vagal dominant throughout their encounter with clients. This capacity is both catalytic for positive change with our clients (i.e., produces co-regulation and secure attachment) while, simultaneously, affording us *de facto* professional resilience – you cannot get (secondarily) traumatized while remaining in a relaxed-muscle body. In addition to these benefits, self-regulation also maximizes our cognitive and motor functioning, helping to optimize our performance with each client. In Phase 0 we also discuss the importance of on-going personal and professional development, consultation, connection/support, and self-care/revitalization.

We are also excited to add to this edition an exploration of the important work of Lawrence Calhoun and Richard Tedeschi (1996) who have been quietly working away for the past 25 years on one of the most important

discoveries in the field of trauma treatment – posttraumatic growth. In their 2013 book *Posttraumatic Growth in Clinical Practice,* the researchers invite the move away from treating the "disease" of PTSD or even the symptoms and, instead, advocate a coaching process of helping trauma survivors suffering from either acute stress or posttraumatic stress to acquire resilience and growth-catalyzing skills, practices, and perceptions. This evidence-based protocol has helped thousands of survivors to lessen the effects of trauma in their lives and begin to find effective living here in the present. Posttraumatic growth and Forward-Facing® trauma therapy (introduced in the previous edition of this book) are both *salutogenic* approaches to the treatment of trauma.

The allopathic – or medical model – of treatment focuses upon the diagnosis of disease and then using prescribed treatments that have demonstrated effectiveness for a particular diagnosis. In contrast, Salutogenic approaches eschew (at least initially) the medical model treatment focus on disease and instead attempt to immediately catalyze and address the impediments to health. With trauma survivors the primary impediment to health seems to be their chronically activated threat response – *it is difficult to heal and repair while we are busy surviving our lives.* By helping trauma survivors to develop skills and practices that interrupt and then minimize the activation of their threat responses throughout the day, we have found their symptoms begin to ameliorate and their sense of comfort and well-being flourish in a relatively short amount of time. In this volume, we suggest that these salutogenic approaches may prove themselves to become increasingly useful in the treatment of trauma, especially in early treatment, as mentioned before, and as part of a generic triage process for everyone.

For many, it will be sufficient to aid individuals to acquire self-regulation skills along with the capacity to face in vivo and imaginal exposure to life stressors. This alone, can be the main step toward a personal and deep shift in self-care and the beginning a life-long process of independent healing. There will be, of course, trauma survivors whose symptoms remain recalcitrant to this self-engaged solution and will need more traditional phased trauma treatment with ongoing imaginal exposure approaches. However, even these clients with high acuity symptoms will benefit moving into this more intensive therapy with the capacity to self-regulate their own autonomic nervous systems (ANS).

This edition also brings to the forefront probably the *most* important emergence in the treatment of trauma over the past decade and that is the polyvagal theory. Although Stephen Porges has been busy developing this work since the late 1980s, it has become increasingly central to working with traumatic stress over the past several years. The polyvagal theory provides a framework to understand the neurophysiology of traumatic stress both for the clinician and the survivor. While the research and depth of understanding is quite complex, it can be tooled into a simple understanding. Specifically, how traumatic stress and the subsequent self-defense behaviors manifest in those suffering with posttraumatic stress. This edition incorporates the use of the polyvagal theory to understand the dual-polar and biphasic nature of traumatic stress, contrasting arousal vs. shut-down. It also provides a platform for understanding the neurobiology of relationships, or as Porges states: "All relationships are a neural exercise" (Porges, 2018, April 23) Teaching clinicians both self-regulation and then co-regulation immediately augments their effectiveness and resilience.

Finally, for this edition we have updated and overhauled our references and citations to provide you with the latest and relevant clinical research for use in your practice. We are extremely grateful to our dedicated readers whose continued interest in our work have allowed us to continue to bring these materials to each of you. As such we are able to continue to carry out our mission of the past 20 years: to help those who help trauma survivors. It is a privilege for us to provide this text. In great appreciation, thank you for joining us in this work.

**Anna B. Baranowsky, PhD, CPsych.**
**J. Eric Gentry, PhD, LMHC, DAAETS, FAAETS**

## Purpose of This Book

This book has been written for the trained clinician and the novice-in-training as a means of enhancing skilled application of cognitive behavioral somatic trauma therapy (CBST). The term *trauma practice* was conceptualized after many years of reflection on the trauma work and training experiences that the authors have encountered. It became clear to us that a practical approach was needed for practitioners who apply themselves in the field of trauma treatment. Recent books and current research on CBT or CBST for trauma stabilization and recovery are focused more on outcome than application and we have made it our mission to produce a practical "how-to" text. In addition, this text draws upon the development and implementation of many trauma training programs that have been ongoing since the fall of 1997 through the Traumatology Institute. We have been training students in trauma

recovery within this CBST trauma therapy framework and have found both a great need for and a warm response to this very practical approach.

This book will provide both the novice and advanced trauma therapist with much of the knowledge and skills necessary to begin utilizing CBST in their treatment of trauma survivors. In addition to presenting a foundational understanding of the theoretical tenets of CBST, this book will also provide step-by-step explanations of many popular and effective techniques of CBST. Some of these techniques include: trigger list development, breath training, layering, systematic desensitization, exposure therapy, storytelling-approaches, assertiveness training, thematic map, and relaxation training. The book is packed with practical approaches that we have used with our clients for many years. In this updated edition, we have replaced some less useful approaches with interventions that have proven more effective with clients and students of the Traumatology Institute. We also include approaches inspired by current research on neuroplasticity (i.e., picture positive, corrective messages from old storylines, and hands over heart space).

The materials in this book are organized and presented from the perspective of the tri-phasic model (Herman, 1992) for the treatment of trauma. In 2000, the International Society for Traumatic Stress Studies (ISTSS) adopted Herman's tri-phasic Model as the standard of care for clinicians working with clients diagnosed with posttraumatic stress disorder (ISTSS, 2000). The expert clinician survey findings of Cloitre et al. (2011, 2012) strongly endorsed a phase-oriented approach for complex PTSD that remains patient centered with attention to prominent symptoms. This is consistent with the trauma practice approach outlined in this book.

These three phases of treatment: Phase I: Safety and Stabilization, Phase II: Working Through Trauma, and Phase III Reconnection are thoroughly explored in this edition. The three phases are the organizing structure and foundation for the trauma practice approach. Specific treatment goals and techniques are offered for each of these three phases of trauma care, making this text a "hands-on" reference and guidebook for clinicians as they navigate through the potentially difficult treatment trajectory with clients who have survived trauma.

With our contemporary look at trauma-informed care, we have already discussed the need to add a Phase 0 as a fundamental element in training trauma focused clinicians. The required prescription for training would include competence, excellence, and mastery. There is a recognition of the crucial element of capacity to self-regulate and then to co-regulate with clients and this demands that the clinicians have inner resources for down-regulating in times of personal strain. It asks that you dedicate yourself as diligently to caring for yourself as you would for your clients.

This edition of *Trauma Practice* also includes the section introducing Forward-Facing® trauma therapy. This form of therapy is an exciting treatment process for rapidly and effectively addressing traumatic stress and all anxiety disorders that do not require accessing and processing survivor's painful trauma memories. Instead, this method teaches and coaches clients to master the regulation of their own autonomic nervous systems (ANS) as the primary focus of treatment. As clients learn and practice these skills, they find their symptoms diminishing and their quality of life maximizing. In addition to mastering self-regulation capacities, the method also assists clients in developing intentional living. The survivor defines for themselves their integrity and then the therapist, through coaching them to confront the perceived threats in their daily lives with regulated bodies, helps them to live principle-based lives with an internal locus of control. This method allows the client to experience immediate and profound treatment effects that quickly lead to an enhanced quality of life. Forward-Facing® trauma therapy also focuses upon helping the client to become more and more purposeful and intentional as they practice self-regulation. The combination of these two factors rapidly accelerates trauma treatment for many survivors.

The authors wish to make a clear statement that this book is only a guidebook and does not act as a substitute for the training and supervised practice necessary to integrate these principles and techniques into practice. The authors have presented the materials found in this book in an e-learning program available or as a two-day intensive training program through the Traumatology Institute (Canada; http://www.psychink.com) and Forward-Facing Institute, LLC (USA; www.forward-facing.com). Please see Appendix 2 for more information on these training courses. Additional trauma training is now available online at psychink.com for those individuals who do not have direct access to face-to-face training programs or the opportunity to bring institute trainers to their locations. We believe that proper training and supervision is required to safely and successfully integrate these powerful techniques into practice with trauma survivors. We offer these principles and techniques based upon the belief that the primary responsibility of the clinician is to "*above all else, do no harm.*" While persons suffering with posttraumatic stress have demonstrated their strength and resiliency by having survived some of the most painful and heinous experiences

known to mankind, it is possible for the well-intended but untrained therapist to engage in treatment with survivors that can actually retraumatize their clients, thus resulting in failed treatment and rendering future treatment even more difficult and painful for the survivor.

For those interested in adjunctive therapy with clients using a tri-phasic approach, visit: http://www.whatisptsd.com. Details of the Trauma Treatment Online Program and the use of adjunctive trauma care programs, systems, and online applications are available for your use with clients.

A further complication within trauma care are personality changes that establish themselves rigidly over time, which form interpersonal skills from a reactive position in the attempt to keep one out of harm's way (Cloitre et al., 2011, 2012). Trauma survivors may have developed concurrent personality disorders and resulting behaviors that may have been useful at the time of the trauma but no longer serve the individual well. Although as clinicians we may aid our clients to resolve the traumatic memories, harness improved self-care skills, and establish systems for reconnecting with meaningful community and activities, our clients may then have to tackle the personality structures or themes that no longer work for them once trauma is extinguished.

## Self-of-the-Therapist

In Friedman's (1996) landmark article entitled "PTSD Diagnosis and Treatment for Mental Health Clinicians," he argues strongly that the development and maintenance of the "self-of-the-therapist" may be one of the most important aspects of treatment with traumatized individuals. We have found, in our own practices and in our training programs, that the ability to develop and maintain a nonanxious presence while working with trauma survivors is a key ingredient to successful treatment outcomes and in maximizing the resiliency of the therapist.

The article of Baldwin (2013) certainly does an excellent job of explaining the underpinnings of nervous system ignition and the brain among trauma survivors and this reinforces our belief that the clinician must be well suited or suitably prepared for exposure to those experiencing PTSD. This will prove helpful not only for the clinician but also for those working with the therapist. Trauma ignition can work both ways and if the clinician is unprepared to bear witness to the trauma content without extreme reactivity neither the client nor the therapist will benefit.

Confronting traumatic material is painful and can be debilitating for the therapist. Many of the techniques presented in this text involve, in one way or another, the confrontation and narration of traumatic experiences by the trauma survivor with support and guidance from the therapist. It is theorized that the ability of the trauma survivor to access, confront, and self-regulate while narrating traumatic experiences may be one of the active ingredients leading to the resolution of traumatic stress. Developing trauma competency is of critical importance in the emerging maturity of any trauma therapist (Gentry, Baranowsky, & Rhoton, 2017). The ability of the therapist to elicit, assist, and self-regulate while the survivor struggles through these narrations is, in our opinion, an a priori requirement for effective treatment. Indeed, we have all worked with posttraumatic clients who have "failed" in previous therapy attempts because they were unable to complete these narratives with their therapists. We believe that a courageous, optimistic, and nonanxious approach, tempered with safety and pacing, to be the key to rapid amelioration of traumatic stress symptoms.

In our training programs, we work diligently toward helping therapists develop the capacity for self-regulation and the maintenance of a nonanxious presence. Research demonstrates that high levels of anxiety can diminish cognitive and motor functioning (Baldwin, 2013; Scaer, 2001, 2014) and this diminished capacity may account for some of the symptoms associated with traumatic stress. It may also point toward some of the difficulties encountered by therapists who work with clients who suffer from traumatic stress. Compassion fatigue resiliency is the focus of the article that you can review at https://psychink.com/blog/2019/06/25/compassion-fatigue-resiliency-a-new-attitude/. Clinician stress when working with trauma survivors is a reality that we all need to reflect on and work through. We hope that you will make a commitment to your own well-being as a trauma care provider.

## Core Objectives

Upon completion of this book readers will be:
- Aware of the underlying principles of cognitive behavioral and somatic trauma therapy (CBST) that are reported to lead to the resolution of posttraumatic stress symptoms
- Aware of the psychophysiology of posttraumatic stress
- Aware of how to apply CBST in accordance with the specific criteria in each of the phases in the tri-phasic model of treatment with trauma survivors
- Able to apply effective trauma stabilization and resolution interventions that best fit the unique requirements of any survivor
- Able to utilize many different CBST techniques to help trauma survivors resolve the effects of their trauma memories and posttraumatic stress symptoms
- Able to utilize CBST techniques to assist trauma survivors in developing more satisfying lifestyles in the present

## Book Description

CBT is one of the most researched and most effective treatments for PTSD and we believe that all skilled traumatologists should have at least rudimentary understanding and skills in this important area of treatment. This book will focus upon the utilization of the principle of *reciprocal inhibition* (exposure + relaxation) as a core knowledge and skill that readers will acquire following a thorough reading and integration of the materials covered in this book. Nearly all of CBST is organized around this principle and we believe it can be found in most *effective* treatments of posttraumatic stress.

This book will begin with a brief outline of the history and the theoretical underpinnings of CBT. A brief discussion of possible physiological pathways to account for the identified behavioral phenomena will be included. This will be followed by an introduction to Herman's (1992) tri-phasic model for the treatment of posttraumatic stress conditions. The tri-phasic approach is recognized as the highly effective approach we have used in the trauma practice approach since we first developed it in 1999 (Cloitre et al., 2011, 2012). This is followed by a thorough exploration of *Phase I: Safety and Stabilization* in the treatment, with an opportunity to practice and learn several skills for use at this stage.

After the reader has learned the skills necessary for the essential development of safety and stabilization with their clients, the book will focus on techniques useful for the successful resolution of traumatic memories in *Phase II: Working Through Trauma*. Readers will learn several specific CBST techniques for assisting their clients with accessing, confronting, and resolving their traumatic memories. These techniques will be presented in a step-by-step process with the goal of skills development. We hope this text will provide readers with a comfort level that will allow them to begin using these interventions in their service to trauma survivors.

In *Phase III: Reconnection*, we will focus on developing skills to assist trauma survivors in further re-integration of skills developed and the resolution of the residual sequelae from their trauma history. Often, even after a survivor has successfully resolved a trauma memory, symptoms such as survivor guilt, distorted and self-critical thinking styles, relational dysfunction, addiction, or painful affect remain unresolved. This last phase of treatment is focused on helping the trauma survivor reconnect with themselves, their families, and loved ones in the present and to connect to their goals for the future. Several approaches will be presented to the reader for their use in helping their clients navigate successfully through this important phase of treatment (Baranowsky, 2000; Baranowsky & Lauer, 2013).

New in this edition, we provide, where possible, audio and video material demonstrating how the different techniques are carried out. These are available via the YouTube links in the text or practitioners can also download them from the publisher's webpage (see Notes on Supplementary Materials, p. 225).

With the completion of this book, the reader will have gained sufficient knowledge and skills to integrate the principles and techniques of CBST into their practice with survivors of trauma.

# Phase 0:
# Foundations of the Trauma Practice Model

*For fast-acting relief from stress, try slowing down.*

Lily Tomlin

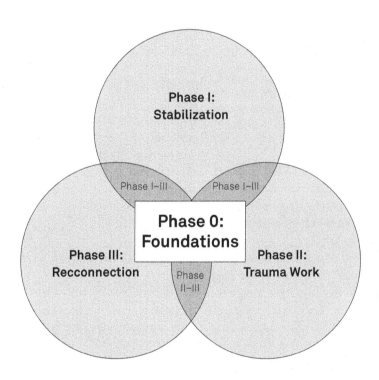

**Summary**

Section 1 provides some of the current theories explaining both the cognitive and physiological underpinnings of the symptoms and successful interventions for the treatment of trauma. The symptoms that manifest from trauma are natural and normal sequelae to exposure to extraordinary events. Understanding the mechanism by which these occur will provide a much better ability to understand the variety of symptoms seen in practice. Understanding how the interventions are logically linked to the mechanism by which symptoms occur should provide a better ability to utilize the techniques presented and increase confidence in their effectiveness with clients. This understanding will help in the creation of on-the-spot interventions to also address the immediate needs of clients.

# Phase 0: Foundations of the Traum Practice Model

We have added a Phase 0 to Herman's (1992) Tri-phasic Model in this edition of *Trauma Practice*. This addition reflects an attempt to identify and promulgate the knowledge and skills necessary for a trauma clinician to meet their clients with competence from the first session throughout the course of treatment and all the way to discharge. We hope this information supports clinicians working with trauma survivors to become increasingly intentional with the ways in which they manage themselves and engage their clients. Recent research is replete with data that suggests the value of what the therapist brings to the process of treatment is much greater than the technical elements of the treatments themselves.

Benish, Imel, and Wampold (2007, p. 746) state:

> *Given the evidence that treatments are about equally effective, that treatments delivered in a clinical setting are effective (and as effective as those in clinical trials), that the manner in which treatments are provided are much more important than which treatment is provided...*

Recent outcome research (Miller et al., 2013, 2020; Llewelyn et al., 2016) has begun to discover what makes psychotherapy optimally effective. It is much less about the treatment method utilized and much more about the relational and technical expertise of the therapist. This process of developing expertise and maximizing outcomes by psychotherapists with all their clients has given birth to a burgeoning field of clinical training and research called *deliberate practice*. Deliberate practice was first discussed by Ericsson (2006) after conducting a study with musicians who were enrolled in an elite training academy in Germany. Through surveys and interviews, Ericsson was able to distill what was common among these students that produced excellence in their playing. These activities were:

1. Observing their own work
2. Getting expert feedback
3. Setting small incremental learning goals just beyond the performer's ability
4. Engaging in repetitive behavioral rehearsal of specific skills
5. Continuously assessing performance

These activities have been utilized in training and supervision programs with psychotherapists and yielded significantly improved outcomes among their clients. Evidence-based psychotherapeutic treatments are effective less because of the technical aspects of the treatment (0–1% of variance) and much more a result of clinician expertise with both the treatment model and maintaining a positive therapeutic experience for the client (5–9% of variance) (Chadwell et al., 2018; Duncan et al., 2010; Lutz et al., 2007; Wampold, 2005). The more deliberate the clinician is in refining technical and relational skills the more effective implementation of evidence-based treatments will become. In addition to relational and technical competence is the requirement for the consistent attuning to our clients, the actual experts of their own struggles. This constant attunement allows us to continually bolster our relationships with them as well as repair any unintentional relational damage done in previous sessions. We strongly advocate integrating feedback-informed practice (Miller et al., 2013, 2015) with all clients in each session.

In addition to developing technical expertise with the clinician's treatment(s) of choice, continual augmentation of relational skills, and the utilization of feedback-informed treatment is highly recommended. This capacity enhances effectiveness with clients across the diagnostic continuum. With this as a starting point, we also wish to add some skills and preparatory activities to evolve a clinician's expertise specifically with trauma survivor clients.

# Preparation for the Therapist

In the 21st Century, therapists who treat trauma and have interest in pursuing excellence in this endeavor must dedicate a significant amount of time and resources toward their preparation. This preparation includes two components: preparation in their professional development and preparation for each and every individual client. Many of these professional preparatory capacities may already be a part of the professional's knowledge and skill set, but if they are not, then some preliminary work will be required to set the work on the right foot before even having contact with their first client. Below is a list of knowledge and capacities that serve as a foundation for the practice of trauma-informed care and the pathway to excellence as a trauma therapist:

- Becoming proficient in the principles and practices of trauma-informed care. Trauma-informed care is:
  - **Understanding** the prevalence of trauma and adversity and their impacts on health and behavior
  - **Recognizing** the effects of trauma and adversity on health and behavior

- **Training** leadership, providers, and staff on **responding** to patients with best practices in trauma-informed care
- **Integrating** knowledge about trauma and adversity into policies, procedures, practices, and treatment planning
- **Resisting** re-traumatization by approaching patients who have experienced adverse childhood experiences and/or other adversities with nonjudgmental support

• The principles of trauma informed care are:
  - Establish the physical and emotional **safety** of patients and staff
  - **Build** trust between providers and patients
  - **Recognize** the signs and symptoms of trauma exposure on physical and mental health
  - Promote **patient-centered, evidence-based care**
  - Ensure provider and patient **collaboration** by bringing patients into the treatment process and discussing mutually agreed upon goals for treatment
  - Provide care that is sensitive to the patient's **racial, ethnic, and cultural background, and gender identity**

In addition to making the principles and practices of trauma-informed care a central and organizing ethos for trauma clinicians, we outline a few additional principles and practices that we believe help articulate competency in the treatment of traumatic stress in the 21st Century. The concepts and factors presented below are offered as an index checklist only (more thorough discussions can be found in Gentry, 2021; Gentry & Dietz, 2020; Gentry et al., 2017; and Rhoton & Gentry, 2021).

• Learn in detail the explanation that trauma is not a psychological pathology but, instead, is the result of an over-adaptative threat detection and threat response system. This includes the ability of the clinician to explain rudimentary components and functioning of the ANS, the human threat response, stress as a threat response with an internal locus of control, and the ways in which this dysregulated ANS (i.e., dysautonomia) can negatively affect a trauma survivor's physical, cognitive, emotional, and spiritual health.

• Possess a thorough understanding of the polyvagal theory (Porges, 2009; Porges & Dana, 2018) that includes the ability to function clinically in the ventral vagal system and to utilize co-regulation as a primary intervention with dysregulated clients.

• Clinicians treating trauma survivors should develop the ability to interrupt our own threat response by integrating both neuroceptive (i.e., top down) and interoceptive (i.e., bottom-up) self-regulation strategies.

• Develop the ability to teachthe above elements to our clients (e.g., threat response, ANS functioning, polyvagal theory, and self-regulation) using simple and straightforward (jargon-less) language.

• Develop a repertoire of common experiences for daily life that illustrate the negative effects of ANS dysregulation and how self-regulation can lessen/eradicate clients' distress in these contexts and restore optimal functioning.

• Be able to use rudimentary motivational interviewing (Rollnick & Miller, 1995) skills to catalyze positive expectancy and engagement; especially in early treatment.

• Evolve away from a flat, dry, disconnected, and objective stance with our clients to one that is warm, engaging, dynamic (broad range and low-intensity affect), uses prosodic voice, while remaining in a regulated ANS (i.e., ventral vagal).

• Be willing to elicit and attune to negative feedback from our clients. We strongly recommend that feedback informed treatment (FIT) (Miller et al., 2013, 2015) should become a central component of treatment with every client in every session.

• Develop an understanding of and an ability to integrate intentionally the active ingredients/common elements of all effective trauma therapies. These minimally include: developing, maintaining, and enhancing a good therapeutic relationship; relaxation and self-regulation skills; exposure protocols (both in vivo and imaginal); and psychoeducational/cognitive restructuring interventions.

• Become well-versed and experienced using multiple methods of trauma resolution, especially for memory processing. We suggest at least one bilateral stimulation approach (e.g., thematic map & release, eye-movement desensitization and reprocessing accelerated resolution therapy, or brainspotting), one narrative/CBST approach (e.g., written narrative, story-book, traumagram, cognitive processing therapy), and one somatic approach (hands over heart space, layering, somatic experiencing, or sensorimotor psychotherapy). Competency in one of these treatment approaches in each of the three categories will provide you with trauma expertise and the ability to address many trauma survivor clients who seeks out treatment. Further complexities may require that you augment your skills to address the treatment of personality disorders (i.e., borderline personality disorder), dissociation, chronic pain, and addictions, which may include internal family systems, dialectical behavioral therapy, hypnosis training; structural or strategic treatment for dissociative disorders and an understanding of contemporary approaches for addiction treatment (i.e., smart recovery, etc).

- Finally, clinicians should develop a library of short (60–90 s) narratives that outline past successful clients' navigation through treatment that outlines both their incremental successes and the challenges during which they struggled in their process toward completing therapy. Judicious sharing of some of these narratives throughout the course of treatment can catalyze positive expectancy, normalize clients' experiences, and point out potential skills they have not yet utilized.

These skills, capacities, and knowledge represent the authors' suggestion not only for developing essential preparatory practices but also for evolving their practice from competence to expertise to mastery in working with trauma survivor clients.

## Exposure in a Relaxed State – Reciprocal Inhibition

Reviewing the work of Patricia Resick (Resick & Schnicke, 1992), Charles Marmar (1990), James Pennebaker (1997), Onno van der Hart (van der Hart & Brown, 1992), Bessel van der Kolk (van der Kolk, 1986; van der Kolk et al., 1996), and the experiences gained from early clinical training, it became apparent that the **type of exposure** used in therapy is very important to effectiveness. If clients are aided in constructing **complete narratives** of their traumatic experiences while in a **relaxed state**, their traumatic stress symptoms (specifically those in Criterion B) could heal at an accelerated rate (van der Kolk, 1986; van der Kolk et al., 1996). By facilitating this important narrative process, not only would the trauma survivor be aided in confronting the traumatic material, but they were being reinforced to structure the intrusive sensory traumata into language. The research supported that effective narrative construction had a powerful ameliorative effect upon the intrusive symptoms of trauma (i.e., flashbacks and nightmares), while virtually every treatment that demonstrated effectiveness with traumatic stress utilized some form of narrative (exposure) paired with some form of relaxation or the use of reciprocal inhibition.

The resolution of intrusive symptoms of PTSD did not mean that PTSD itself was resolved. Early on, that was the primary focus of treatment: to resolve the flashbacks and nightmares. There was an implicit belief in the field that, if you were able to desensitize and reprocess the memories, present-day discomfort, anxiety, and distress would spontaneously ameliorate. By 1997, just before publishing the first edition of *Trauma Practice*, the authors worked diligently on strategies for addressing the impact of compassion fatigue. During this time, we reflected and tested out the integration of approaches that addressed self-regulation of the autonomic nervous system (ANS) as the central ingredient to both resolving and preventing work-related stress. Several published works describe the effectiveness of these interventions for the symptoms of compassion fatigue treatment and its prevention (Cocker & Joss, 2016; Craigie et al., 2016; Flarity, Jones Rhodes, & Reckard, 2016; Flarity, Nash et al., 2016; Potter et al., 2010, 2015; Flarity, Holcomb & Gentry, 2014; Flarity et al., 2013; Rank et al., 2009; Baranowsky et al., 2005; Gentry et al., 2002; Gentry, 2002; Gentry, et al., 2004; Potter, Berger, et al., 2013; Potter, Deshields, & Rodriguez, 2013; Rank et al., 2009).

As a result, we have identified self-regulation as the primary component of symptom resolution for work-related stress. The self-regulation component of the trauma practice approach has been firmly situated within the somatic range of self-response since the first edition in 2001 (i.e., layering, hands over heart space, expanding emotions, etc). Peter Levine brought forward somatic therapy as a form of treatment that focused on body sensations and the interwoven memory and emotion processing. Although we did not use that language at the time, exercises that address the somatic experience directly have certainly been integrated within *Trauma Practice* since the first edition. With this in mind, we have updated the book to fully embrace this language and extended the subtitle to "Cognitive-Behavioral-**Somatic** Therapy."

Further refining this work, there have been eleven peer-reviewed journal articles that described the effectiveness of the Forward-Facing® professional resilience approach in significantly lessening work-related stress symptoms, while simultaneously enhancing professional resilience.

The Forward-Facing® approach (Gentry & Dietz, 2020) has demonstrated effectiveness in both lessening compassion fatigue symptoms (i.e., secondary traumatic stress and burnout) while also enhancing resilience and work satisfaction for care professionals. This effectiveness is based upon teaching care providers a set of skills that function as an "immune system" to the potential for toxicity in a demanding healthcare work environment, and they include:

1. Self-regulation of the ANS through neuroception, interoception, and acute relaxation

2. Intentionality
3. Perceptual maturation
4. Connection and support
5. Self-care and revitalization

With increased understanding of central nervous system (CNS) functioning and especially the role of perceived threat and sympathetic dominance in the etiology of traumatic stress symptoms, the importance of relaxation became even more relevant in treatment application. Integrating the work of Babette Rothschild (2000), Bessel van der Kolk (2015); Peter Levine (1997, 2010), Pat Ogden (2000, 2006); and Robert Scaer (2005, 2014) along with our own developments on self-regulation, it became apparent that individuals who learn to maintain a regulated ANS (i.e., confronting perceived threat with acute relaxation), experienced symptom resolution.

*You cannot experience distress, posttraumatic stress, or any kind of stress while in a relaxed-muscle body (relaxed somatic state).* When a trauma survivor learns and develops mastery in confronting perceived threats of their life in a relaxed-muscle body, they no longer met the diagnostic criteria for PTSD. They no longer suffer physiologically when confronting a frightening world with an internally self-regulated ANS.

## Meaningful Human Care and Connection

Although exposure and relaxation are essential treatment elements to address traumatic stress (i.e., reciprocal inhibition) more is needed to resolve complex trauma history fully. In 1999, Hubble, Duncan, and Miller released a text of major importance: *The Heart and Soul of Change.* This book was chock-full of paradigm-shifting information, and one of the most important truths came from their systemic review of meta-analytic studies in psychotherapy. They'd found that the most important predictor of positive outcomes had nothing to do with the therapy itself but rather what happened *outside* of therapy, which accounted for over 40% of positive outcomes. Of the 60% that therapists could influence, 30% was contingent upon the development and maintenance of a good therapeutic relationship, while the remaining 30% was split equally between positive expectancy and techniques/models. There was a good argument that the process of developing expectancy/hope/placebo was also a relational function, and it is possible that the degree to which clinicians could influence positive outcomes for clients would be even more highly contingent on relational factors, thus leaving less contingent on technical and/or philosophical factors.

The important conclusion is that **people heal people!** Neither trauma practice, somatic therapy, EMDR, CBT, or psychopharmacology accounts for most of the magical transformations that happened inside our offices (or on our computer screens). It is the quality of relationships that you build with your clients that is the most effective approach. With the development of a solid foundation of a good therapeutic relationship, clinicians can then deliver these effective treatments and enjoy positive outcomes. Said differently: Evidence-based treatments do NOT heal traumatic stress ... it is the **effective delivery** of these treatments that account for the change, growth, and healing. With this effective delivery, we have the privilege to witness remarkable trauma recovery.

One of the primary factors in the navigation of significant traumatic events is meaningful human care and connection. Most of us can recall a time when the presence of a caring, supportive other has been a crucial element in safely navigating a devastating life event. Whether this came in the form of a loving family or friend or a caring professional, this can make a huge difference in the outcome trajectory, emotionally and even physically. Look at this from your own personal perspective: How big a role does your medical professionals' interactions with you regarding your diagnosis and ensuing treatment play into your overall healing? It is then easy to see the inherent importance of the therapeutic role of relationships in mind, we must build client connections that reinforce successful narrative co-construction and teach self-regulation.

The findings of Hubble et al. (1999) have been thoroughly integrated into present-day clinical practice. We can extract from these findings that there are three common primary "active ingredients" indigenous to treatments demonstrating effectiveness for the treatment of traumatic stress that clinicians can use to augment their practice. These three active ingredients were: therapeutic relationship, relaxation, and exposure. A final fourth ingredient was also found in the meta-analysis of PTSD findings by Hubble et al. This fourth ingredient is the process of teaching clients different (healthier and more satisfying) ways of perceiving themselves and the world. Alternately referred to as "psychoeducation" or "cognitive restructuring." This crucial component can then added to the list of generic factors for effective trauma treatment.

The four active ingredients for treating traumatic stress can thus be listed as follows:

1. Therapeutic relationship: A secure, collaborative, and dynamic relationship between helper and survivor

2. Relaxation/self-regulation: The ability to regulate one's own ANS by confronting perceived threats with a relaxed-muscle body or somatic processing
3. Exposure/narrative: The ability to sequence the micro-events of a trauma into a narrative, and then share that narrative with a safe other while maintaining a relaxed body (reciprocal inhibition)
4. Psychoeducation/cognitive restructuring: Evolving shame and fear-based perspectives of self and the world into self-compassionate and intentional perception (or resolving themes)

When individuals are provided an opportunity to complete all four therapeutic tasks, they can work through their PTSD in a profound way. Furthermore, unless the client has an organic condition, it is possible that they may no longer meet diagnostic criteria for any psychiatric disorder.

Building and maintaining a strong therapeutic relationship, teaching survivors how to relax their bodies (especially in the context of a perceived threat), helping them construct complete chronological narratives of their traumatic experiences, and helping them evolve their perceptions of themselves and the world (the completion of these four tasks can heal traumatic stress). Four tasks = trauma recovery. *Simple.* Not easy, but simple. It may take years of work through countless sessions to accomplish all four of these tasks, but deliberate and intentional focus upon the completion of these tasks has been proven through research and anecdotal practice to be an incredibly effective, useable, and gentle approach for healing trauma.

Two recent publications (Gentry et al., 2017; Rhoton & Gentry, 2021) represent the evolution of the development of a generic therapeutic approach for traumatic stress that infuses the elements essential to effective trauma treatments.

## The Evolution of PTSD Treatment and the "Active Ingredients"

In 1980, the American Psychiatric Association conceptualized the diagnostic criterion for PTSD. Since then, researchers and counselors have labored to develop and refine reliable, effective treatments for survivors of trauma.

In 2010 and 2017, a significant milestone was achieved with the publication by the Department of Veterans Affairs (VA) and the Department of Defense (DoD) of treatment guidelines for PTSD and acute stress disorder, which presented solid evidence that trauma-focused treatment worked well for clients suffering from trauma-related symptoms.

Using 56 professional reviewers, the VA and DoD created a comprehensive clinical practice guideline for the management of posttraumatic stress disorder that may still be the most comprehensive documentation for understanding effective treatment of posttraumatic conditions to date. Its authors conducted a thorough literature review regarding psychotherapeutic and psychopharmacological treatments that had demonstrated effectiveness in studies from 2002 to 2009, evaluated the evidence for each method, and assigned them to categories based upon the strength of evidence. The methods most strongly recommended were evidence-based trauma-focused psychotherapeutic interventions that include components of exposure and/or cognitive restructuring; or stress inoculation training (US Department of Veterans Affairs & Department of Defense, 2017).

The authors of this guideline promulgated that the cornerstone of trauma recovery is the use of evidence-based trauma-focused interventions, which were found to be more effective with clients and were strenuously indicated over nonspecific treatment, and were up to 86 % better than no treatment at all. Not surprisingly and in line with the recognition of the human relationship, in an analysis of seven existing guidelines for treating PTSD, a panel of expert authors indicated that current evidence was insufficient to drive most of the recommendations made by the guidelines (Forbes et al., 2010; Berliner et al., 2019).

While the authors supported the use of the evidence-based and recommended first-line treatments for posttraumatic stress, they concluded that these treatments could not resolve traumatic stress by themselves, and that they remain embedded in broader clinical care. They identified therapeutic alliance, assessments, case formulation, and treatment planning as essential components of all therapeutic work and argue that it is unrealistic to expect any clinician to adhere to Level I empirical data and recommendations when attending to the diverse needs of clients (Forbes et al., 2010; Berliner et al., 2019). This passage underlines the importance of a trauma counselor's good clinical judgment. Essentially, this is not taking a "one size fits all" approach to treatment, in conjunction with the identification and implementation of certain common factors found in all evidence based treatments (EBTs) in a myriad of contexts.

In 2008, Benish, Imel, and Wampold published a meta-analytic study that directly compared evidence-based trauma-focused treatments to determine which, if any, were better than the others. They reported that, "the primary analysis revealed that effect sizes were homogenously distributed around zero for measures of PTSD symptomology, and for all measures of psychological functioning, indicating that there were no differences between psychotherapies" (Benish et al., 2008, p. 746) In other words, they found no discernible differences in the levels of relief provided by the trauma-focused treatments. This study has been replicated elsewhere with similar results (Schynder et al., 2015; Murray et al., 2014, Forbes et al., 2010, Powers et al., 2010 Bisson et al., 2007, Foa et al., 2007).

Prior to the study by Benish et al., (2008) models and methods of treatment competed to be considered evidence-based and the best therapy for PTSD. This competitive climate led many clinicians and academics to become strictly faithful to certain methods, which fractured the field of traumatic stress treatment into separate and distinct groups. However, the findings of Benish et al. indicated that while trauma-focused therapy worked, the outcome had little to do with the particular method employed and this was a revelation. Instead of asking which treatment was better, the question became "What makes all of these treatments effective?"

As it was recognized that common elements central to change could be extracted from the effective treatments, further important questions arose: "How do trauma counselors integrate what works across these models into treatment with all survivors of trauma?" and "How do educators train clinicians to become effective at treating traumatic stress instead of simply implementing evidence-based practices?" Benish et al. (2008) suggested that clinicians' mastery and implementation of these common factors within their own forms of treatment, whatever they may be, would be the most effective approach to a lasting alleviation of PTSD symptoms.

Miller et al., (2013) also argued that the primary factors accounting for change among clients were not model-specific. Citing previous studies (Duncan et al., 2010; Lutz et al., 2007; Wampold, 2005) along with their own study, they reported that the variance of outcomes attributable to specific treatments was a very low (0–1%). This contrasted sharply with therapeutic alliance (5%) and therapist variables (5–9 %) explaining more of the variance in outcomes. The same authors reported that the nonspecific common factors in effective treatments were much more potent for achieving client outcomes than any specific model or method of treatment. This nascent shift away from EBTs and toward empowering counselors with what actually works was representative of a movement in a new direction for the field of trauma treatment.

This was a promising adjustment, as EBTs weren't always representative of a treatment's effectiveness for the general population. Those who participated in them were often college students and received payment for their involvement, yet there was still a prevailing dropout rate that hovered around 30% and resulted in a selective data set. While those EBTs could appear effective, they were often done in a laboratory and had little resemblance to what actually happens in consumer-driven psychotherapy.

Nonetheless, the noteworthy research conducted by Keating and colleagues (2021) in a private practice setting seems to address this issue well, while demonstrating that the trauma practice approach produces statistically significant outcome within this the rarely researched setting of private practice.

However, highly manualized approaches often diminish treatment appropriateness for veterans or other trauma survivors, who seem to flourish more with a personalized approach. With field maturity, it became increasingly evident through continued research that the mental health culture needed to construct and embrace psychotherapies that were fitted to the individual client, rather than demanding those with diminished capabilities to conform to the therapy's strict and exact requirements.

In 1995 and 1996, Figley and Carbonell (Carbonell & Figley, 1996; Carbonell & Figley, 1999; Figley et al., 1999) hosted a clinical demonstration project at Florida State University designed to identify and extract the active ingredients from several treatments for traumatic stress. At that time, developers and practitioners of novel therapies were invited to demonstrate their treatments with volunteer clients before a live audience (Gallo, 1996). The project showcased methods such as EMDR, TIR, TFT, vsualkinesthetic dissociation, and other energy-focused treatments. It also provided a forum for attendees to discuss the factors that were common in all of them. Attendees found that all the treatments coupled some form of exposure with some type of relaxation to help survivors desensitize the negative effects of their traumatic memories (Gallo, 1996). Known as reciprocal inhibition and pioneered by South African psychiatrist Joseph Wolpe in 1958, the pairing of exposure and relaxation had already been widely accepted as a central factor to effectively treating trauma, thus exhibiting its appropriate role as one of the active ingredients.

In 2011, Cloitre et al., surveyed 50 expert trauma clinicians and found that 48% endorsed phase-based or sequenced therapy as the most appropriate treatment approach, with interventions tailored to specific symptom sets. First-line interventions they matched to specific symptoms included:

1. Emotion regulation strategies
2. Narration of trauma memories as an exposure process
3. Cognitive restructuring
4. Anxiety and stress management
5. Interpersonal skills development

The survey results provided a strong rationale for conducting research focused on the relative merits of traditional trauma therapies and sequenced multicomponent approaches applied to different population. Echoing similar sentiments, the 2017 and 2010 VA/DoD Clinical Practice Guideline (Management of Post-Traumatic Stress Working Group, 2010; Management of Post-Traumatic Stress Disorder Working Group, 2017) also pointed out exposure, cognitive restructuring, anxiety management, and psychoeducation as key components of recommended EBTs, and emphasized the importance of the therapeutic relationship in treating trauma survivors.

The efforts taken above have led to the identification of active ingredients (for effective treatment) along with a generic clinical structure for addressing posttrauma conditions that integrate the four common elements for successful trauma treatment in a phasic model (Gentry et al., 2017; Rhoton & Gentry, 2021). By utilizing the phasic structure of this model, counselors will be able to efficiently complete these four therapeutic tasks while still employing the evidence-based trauma resolution methods of their choice (see Video 1 available in the supplementary material for this book, p. 226, or Baranowsky, 2020, December 5, *Recovery Now Trauma* – audio recording https://youtu.be/DvzwJ614frM). In the same way that generic medication still produces the same outcome as a name brand, we're proposing a model that is malleable, easy to personalize to each particular client, and equipped to navigate a wide range of clinical challenges effectively.

## The Four Active Ingredients

We believe health professionals who treat trauma can greatly benefit from developing understanding and skills associated with each of these active ingredients. By developing expertise in delivering these common factors of effective treatments, the clinician is rewarded with a de facto generic treatment that embraces the best of what all trauma treatments have to offer. Skilled application and delivery of these four ubiquitous components will provide the clinician with a pathway forward when the evidence-based protocols are not well-tolerated or ideal for the client. Moreover, the implementation of the active ingredients as a primary focus of treatment allows the practitioner to deliver a treatment that is tailored to the survivor's informational processing and relational style. Thus, treatment can be designed to fit the individual instead of requiring the survivor to fit themselves to the treatment manual.

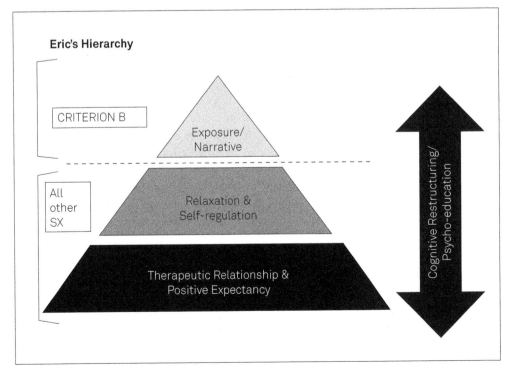

**Figure 1.**
The active ingredients

As was previously illustrated, these active ingredients have been identified as the essential components of effective treatment for traumatic stress by scores of researchers in hundreds of publications on four continents over two decades of scientific investigation.

Figure 1 illustrates the orientation for the clinical delivery of these active ingredients throughout the treatment trajectory. We begin with the development, maintenance, and continued enhancement of the therapeutic relationship. With the solid foundation of a therapeutic alliance established, we then transition to helping our clients develop and master the ability to interrupt their physiological involuntary threat response and to regulate their own autonomic nervous system. With this skill firmly established, we can then begin the exposure process to catalyze reciprocal inhibition and desensitize trauma responses. We prescribe in vivo exposure to environmental cues associated with past trauma paired with self-regulation as primary method of exposure. However, survivors with self-regulation skills are also poised to optimize imaginal exposure protocols (e.g., EMDR, PE, CPT, etc.), if the clinician chooses this route of exposure. Finally, cognitive restructuring/psychoeduction is ubiquitous throughout the course of treatment and is likely included in most sessions. Each of these active ingredients and their utility in the treatment process is further explored in the following sections.

## 1. Therapeutic Relationship and Positive Expectancy

Establishing, maintaining, and enhancing an excellent therapeutic relationship through the use of feedback-informed treatment (FIT) (Duncan et al., 2004; Seidel, 2012; Miller et al., 2013, 2020; Miller et al., 2015; Miller et al., 2016).

Since Hans Eysenck's formative research on variables leading to effective treatment outcomes in 1952, evidence has supported the therapeutic relationship as one of the most important factors leading to positive outcomes (Barlow et al., 2013; Norcross, & Lambert, 2018). It continues to emerge in meta-analyses and deconstruction studies as a crucial component of effective treatment (Arnow et al., 2013).

In 2011, Knerr et al., discovered that to develop, maintain, and enhance therapeutic relationships, counselors should possess the following traits:
- A strong, differentiated self-concept
- An ability to regulate their own emotions and behaviors

- An awareness of their own beliefs, preferences, and needs
- An ability to manage stress
- An ability to maintain relaxation when working with clients

These last two traits are especially crucial in the co-regulation of a distressed client's ANS. Specifically, the relaxed state of a mental health professional can help reduce a state of nervous system arousal in clients.

A meta-analysis by Karver et al., in 2006 found several other counselor skills that contributed to clinical success with adolescents and their families:
- Interpersonal skills such as empathy, positive regard, warmth, and genuineness
- Engaging clients in treatment
- Delivering information clearly and concisely
- Giving a believable and reasonable rationale for information

In 2014, research was done by Fife et al. exploring integrations of multiple models of client treatment, and their findings suggested that three factors related directly to treatment outcomes:
- The creation of a therapeutic alliance
- The ability to employ interventions that fit the client
- The counselor's personal character or way of being

These studies all suggest that effective counselors are emotionally mature and self-regulating individuals who exhibit compassion and charity with their clients.

The most important occurrence in the psychotherapy field over the past decade has been the emergence of FIT (Anker et al., 2009; Duncan, Miller, & Sparks, 2004; Miller, Hubble, Chow, & Seidel, 2013; Prescott et al., 2017; Black et al., 2017). FIT significantly evolves and accelerates the way in which counselors develop, maintain, and enhance therapeutic relationships. Before FIT, counselors would likely attempt to apply the characteristics recommended by Carl Rogers in 1966 to enhance a therapeutic relationship: empathy, warmth, compassion, authenticity, and so forth. Put in Rogers' own words from the *American Handbook of Psychiatry*:

Genuineness in therapy means that the therapist is his actual self during his encounter with his client. Without facade, he openly has the authentic feelings and attitudes that are flowing within, at the moment. This involves self-awareness; that is, the therapist's feelings are available to him to his awareness – and he is able to live them, to experience them in the relationship, and to communicate them if they persist. The therapist encounters his client directly, meeting him person to person. He is being himself, not denying himself.

Since this concept is liable to misunderstanding, let me state that it does not mean that the therapist burdens his client with overt expression of all his feelings. Nor does it mean that the therapist discloses one's total self to the client. It does mean, however, that the therapist does not deny what is felt or experienced within the therapeutic relationships and allows this to be known when therapeutically beneficial to the client. It means avoiding the temptation to present a facade or hide behind a mask of professionalism, or to assume a confessional-professional attitude.

It is not simple to achieve such reality. Being real involves the difficult task of being acquainted with the flow of experiencing going on within oneself, a flow marked especially by complexity and continuous change. (1966, p. 185)

Though a steppingstone in the right direction, this rather "cookie cutter" approach to relationship building has been demonstrated to be significantly less effective in generating positive outcomes, as counselors frequently overestimate the quality of relationships with their clients (Carlson et al., 2000).

In 2013, the International Center for Clinical Excellence reported that FIT was included in the Substance Abuse and Mental Health Services Administration's (SAMHSA) National Registry of Evidence-Based Programs and Practices (Prescott et al., 2017) and that it as much as *doubled* clinician effectiveness. Not only does FIT provide a structured, empirically validated method for enhancing therapeutic relationships and improving outcomes, but it funnels counselors into a process of developing deliberate, collaborative practice with their clients as a pathway for maturation. For these reasons, we strongly advocate that FIT become a required component of trauma-focused counseling.

Additionally, Lambert's 1992 study found that another determining factor of a therapy's effectiveness is the client's positive expectancy for change. Preparation and hope building can capture up to 45% of what influences the outcomes of therapy, while self-of-the-therapist and a healer's personal maturation and style can significantly impact the quality of the therapeutic relationship being built. Lambert suggested four common factors that positively promoted beneficial therapeutic outcome, and they were:

a) Extra-therapeutic change factors
b) The client–therapist relationship
c) Technique or mechanical factors of a model of treatment
d) Expectancy factors

## 2.  Relaxation and Self-Regulation

Teaching survivors to monitor and regulate autonomic arousal through ongoing relaxation.

With a good therapeutic relationship established, the next task of treatment is to help clients learn the workings of their ANS and the importance of regulating this system. Virtually every effective treatment for posttraumatic stress, especially CBST, includes some strategy for achieving and maintaining relaxation (Ford & Russo, 2006). This isn't really a new concept. Hippocrates promoted having a relaxed body that was well-rested and adequately nourished, with an emphasis on balance between a person and their environment. It is fascinating that methods that work can be repeatedly ignored or lost because of the popular trends of the moment, only to (hopefully) resurface decades, centuries, or even millennia later.

In 1958, Joseph Wolpe discovered that when people with anxiety disorders confronted things that made them anxious while keeping their bodies relaxed, they were able to resolve their symptoms of anxiety. This process, known as reciprocal inhibition, is now the primary tool for desensitizing trauma memories in effective treatments of PTSD.

In a sense, psychoeducation regarding the body puts clients in the driver's seat of their physiological "vehicle." As they become increasingly skilled at recognizing changes in their physiology, they have an easier time tying the changes in their body to the changes in their emotions, thinking, and behaviors as an organic response to that changed state. This allows them to step away from the notion of being ill, feeling "crazy," or mentally disordered, and return self-control to the individual.

Many cognitive behavioral treatments such as prolonged exposure (PE), trauma-focused cognitive behavioral therapy (TFCBT), and stress inoculation training (SIT) explicitly prescribe teaching relaxation strategies before addressing traumatic memories with clients (Foa et al., 2009). Techniques such as diaphragmatic breathing, guided visualization, progressive relaxation, and autogenics are supported for use in treatment manuals and CBT protocols (Foa & Kozak, 1998). EMDR (Shapiro, 1995) integrates a safe place exercise into the preparation phase of treatment to help clients develop a capacity for relaxation, while the bilateral stimulation central to EMDR may produce a modicum of relaxation as well. Additionally, hypnotic protocols use hypnotic induction as a relaxation strategy to prepare the survivor to confront, integrate, and desensitize trauma memories (Corrigan, 2002). With all of this evidence, it is undeniably clear that developing skills for relaxation is key to effective treatment of traumatic stress.

One result of recent upheavals in healthcare services has been the systematic and institutional attempt to take the trauma-informed approach. With this evolution away from "What's wrong with you?" toward "What happened to you?" (Bloom, 2013), more care is taken to understand the effects of past trauma on current physical symptoms. One adaptation that prior trauma produces is a sensitive and overly active ANS (Ford, 2005). This means that trauma survivors perceive a more frequently and intensely dangerous world than those without a history of trauma. Increased perceived threat, coupled with an overly developed threat response system, is at the core of the survivor's dysregulation (Ford & Blaustein, 2013).

Training clients to perform ongoing monitoring and self-regulation of their anxiety symptoms can serve as both a treatment and resiliency tool (Gentry & Dietz, 2020). Developing this capacity for self-regulation can ameliorate distress associated with anxiety disorders and lessen symptoms across the mental disorder spectrum (Shah et al., 2014).

## 3.  Exposure/Narrative and Reciprocal Inhibition

Using exposure and/or narrative approaches to integrate and desensitize repressed, suppressed, and dissociated traumatic memories and memory fragments.

As previously mentioned, reciprocal inhibition is at the center of effective treatments for PTSD. It desensitizes hyperarousal effects and integrates dissociated, suppressed, or repressed trauma memories (Rauch et al., 2012). There is also evidence that exposure therapy helps trauma survivors regain optimal brain functioning (Roy et al., 2014).

The Category A treatments for PTSD identified by the Management of Posttraumatic Stress Working Group in 2010 are primarily exposure-based methods, while treatment manuals for prolonged exposure (Rothbaum et al., 2007) and cognitive processing therapy (CPT; Resick et al., 2006) articulate exposure as a central component of their effectiveness. CPT has become a more popular way to treat trauma in the past decade, especially among mental health providers working with combat veterans; it facilitates exposure by helping survivors construct and reconstruct narratives of their traumatic experiences. Increasingly, clinicians and researchers are advocating the use of narratives to help survivors confront, desensitize, and integrate charged trauma memories (Adenauer et al., 2011).

Exposure interventions focus on safely working through unresolved traumatic memories without overstimulating clients, and outcome research (Cloitre et al., 2012) has consistently demonstrated the effectiveness of exposure-based methods in lessening trauma-related symptoms and improving a client's quality of life over time.

Five criteria (Gentry & Schmidt, 1999; Baranowsky, Gentry, & Schultz, 2005) establish when a client is ready to begin exposure work:

1. Resolution of real danger (i.e., survivor is physically safe)
2. The ability to distinguish being safe from feeling safe
3. Demonstration of ability to self-regulate while confronting both environmental perceived threats and imaginal exposure to traumatic memory/memories
4. Ability to self-rescue from abreaction
5. A negotiated contract and informed consent for resolution of trauma memories

## 4.  Cognitive Restructuring and Psychoeducation

Restructuring cognition, with a focus on psychoeducation about the neurological, physical, and psychological effects of trauma.

Psychoeducation is a primary tenet of CBT and an early intervention in treating PTSD (National Association of Cognitive Behavioral Therapy). It can serve to establish the credibility of the counselor, generate positive expectancy, make treatment seem immediately helpful to the client, frame and reframe the symptoms, and prepare the client for their next steps. Psychoeducation is a central element of effective treatment, and can also significantly enhance outcomes, jumpstart cognitive restructuring, and lessen the debilitating posttraumatic shame and guilt many survivors carry (Yeomans et al., 2010; Beck et al., 2011).

Effective cognitive restructuring can be administered in brief discussions when the client has questions, and more systematically as a formal activity. This approach can also be delivered to either individuals or groups. Because people with PTSD often have difficulties with concentration and memory, it is important to repeat information and provide it in writing. For an example of client-friendly discussions on this topic, read Baranowsky and Lauer's (2013) *What Is PTSD: 3 Steps to Healing Trauma*.

PTSD-related education can cover topics such as:

1. Emotional and physical PTSD symptoms
2. Positive and negative coping skills and their differences
3. Recovery as an ongoing daily gradual process
4. Treatment options, including EBTs (Wampold et al., 2010)

While we recognize that there are some slight conceptual differences between psychoeducation and cognitive restructuring (i.e., that psychoeducation is the *process* and cognitive restructuring is the *outcome*), we believe they are similar enough to be combined into one category. There is very little, if any, cognitive restructuring that happens without educating clients on how to perceive themselves, their past, and their world differently. For this reason, we use the terms interchangeably to define this process of teaching clients to evolve their perceptions. Probably the most important goal of cognitive restructuring/psychoeducation with survivors of trauma is to help them to see their symptoms as adaptations instead of afflictions. This simple process goes a long way toward ameliorating some of the debilitating shame that plagues our clients in early treatment.

These four active ingredients represent a core foundation of competency for both new and seasoned trauma therapists. Developing insight into the ways in which all other treatments incorporate and catalyze these four components of PTSD treatment can provide the clinician greater insight into the mechanisms that resolve symptoms and heal the lives of trauma survivors. An a priori understanding of how and why these factors ameliorate symptoms and improve functioning in the lives of our survivor clients can greatly augment a clinician's deliberate practice with any treatment approach. For these reasons, we advocate this approach for those that treat people with posttraumatic stress as they intentionally develop their understanding and implementation of these active ingredients as a framework for augmenting their effectiveness and comfort in working with the clients who present with trauma histories at their practices. In the following sections we will explore the ways in which traditional evidence-based treatments for traumatic stress utilize and deliver these active ingredients.

# The Main Therapeutic Approaches, Research, and Guidelines

## 1. Behavioral Therapy

The origins of many current practices used to treat posttraumatic stress disorder (PTSD) and other posttraumatic conditions can be traced to a developmental history that includes behavioral therapy (BT). This is because BT, with its roots in classical and operant conditioning (i.e., Pavlov, 1897/1902, 1927/2015; Skinner, 1938), demonstrated a good outcome in addressing problems associated with fear and anxiety. It is interesting to note that practitioners of strict BT were uninterested in the events that occurred inside the minds of their clients. This was considered a black box that was not relevant to the outcome of behavioral interventions. A practitioner of pure BT was concerned primarily with the observable and manifest occurrences (or behaviors) in the lives of their clients and the specific antecedents that elicited those behaviors. They were not interested in what one thought of the events or how one interpreted or gave meaning to the events.

From the perspective of BT, the symptoms of posttraumatic stress occur in a two-step process that involves first classical conditioning and then operant conditioning. These two theories of conditioning explain why certain behaviors (in this case, symptoms of trauma) are likely to reoccur. From the 1890s to early 1900s, Pavlov investigated gastric function in dogs and reflex responses that eventually led to his theory of classical conditioning. He was awarded the Nobel Prize for this research in 1904. In classical conditioning, an unconditioned stimulus (UCS) such as meat powder is presented to an animal and it elicits salivation. This is a normal reaction to food and is called the *unconditioned response* (UCR). When the meat powder is paired with another (conditioned) stimulus (CS) such as a bell, time after time, eventually the bell will also elicit salivation. So, although the bell is at first just peripheral sensory information to the meat powder, it is eventually associated as a signal that meat powder is present and elicits the physiological response of salivating, which is now called the *conditioned response* (CR). To unhook this response of salivation to the sound of the bell is called *extinguishing the behavior*. This involves presenting the bell many times without the associated meat powder. Eventually the bell no longer produces salivation. To see an interactive example of how this works, visit https://educationalgames.nobelprize.org/educational/medicine/pavlov/

Operant conditioning suggests another mechanism to explain behaviors. In operant conditioning, the subject operates on the environment by performing behaviors. If the behaviors result in a favorable outcome (i.e., are reinforced), the subject is more likely to perform those behaviors again. Reinforcement of favorable outcomes might include actually getting something for the behavior (e.g., a pellet of food, a smile, etc.) or removing a noxious condition (e.g., a blaring noise or anxiety). The first is called *positive reinforcement* and the second is called *negative reinforcement*. Either forms of reinforcement increase the likelihood of behaviors to occur. In operant conditioning, one way to make behaviors less likely to occur is to remove all reinforcement for the behaviors.

In the case of PTSD, the first form of conditioning that occurs is classical. In this instance, a traumatic event (the UCS) produces fear/anxiety/arousal (the UCR). This is a normal reaction to trauma, and it is a very powerful response associated with the survival mechanism. The brain is hardwired to attend to all information associated with survival and registers much of the sensory information peripheral to the traumatic event. Like the bell in Pavlov's experiments, this peripheral sensory information is the CS (i.e., all the sensory input peripheral to the traumatic event). However, unlike Pavlov's bell, which takes many pairings of the bell and meat powder to produce salivation, the association of the UCS/CS (traumatic event/all other sensory information) to fear/anxiety/arousal happens instantly. This is an example of one-trial learning. From that time forward, anytime the CS (any sensory information that was associated with the original event) occurs, a CR (fear/anxiety/arousal) can potentially occur. This becomes problematic when, subsequent to a seemingly random sensory experience, this fear/anxiety/arousal response occurs. The brain has no specific event to associate to the fear response and begins to generalize it to more normal events not originally associated with the traumatic event. This makes the symptom picture seem very complex.

A simple example of this would be the anxiety associated with an automobile accident. The accident itself is the UCS, which generates a considerable amount of fear and anxiety (the UCR). For illustration purposes, say the accident occurred in heavy traffic with a high concentration of exhaust fumes in the air, at a stop light, at dusk. These would be considered the conditioned sensory stimuli (CS). If the accident resulted in a severe response, these conditioned stimuli (e.g., fumes, stop lights, and dusk) might then produce the fear and anxiety associated with the original accident, even when there is no current threat of accident. The fear and anxiety produced by the CS are now referred to as the conditioned response (CR). Now, as exposure to traffic, exhaust fumes, stop lights, and dusk occur, the individual can be retriggered to the traumatic memory and associated physiological, behavioral, and emotional responses associated with the accident itself. Other sensory information can also generalize to the accident and become associated with the anxiety. For instance, the driving anxiety may recur in a different vehicle under new circumstances that do not include any dangerous events but illicit feelings of fear and emotional distress. The different vehicle, daylight hours, and driving in general are all potentially added to the list of conditioned stimuli and may subsequently evoke anxiety as well.

The problematic behaviors associated with PTSD, such as avoidance, social isolation, anxiety-provoked reactions (e.g., anger, startle response), self-medication through substance abuse, etc. are behaviors that are meant to reduce the anxiety associated with the event (or subsequently associated events). When the fear/anxiety/arousal response occurs, the individual performs behaviors meant to help alleviate the anxiety. These behaviors are maintained through an operant conditioning model, where the anxiety and arousal brought about by the conditioned stimuli are reduced by the problematic behavior. The behaviors are negatively reinforced and, thus, more likely to occur.

To continue with our accident example, the person who had the accident may begin to experience anxiety in heavy traffic, and/or when smelling exhaust fumes, and/or at stop lights, and/ or at dusk while driving. To avoid this anxiety, this person may cease driving in any or all of the above conditions. When the person stops driving, the anxiety decreases. From the operant conditioning model, a noxious stimulus has been removed. This is negative reinforcement and the behavior of stopping, or even not venturing out, will be more likely to occur.

Figure 2 is a simple diagram of the first step in the creation of posttraumatic stress. This is the classical conditioning of the fear/anxiety/arousal response.

In this simple learning theory model (Mower, 1960), the traumatic event (UCS) produces a fear response (UCR) and when the survivor experiences stimuli that have come to be associated with the event (CS), the fear returns to plague the survivor in the form of intrusive symptoms (e.g., nightmares and flashbacks) and arousal symptoms taking the form of rapid heart rate, shallow breathing, muscle tension, etc. (CR).

The second step explains the manifestation and maintenance of many of the problematic behaviors associated with posttraumatic stress such as avoidance, substance abuse, anger, etc. This step is an example of operant conditioning wherein a problematic behavior is reinforced by the removal of fear/anxiety/arousal (see Figure 3).

In other words, as the survivor is continually confronted with this fear, they begin to develop behaviors to help alleviate the arousal and anxiety associated with the stimuli (CS). These behaviors are likely to include avoidance of the objects, people, and events that trigger remembrances of the traumatic event and the negative emotions associated with them. The behaviors may also include those meant to dull the intensity of the emotions

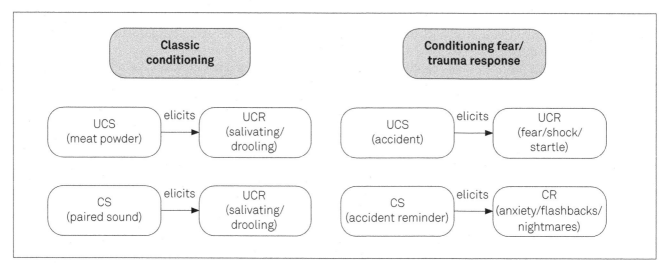

**Figure 2.**    Classical conditioning of the fear/anxiety/arousal response.

such as substance use or emotional withdrawal. From the BT perspective, this ever-widening circle of arousal and avoidance is thought to be the essence of PTSD.

The actual practice of BT involves carrying out a *functional analysis* of the survivor's environment to help identify stimuli and reinforcers that elicit and maintain problematic behaviors. However, the essence of the resolution of PTSD using BT requires that the survivor begin to confront, rather than avoid, the traumatic memory and the triggers associated with the trauma. This confrontation may be of the actual memory and/or the triggers associated with the trauma. The survivor is given skills to help them address the fear/anxiety/arousal and challenged to remain engaged in these confrontation/exposure situations until the fear diminishes and symptoms are, ultimately, extinguished.

For the trauma survivor, confronting their memories of abuse, horror, terror, and pain are often like riding a dangerously bucking bronco. The memories elicit the fear/anxiety/arousal associated with the original event and create a huge disincentive to do the work. It is a challenging process that demands skill, patience, and assistance from both the client and the therapist. Nonetheless, just as the horse adjusts to the rider and the dog stops salivating over time (when a bell is rung and meat powder is never produced), a trauma survivor can also learn to experience a trauma memory without eliciting the response of fear/anxiety/arousal. The behavioral therapist assists the trauma survivor by structuring the treatment process in a way that allows them to gain mastery over this response.

In 1958, Joseph Wolpe, a behavioral therapist and researcher, developed the theory of reciprocal inhibition (Wolpe, 1958) to explain and direct the treatment of anxiety and phobia symptoms. The theory of reciprocal inhibition holds that when exposure to an anxiety-provoking stimulus is paired with the relaxation response (i.e., the individual is able to keep the muscles in their body relaxed) and the client is able to maintain this relaxation, then the conditioned response to the fear-provoking stimulus is extinguished (see Figure 4). There are sound physiological and neurological reasons to explain the one-trial learning of classical conditioning. The reasons why

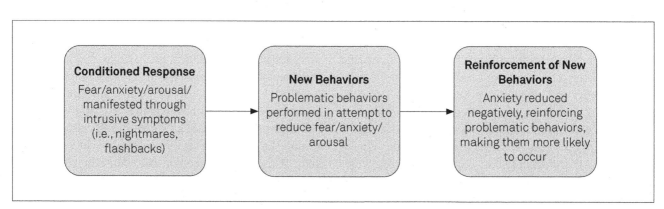

**Figure 3.**    Operant conditioning: Problematic behavior is reinforced by removal of fear/anxiety/arousal.

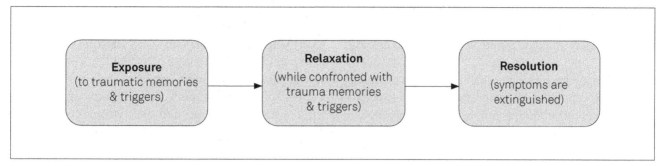

**Figure 4.**    Theory of reciprocal inhibition.

reciprocal inhibition works with trauma survivors specifically will be discussed in the Section 5: Psychophysiology of Trauma.

Reciprocal inhibition, the pairing of exposure and relaxation, is at the heart of all BT for symptoms of anxiety. Some BTs (e.g., *in vivo* exposure or flooding) begin with exposure and push their way through the anxiety, hopefully to a point where the client is relaxed in the face of exposure. However, these techniques have the potential for retraumatizing the client if the individual is not able to fully maintain relaxation throughout the exposure exercise or, if there is insufficient time to resolve or habituate to the trauma memory, leaving the trauma memory work incomplete. It is not until relaxation occurs in the face of exposure that symptoms subside. It is our opinion that relaxation is a necessary ingredient to symptom resolution and better learned before and experienced during exposure than experienced after the process of being overwhelmed by anxiety. Thus, we identify reciprocal inhibition as a necessary ingredient in effective treatments of PTSD. Most of the learning involved in this book will focus on teaching you, the reader, skilled application and utilization of reciprocal inhibition. You will learn techniques to help client's approach and confront their traumatic material. You will also learn techniques for assisting them in developing and maintaining the capacity to harness calm during this exposure. The ability to assist the client in maximal attenuation of this process, also known as *titration*, can rapidly accelerate the treatment of PTSD and is the artful skill of the traumatologist.

Present-day practitioners of strict BT are still primarily interested in behaviors and a functional analysis of the specific life occurrences that elicit dysfunctional behaviors. However, as you might expect, they have come to believe that the mind may mediate some of these events. While they still help their clients focus on their problematic behaviors (or failure to practice positive behaviors) and assist them with stopping or eradicating these problematic behaviors and/or learning and practicing new,

more fulfilling behaviors (Hersen & Gross, 2008), some of these interventions are now decidedly cognitive.

The BT process known as *direct therapeutic exposure*, which was commonly utilized with Vietnam veterans, is an example of this procedure. In this process, a functional analysis of the client's life is performed wherein a number of factors are assessed. These include, but are not limited to, safety, secondary gain, resources, other life traumas, triggers, and reinforcers. Target behaviors are also identified. Then, a considerable amount of psychoeducation occurs. The client is taught relaxation techniques, learns coping skills, is specifically taught the two-step process of symptom generation to normalize the experience, and has the process of exposure in therapy explained. After the client has demonstrated adequate stabilization, they begin the process of remembering what happened with full affect. The client is encouraged to stay with the process until the anxiety lessens. This may mean repeating the memory process several times. Once they have finished, the therapist assists in returning them to a state of relaxation. The therapist then processes the information, helping the client create new meanings and beliefs about the experience. In other words, they begin the process of cognitive restructuring. The exciting part of this work is seeing client transformation through exposure and then habituation, resulting in extinction of the trigger or the traumatic memory. When it comes to extinction of traumatic memories, the result is a lessening of reactivity when exposed to trauma reminders in the future. Although this process is explained above, the trauma practice approach allows for alternative methods to achieve the desired outcome.

## 2. Cognitive Therapy

In the 1960s and early 1970s, and, many would say, in reaction to BT's clinically sterile fascination with only manifest behaviors, clinical and research psychologists became progressively more interested in what was happening *inside* the client who was struggling with symptoms of anxiety and depression. Scientists like Ellis (Ellis & Harper, 1961) and Beck (1967, 1976) began to investigate the importance of a client's thoughts, and the meanings, beliefs, and interpretations they attached to events, for both the understanding and treatment of psychological disorders and their symptoms.

A cognitive therapist would be quick to point out that not everyone who experiences the same traumatic event develops posttraumatic symptoms, and those who do experience a vast array of different consequences from the same event. From the perspective of cognitive therapy (CT), this difference was due to the survivor's beliefs, meanings, interpretations, and other *internal* events and reactions to the traumatic experience. Cognitive therapists believe that certain (traumatic) events, especially during developmental periods, can result in the entire belief system, or schema, becoming distorted. These distorted schemas continue to shape and misshape the world for many trauma survivors. Treatment is oriented toward identifying the distorted beliefs that survivors attach to painful or traumatic experiences and helping the survivor renegotiate these beliefs and meanings toward healthier and adaptive ones. This process of assisting a client in changing or re-scripting their distorted thoughts of themselves and their world is called *cognitive restructuring*.

A common example of this technique is a client who had been molested in childhood. Because her abuser used words like "sexy" and "pretty" during the abuse, she came to believe that it must have been something about her looks that caused her abuser to molest her. To ensure that it did not happen again, she began to overeat obsessively, in the mistaken belief that being overweight would make her less "sexy" and protect her from being molested again. As the years pass, she may no longer remember the first thought of making herself less attractive. However, subsequent attempts to lose weight are not only unsuccessful, they also result in a considerable increase in anxiety. Treatment would involve identifying the distorted belief about why she was abused in the first place and help in restructuring her belief system to allow her to create a healthier way to be safe.

Cognitive therapists assist clients to first identify their distorted thoughts and beliefs and then help them substitute new, more satisfying beliefs. Techniques like thought stopping, positive affirmations, rehearsal, and the triple column technique (Burns, 1980) are all frequently utilized in CT to assist the client in shifting these thinking patterns.

There exists a debate among cognitive therapists about whether or not it is important to gain insight and understanding into the causes and events that gave rise to distorted thought patterns. Some believe that focusing treatment energy and resources on assisting the client in developing more satisfying beliefs, thoughts, and lifestyle in the present is the most crucial ingredient to therapy. Others believe this minimizes the importance of revisiting the traumatic events and the meanings ascribed to them; such therapists spend more time identifying the specific distorted thoughts that arise from the events.

For reasons to be discussed shortly, we believe helping the trauma survivor develop more satisfactory living skills in the present, including the ability to utilize positive thinking and beliefs, is a necessary ingredient for symptom resolution and should be included in any treatment of trauma. This is consistent with the DSM-5 (American Psychiatric Association, 2013) Criterion D that addresses the importance of mood and cognition after exposure to trauma. We will utilize many techniques drawn from CT to teach methods for assisting the trauma survivor in developing this present-day stabilization and satisfaction. However, we will also utilize CT techniques to teach readers of this book to assist trauma survivors in confronting and resolving their traumatic memories. These procedures involve a combination of both CT (helping the survivor resolve their thoughts and meanings about the trauma, themselves, and the world) and the techniques of BT (helping the trauma survivor confront and resolve the traumatic memory using reciprocal inhibition). This combination results in a powerful collection of techniques known as *cognitive behavioral therapy* (CBT) and is one of the main focuses of this book.

## 3. Cognitive-Behavioral Therapy

CBT is one of the most utilized, researched, and consistently effective treatment for the symptoms of posttraumatic stress currently used by clinicians who treat trauma survivors (Foa & Meadows, 1997). Trauma focused CBT has been strongly recommended as a treatment that should be prioritized among the front line of options for PTSD treatment by the APA and the VA/DoD (Management of Posttraumatic Stress Disorder Work Group, 2017; Watkins et al., 2018; see Table 4 and Box 1. CBT combines aspects of BT and CT, so it includes both the explicit and observable, as well as the implicit and internal behaviors. Many writers have acknowledged the "cognitivization" of BT over recent years and a blurring of boundaries between CT, BT, and CBT.

We believe that it is paramount to the professional development of any trauma-care practitioner to integrate a broad tri-phasic approach utilizing approaches that address the mind, body, beliefs, emotions, and behaviors (Gentry et al., 2017).

Follette, Ruzek, and Abueg (1998) wrote:

As the field of behavioral therapy has evolved, it has generated a large number of both broad and specific theories that sometimes complement one another and sometime compete for explanatory relevance. Indeed, there has been much debate about whether such a range of theoretical formulations can or should be accommodated under a single rubric of "behavioral therapy" or "cognitive-behavioral therapy," when alternative formulations sometimes do violence to the core assumptions and conceptual underpinnings of one another. With the growth in trauma-related cognitive-behavioral research and treatment, these same controversies are present. However, we believe there is some movement toward rapprochement among these differing perspectives (pp. 4–5).

For the purposes of this book, we will integrate the principles and techniques of BT and CT together and identify these principles and techniques as CBT trauma therapy. Updated in this edition, we include the *somatic* in exchange for the term body and integrate this into the CBT framework to result in cognitive-behavioral-somatic therapy approach (CBST).

Conclusions or assumptions are often at the root of PTSD and if we can make good sense of an event or challenge distorted cognitions (beliefs) we may be able to change old beliefs, such as "I am never safe" to "I am safe in this moment right now!" Any thorough approach to trauma therapy must include a focused effort to challenge distorted cognitions that negatively impact the client's life, limiting activities, outlets, and life pleasures. These include:

- Identifying distorted beliefs
- Identifying the root of the distortion (when did the belief first surface? what happened at that time?)
- Extinguishing the old belief (often through various exposure and/or challenging exercises)
- Developing new more adaptive and intentional schemas or belief systems (e.g., I am doing my best)

Reflecting on the concept of *neuroplasticity* helps us to see how negative thoughts and beliefs can undermine our recovery. Doidge (2007) comments that "neurons that fire together wire together" (p. 174) and this idea is critically important for our understanding of the impact of traumatic stress. By learning how to rewire our brains to engage corrective messaging (i.e., I am safe now, etc), to engage reciprocal inhibition approaches, and to harness calm, we can short-circuit chronic re-ignition over lower-level reminders of a traumatic event. It's also been shown that

**Box 1.** Active ingredients found in different CBT trauma therapy research

**2010 VA/DOD Clinical practice guideline for management of post-traumatic stress (Bernardy & Friedman, 2012)**

- Psychoeducation
- Exposure
- Anxiety management
- Cognitive restructuring

**The ISTSS expert consensus treatment guidelines for complex PTSD in adults (Cloitre et al., 2012)**

- Emotion regulation strategies
- Narration of trauma memory
- Cognitive restructuring
- Anxiety and stress management
- Interpersonal skills

**Australian Government, National Health and Medical Research Council (n.d.)**

- Therapeutic alliance
- Psychoeducation
- Emotional regulation and coping skills
- Some form of exposure to memories of traumatic experiences
- Cognitive processing, restructuring, and /or meaning making
- Tackling emotions
- Altering memory processes

**European Union Traumatic Stress Network (Schnyder et al., 2015)**

- Psychoeducation
- Emotion regulation and coping skills
- Imaginal exposure
- Cognitive processing and restructuring
- Meaning making
- Dealing with emotions
- Resolving memory processes

**Common Elements Treatment Approach (CETA) – Johns Hopkins University (Murray et al., 2014)**

- Relaxation
- Cognitive coping
- Exposure to trauma memories
- Direct therapeutic (in vivo) exposure
- Cognitive restructuring
- Behavioral activation
- Problem-solving

stress can reduce hippocampal neurogenesis (Fuchs & Flügge, 2014) but that this can be reversed. A literature review by Shaffer (2016) suggests that sleep, aerobic activity combined with cognitive exercises, meditation, and cognitive behavioural techniques are among those that promote neurogenesis and positive neuroplasticity in the brain. A gratitude vs resentment study by Kyeong et al. (2017) also demonstrates that cognitive exercises such as gratitude can have a positive effect on brain physiology, while resentment can have the opposite impact, and suggests that gratitude may be able to play a part in recovery from PTSD. Neuroplasticity is covered later in this chapter in greater detail.

## 4. Cognitive-Behavioral Therapy Research

### Expert Guidelines

There are a considerable number of CBT techniques available to address the symptoms of PTSD (see Tables 1 and 2). Choosing which is the most appropriate might seem confusing. When selecting the most appropriate therapeutic intervention to utilize with specific client groups it is important to look to both research *and* expert consensus to guide us. Although research can provide us with information about the factors associated with recovery, there are several reasons why the use of expert guidelines can also be useful in your day-to-day practice.

First, research does not always generalize easily into clinical practice and research studies often fail to reflect the complexities of the cases that we must address in our caseload. Second, systematic studies frequently fail to answer all the questions that arise in clinical practice in a comprehensive and effective manner. Third, research can be a tedious and time-consuming practice that does not move as quickly as meaningful and efficacious clinical innovation. This does not mean we discard the excellent research that highlights strong clinical methodology, but that we supplement it with the best methods endorsed by expert consensus. This type of "research in motion" is certainly the lifeblood of all new and useful approaches.

**Table 1.**    Preferred psychotherapy techniques for different PTSD target symptoms

| Most prominent symptom | Recommended techniques | Also consider |
|---|---|---|
| Intrusive thoughts | Exposure therapy | Cognitive therapy<br>Anxiety management<br>Psychoeducation<br>Play therapy for children |
| Flashbacks | Exposure therapy | Anxiety management<br>Cognitive therapy<br>Psychoeducation |
| Trauma-related fears, panic, and avoidance | Exposure therapy<br>Cognitive therapy<br>Anxiety management | Psychoeducation<br>Play therapy for children |
| Numbing/detachment from others/loss of interest | Cognitive therapy | Psychoeducation<br>Exposure therapy |
| Irritability/angry outbursts | Cognitive therapy<br>Anxiety management | Psychoeducation<br>Exposure therapy |
| Guilt/shame | Cognitive therapy | Psychoeducation<br>Play therapy for children |
| General anxiety (hyperarousal, hypervigilance, startle) | Anxiety management<br>Exposure therapy | Cognitive therapy<br>Psychoeducation<br>Play therapy for children |
| Sleep disturbances | Anxiety management | Exposure therapy<br>Cognitive therapy<br>Psychoeducation |
| Difficulty concentrating | Anxiety management | Cognitive therapy<br>Psychoeducation |

Adapted and reprinted with permission from "The expert consensus guideline series: Treatment of posttraumatic stress disorder" by E. B. Foa, J. R. T. Davidson, & A. Frances, 1999, *The Journal of Clinical Psychiatry, 60,* p. 15. © 1999 Physicians Postgraduate Press. (See also American Psycholgoical Association, 2017; Cloitre et al., 2011, 2012.)

Sources of expert guidelines we can consider include the "ISTSS Expert Clinician Survey on Best Practices" (Cloitre, et al., 2011, 2012), the "APA Clinical Practice Guideline for the Treatment of PTSD" (APA, 2017), and the "Expert Consensus Guidelines Series: Treatment of Posttraumatic Stress Disorder" (Foa et al., 1999). These articles present recommendations from approximately 50 expert trauma clinicians offering opinion based on their experience and approximately 57 medication experts who make recommendations based on their experience treating PTSD. Dr Baranowsky, Eric Gentry, and Robert Rhoton have also written a recent paper compiling research on these best practices from meta-analyses on effective trauma care in which we provide guidelines on trauma competency and a phasic structure for trauma care (Gentry et al., 2017). In this paper, we outline four common elements identified by a meta-analysis on the research to be important for effective treatment of PTSD: Cognitive restructuring and psychoeducation, a deliberate and continually improving therapeutic relationship, relaxation/self-regulation, and exposure via narrative (2017). We propose that these four ingredients can act as critical competencies and baseline standards for trauma counselling. For further elucidation please refer directly to the source documentation referenced in this book.

Cloitre et al. (2011) integrate expert opinion from 50 PTSD experts. Phase-based approaches were endorsed by 84% of those sampled while the need for symptom-specific interventions was also identified as important.

Primary interventions included emotional stabilization, cognitive restructuring, anxiety and stress management, trauma narrative processing, and development of interpersonal skills. Secondary approaches included mindfulness and meditation type approaches for symptom management. Table 1 and Table 2 integrate still-relevant findings from the earlier Expert Consensus Guidelines, which continue to form a meaningful foundation for this work (Foa et al., 1999).

## International Society for Traumatic Stress Studies (ISTSS) Practice Guidelines

CBT is the most widely researched treatment approach identified in the literature. *Effective Treatments for PTSD: Practice Guidelines From the International Society for Traumatic Stress Studies* (Foa et al., 2009; Foa et al., 2000), provides an excellent historical review of CBT research for treating posttraumatic stress. Shubina (2015) and Watkins et al. (2018) provide a more contemporary review of the use of cognitive-behavioral therapies in treatment. The focus of this review addresses a number of brief CBT interventions. These include: exposure therapy (EX); systematic desensitization (SD); stress inoculation training (SIT); cognitive processing therapy (CPT); cognitive therapy (CT); assertiveness training (AT); biofeedback (BIO); relaxation training (RLX); dialectical behavior therapy (DBT); acceptance and commitment therapy (ACT), and various combinations of those listed above.

**Table 2.**   Selecting psychotherapy techniques based on effectiveness, safety, acceptability, and speed of action

| Technical approach | Recommended techniques | Also consider |
|---|---|---|
| Most effective techniques | Exposure therapy<br>Cognitive therapy | Anxiety management |
| Quickest acting techniques | Exposure therapy | Anxiety management<br>Cognitive therapy<br>Psychoeducation |
| Techniques preferred across all types of trauma | Cognitive therapy<br>Exposure therapy<br>Anxiety management | Psychoeducation |
| Safest techniques | Anxiety management<br>Psychoeducation<br>Cognitive therapy | Play therapy for children Exposure therapy |
| Most-acceptable techniques | Psychoeducation<br>Cognitive therapy<br>Anxiety management | Play therapy for children |

Adapted and reprinted with permission from Foa, E. B., Davidson, J. R. T., & Frances, A. The expert consensus guideline series: Treatment of posttraumatic stress disorder. *The Journal of Clinical Psychiatry*, 1999, 60, p. 17. © 1999 Physicians Postgraduate Press. (See also American Psychological Association, 2017; Cloitre et al., 2011, 2012.)

**Table 3.**    CBT research synthesis

| Inter-vention | Number of studies reviewed | AHCPR rating | Gold standards for clinical studies | Summary |
|---|---|---|---|---|
| ACT | 0 | N/A | N/A | Theoretically based approach relating to avoidance of trauma content resulting in lack of processing and avoidance/intrusion distress (Cahill et al., 2009). Complementary to exposure-based therapies and can be used to address comorbidities to PTSD that are relevant to trauma survivors, such as depression. (Scarlet et al., 2016). Shows potential for treatment for PTSD but more research needed (Bean et al., 2017). |
| AT | 1 | Level B | Moderate adherence to 3 of 7 standards. | "Has not received strong support" (Rothbaum et al., 2000). |
| | 1 | Level B | Moderate adherence to 4 out of 7 standards. | "Significant improvement pre- to posttreatment" (Cahill et al., 2009). |
| BIO | 1 | Level A | Meets 4 of 7 standards. | "BIO has not received support" (Rothbaum et al., 2000). |
| CPT | 1 | Level B | Meets 4 of 7 standards. | "Effective" (Rothbaum et al., 2000). Modify to various trauma populations. |
| | 1 | Level B | Meets 4 of 7 standards. | "Intervention was superior to waitlist on measures of PTSD, depression and dissociation" (Cahill et al., 2009). Strongly recommended for treatment of PTSD (American Psychological Association, 2017; VA/DoD Clinical Practice Guideline Working Group, 2017). |
| CT | 3 | Level A to C | Mixed results. | "CT ... effective in reducing ... symptoms" (Rothbaum et al., 2000). Strongly recommended for treatment of PTSD (American Psychological Association, 2017). |
| EX | 12 | Level A (8 studies) Level B – (4 studies) | Mixed results. Several met all 7 standards while some met notably fewer. | "Compelling evidence ... quite effective" (Rothbaum et al, 2000). |
| | 26+ | Level B | Moderate adherence to 4 of 7 standards. | "Statistically superior to control group" (Cahill et al., 2009). |
| DBT | 2 | Level A & B | Mixed results. Rigor of studies varies. | "Statistically superior to control group ... (TSI)" (Cahill et al., 2009). |
| RLX | 1 | Level A (1 study) | Met all 7 standards. | Combination of EX plus CT was superior to FLX on PTSD posttreatment (Cahill et al., 2009). |
| SD | 6 | Level A through C Most B or lower | None met all 7 standards. | Methodological problems and failed to receive strong research-based support (Rothbaum et al., 2000). |

**Table 3.**    Continued

| Intervention | Number of studies reviewed | AHCPR rating | Gold standards for clinical studies | Summary |
|---|---|---|---|---|
| SIT | 4 | Level A (2 studies) Level B (2 studies) | Mixed results. Rigor of studies varies. | "Found SIT effective" (Rothbaum et al., 2000). Focus only on female sexual assault survivors. Recommended for treatment of PTSD (US Department of VA and Department of Defense Clinical Practice Guideline Working Group, 2017; Lancaster et al., 2016). |

(See also Foa, Keane, Friedman & Cohen, 2009; Shubina, 2015; Watkins et al., 2018)

Each of the many research studies reviewed were subsequently organized based on type of treatment, adherence to the Gold Standards Rating and the Agency for Health Care Policy and Research (AHCPR) ratings (see Column 3 in Table 3). These standards rate research based on a seven-point system that categorizes their level of methodological rigor. Studies can be categorized as Level A: very well controlled or methodologically rigorous; Level B: less well controlled or moderately rigorous methodology; Level C or lower: not well controlled or weak studies. Table 3 is a synthesis of the various literature reviews of the current research. A literature review by Kar (2011) also points to a robust evidence base for CBT as a safe an effective intervention for the treatment of chronic PTSD, but that nonresponse to CBT for PTSD can be another potential outcome in cases due to presence of other factors such as additional diseases or medical conditions. A study by Jonas et al. (2013) showed that 61–82% of patients who were diagnosed with PTSD lost that diagnosis after being treated with CBT. These results of recovery were 26% higher than those in a waitlist or supportive counselling group.

It is clear that the CBT outcome results in this review are mixed. Nevertheless, CBT stands out in the literature as more efficacious than any other single approach in the psychological treatment of trauma. To understand this discrepancy, it is necessary to recall the limitations of research based on this review. First, we are always limited to the research currently available – methods may be clinically "effective" but not yet supported by research; second, studies available may have been conducted using poor methodologies; third, we cannot necessarily generalize the utility of a well-studied approach for one population based on another (e.g., exposure therapy for PTSD based on research for depressed married females). Therefore, it is useful to refer back to the expert guidelines discussed earlier and with more contemporary ones as

illustrated in Table 4. It is also important to recognize that some of the most effective approaches, such as exposure therapy, require a skilled practitioner to implement because the possibility of retriggering can occur if the client has not been adequately taught to initiate stabilization and self-care if symptoms become overwhelming.

## 5. Psychophysiology of Trauma

The hows and whys of posttraumatic stress, subsequent symptoms, and symptom resolution can be understood in relation to the events that occur in the brain during and after a traumatic event. What follows is a *brief* description of the sequence of events during and after a trauma. This information is extremely useful when educating survivors and explaining that their symptoms are natural responses to extreme events. For a more complete understanding of the neurological sequence involved in trauma, see Scaer, 2006, 2014; van der Kolk et al., 1996; Rothschild, 2000; Center for Substance Abuse Treatment, 2014; Dumovich & Singh, 2021).

When a person experiences a traumatic event, the information is registered in the brain along two pathways. The first and quickest path sends sensory information (e.g., scent, related objects, sounds, sights, etc.) to the amygdala, where a fear response is triggered and the information is cataloged as important for survival. From the amygdala, the information proceeds to other areas of the brain (i.e., the stria terminalis and the locus ceruleus) responsible for preparing the body for flight or fight and a subsystem of the ANS (the sympathetic nervous system) is activated. The information is eventually stored in the hippocampus as a memory important for survival. Thereafter, anything that stimulates that sensory memory trace will also potentially stimulate the body to prepare for survival (fear/anxiety/arousal). In other words, when an

**Table 4.**    Clinical practice guidelines for treatment of PTSD

| Clinical Practice Guideline | Methodology | Strongly recommended therapies | Recommended therapies |
|---|---|---|---|
| American Psychological Association (2017) | Independent systematic review; RCTs published from 5/25/12–6/1/16; Expert review | Cognitive behavioral therapy, cognitive processing therapy, prolonged exposure, cognitive therapy | Brief eclectic psychotherapy, EMDR, narrative exposure therapy |
| VA/DoD Clinical Practice Guideline Working Group, 2017 | Independent systematic review; RCTs from 1/1/09–March 2016; Expert review | Cognitive processing therapy, prolonged exposure, EMDR, specific CBT for PTSD, brief eclectic psychotherapy, narrative exposure therapy, and written narrative exposure | Stress inoculation training, present-centered therapy, interpersonal psychotherapy |

Reprinted with permission from "Treating PTSD: A Review of Evidence-Based Psychotherapy Interventions" by L. E. Watkins, K. R. Sprang, & B. O. Rothbaum, 2018, *Frontiers in Behavioral Neuroscience*, 12, Article 258. © 2018 CC BY 4.0 https://doi.org/10.3389/fnbeh.2018.00258

individual is exposed to related cues to the memory (e.g., scent, related objects, sounds, sights, etc.), these sensory reminders reignite the associated strong feelings. The memory of the traumatic event itself may or may not be recalled. This can leave the individual feeling as if they are in danger but not necessarily knowing why (Kirmayer et al., 2007; Center for Substance Abuse Treatment, 2014).

This variability in memory can be understood by following the second pathway for information processing. This second and much longer path for the information proceeds through the thalamus, which routes sensory information to appropriate parts of the neocortex to be analyzed. This information is processed through various areas in the neocortex where language is used to organize and generate responses (a declarative memory is formed), associations to other information are made, and meaning is created. It is then routed to and stored in the hippocampus. The neocortex also contains inhibitory areas that are capable of inhibiting or turning down the survival/fear response generated by the information passed through the amygdala. In other words, the neocortex can potentially change the meaning of the original memory trace and alter or modulate the survival response (Kirmayer et al., 2007); Schumann et al., 2011; Sato et al., 2016).

Under conditions of extreme stress, the brain produces stress hormones such as cortisol that interfere with the consolidation of the information from the neocortex. This also interferes with the possible inhibitory responses that would ameliorate the anxiety of the survival response. Memories that are formed under conditions of trauma often become fragmented. They remain out of context

and are thus left unincorporated and unassociated with other memories. The result is that, whenever the memory trace is stimulated, the body reverts to survival mode, which is experienced as anxiety. Because the traumatic memories are often unconsolidated, it is sometimes difficult for a survivor to make the link between earlier traumatic experiences and the current feeling of anxiety. The individual then begins to perform behaviors to relieve the anxiety. If these behaviors work to relieve the anxiety (i.e., remove a noxious condition), they are negatively reinforced to occur again.

These information storage pathways account for the symptoms discussed in the previous example of the person who was involved in an accident. During this accident, a large number of sensory cues were recorded, such as the smell of exhaust fumes, heavy traffic, and dim light. This sensory information is recorded in such a manner that, even without actually remembering the original accident, the person in the accident might find themselves becoming extremely anxious at the smell of exhaust fumes or by being in heavy traffic at dusk. Because they do not necessarily begin to consciously recall the original event, they will try to make sense of their feelings using information from the current moment. This is often a confusing task, especially if there is nothing particularly threatening in the current moment. They may just assume they are having an anxiety attack and attribute it to a physiological problem. Or they may simply begin to perform behaviors to reduce their anxiety, such as self-medicating with drugs or alcohol or avoiding driving.

The initial neurological response of the brain is likely the mechanism by which the classical conditioning of the traumatic response is accomplished. In one-trial learning, the sensory stimuli are sent to the midbrain and recorded as a threat to survival. The brain attaches the emotions of fear and anxiety to these stimuli and prepares the body for flight or fight. Very little cognitive processing occurs at this stage because the neocortex has been flooded with cortisol and other corticosteroids that interfere with memory consolidation. The fact that memories are unconsolidated and unconnected results in the failure to normally resolve the fear/anxiety/arousal response. In other words, the brain has failed to unhook the sensory information from the fear/anxiety/arousal response. Later behaviors are operationally learned as a way to alleviate this fear/anxiety/arousal.

A video about this topic titled "The Emotional Brain Lays a Landmine of Frightening Memories. Ask Dr Anna S.2.E.40," (see Video 2 in the supplementary material or Baranowsky, 2015, November 11, https://youtu.be/sL-kJSleE_c) helps explain some of the ways in which these traumatic memories can be stored in our body and nervous system after trauma, and how it can be both of benefit and detriment to health after trauma. This video can be shared with trauma survivors to help them understand the physiological processes that might be causing them to feel heightened anxiety, and through this understanding we can help to loosen the hold and grip these processes have over the life and recovery of trauma survivors.

Subsequent stimulation of this memory trace will potentially reactivate the survival routines until the neocortex has been allowed to process the information and inhibit the response. Relaxation in the face of exposure facilitates access to neocortical functions (declarative memory, meaning generation, and anxiety inhibition). Research suggests that this may be mediated by a decrease in cortisol under conditions of relaxation (Benson, 1997; Luecken et al., 2004) Emerging research has also shown mindfulness-based interventions can help to normalize cortisol levels (Bergen-Cico et al., 2014; Kim et al., 2013) and reduce circulating inflammatory cytokines (Gallegos et al., 2015). Strictly behavioral interventions pair the memory trace with responses (relaxation, self-soothing) that are inconsistent with the survival mode (fear/anxiety/arousal), expanding the response set. Cognitive interventions specifically work to pair the memory trace with more fully processed (and hence more meaningful) information that has the ability to inhibit the survival response.

Recall the client who experienced an automobile accident. The sensory stimuli are sent to the midbrain and recorded as a threat to survival. The brain attaches the emotions of fear and anxiety to these stimuli and prepares the body for flight or fight. As expected, little cognitive processing occurs at this stage, and the neocortex becomes flooded with cortisol and other corticosteroids, essentially inhibiting the ability to consolidate and fully store memories. Future reminders of the memory will reignite the poorly stored memory trace of the event, resulting in survival strategies being engaged. Survival responses will continue to occur until neocortical processing of the traumatic memory has adequately allowed for re-storage of the memory, while concurrently extinguishing the emotional distress associated with the memory. An *in vivo* (on-site) behavioral intervention would teach relaxation techniques and then pair relaxation with the sensory stimulus. In this example, a client would be relaxed and then perhaps be taken into traffic or allowed to smell exhaust by the roadside until they become anxious. The client would then initiate relaxation exercises until the symptoms of anxiety begin to reduce. This can occur either *in vivo* or after departing from the anxiety-provoking situation. This might require many exposures until the client is no longer anxious in the presence of fumes or traffic. Cognitive interventions also require teaching relaxation techniques and re-experiencing the event. However, these would more likely involve the client intentionally remembering the traumatic event under conditions of relaxation, rather than direct exposure to traumatic stimuli. Initial sessions would involve discussions of memories peripheral to the actual trauma and subsequent beliefs about the event. Eventually, trauma reduction sessions would involve the direct memory of the event (again, under conditions of relaxation) and the ability to describe the event without anxiety. Finally, cognitive restructuring would address distorted beliefs and behaviors previously learned and used to keep safe.

## Epigenetics

What were the conditions in which your mother carried you as a fetus? Did you grow up in a household filled with love and kindness or anger and fear? Did you feel safe walking to school as a child, or did you hide when you saw the school bully coming toward you? Was life kind to your parents and their parents – offering opportunities and support; or cruel – consistently exposing them to loss, grief, and pain? These are the questions we might ask if we were to dig more deeply than the current day exposure to a car accident or an act of violence. The research on Epigenetics suggests that we may be born with DNA that results in a higher degree of vulnerability as a result of our genes or even what our parents or grandparents experienced in their lifetimes (Wolynn, 2016; Youssef et al., 2018). This certainly helps us to understand why one person or group might tolerate a traumatic event better than another given similar circumstances (Dudley et al., 2011; Heinzelmann & Gill, 2013; Nestler, 2012; Radley et al., 2011, Bezo & Maggi, 2018; Yehuda & Lehrner, 2018, Yahuda, 2016).

To further unpack how epigenetics can impact health, please watch a video interview with Mark Wolynn, author of the book *It Didn't Start with You: How Inherited Family Trauma Shapes Who We Are and How to End the Cycle* (2016). This interview (Baranowsky, 2017, July 19) also explores pathways towards healing and recovery from inherited family trauma and can be found in Video 3 in the supplementary material (p. 226; or at https://www.youtube.com/watch?v=WzQ5FM3hCgo).

The adverse childhood experiences study (ACE; Felitti et al., 1998) is a 20+ year ongoing study exploring the effects of aversive childhood experiences upon the lives of adult survivors of these experiences. There have been dozens of studies generated from this first study that showed traumatic experiences in early life correlate strongly with negative health and mental health outcomes. Early death, chemical dependency, cardiovascular diseases, obstructive pulmonary diseases, AIDS and other sexually transmitted diseases, smoking/tobacco use, unwanted pregnancy, and mental illness diagnoses are all closely related to childhood aversive experiences. In addition to the pain and difficulty that these early life experiences cause the survivor, it has become clear that trauma perpetrated upon children produces adults who are extreme utilizers of health resources. This drain on healthcare resources by adult survivors of childhood trauma has begun to focus many service providers and researchers, including the Centers for Disease Control, towards early detection of trauma and developing strategies for prevention of traumatic stress in adult survivors.

While the epigenetics of unresolved trauma have been and are currently passed along to subsequent generations, causing a myriad of negative effects, the reverse of this is also true. The authors applaud the work of the ACE study (see http://www.acestudy.org) and other trauma prevention initiatives. This work has made us hopeful about what this means for our future. As we begin to raise children free from the trauma of abuse and neglect, they will grow into healthier adults who will significantly lessen the perpetration of trauma upon their children. As we assist others in healing their trauma, we are building a better world for our children and grandchildren. Thanks to the work currently being done around the globe on lessening the effects of trauma we can, maybe the first time in history, visualize a world in which health and connection instead of trauma and fear are the dominant principles of our future world.

## Neuroplasticity

We now know that the brain is not static but can be changed by the experience of trauma. It is also clear from the current research on neuroplasticity that, with the right exercises and massed practice (or regular corrective exercises or interventions), we can relearn or retrain our brain to overcome traumatic events (Doidge, 2007; Pickersgill et al., 2015; Krishnamurthy et al., 2016). We are truly excited by this new research and feel that it reinforces many of the approaches for stabilization and daily practice that we have encouraged our clients to follow for years. It also opens up our minds to the possibility of even greater posttraumatic growth and recovery beyond what we had originally hoped or anticipated for those we care for (Kays et al., 2012).

Huttenlocher (2002) on neuroplasticity explains that: "An important factor that needs to be stressed is the fact that malleability of the nervous system does not end with maturity. It has been shown to persist to some extent until old age" (p. 9).

What an extremely hopeful concept this is. This reinforces the idea that even many years after a traumatic event, we can still apply correct approaches to reduce suffering among those trauma survivors we assist, because essentially humans remain malleable.

Although principles related to CBT lay a foundation for our trauma practice approach, research on neuroplasticity and positive psychology helps to guide us in developing new approaches that integrate well within the given model. You will find examples of this throughout the book.

The idea that "neurons that fire together wire together" (Doidge, 2007) relates to frequent response sequences, thoughts, or behaviors that create powerful connections or pattern habits that lead to more of the same. This is true whether it is a negative fear response or a tendency to see the bright side of things. Consequently, in order for us to function better after trauma, we need to retrain our brains so that our neurons fire together in a new more adaptive way and are less inclined to fire around reminders of a stressful past. The latter would result in chronically high levels of emotional and physiological strain (Krishnamurthy et al., 2016; DeFina et al., 2009; Neumeister et al., 2007).

In line with neuroplasticity research, we strongly believe that those we serve and care for are not forever damaged by trauma but injured with the very real possibility of recovery. Intentional and deliberate choice followed by consistent action using the right approaches over time (or "massed practice," as termed by Taub, 2000) has the power to change the impact of trauma moment by moment. Massed practice is another concept brought to us through the field of neuroplasticity and offers up the powerful idea that we have the capacity to retrain our brains over time. We believe this perspective is currently re-invigorating the field of after trauma care to include the notion of healing.

We like the phrase "practice is not a luxury item" and use it regularly to introduce the importance of daily practice to reinforce learning and retrain our brains (Taub, 2000). This massed practice approach is at the core of the 30-day video stabilization program, which utilizes this concept with the clients we work with every day in our practice. The first 10 days of the 30-day video stabilization program is freely available at http://www.whatisptsd.com/find-calm/

## The Polyvagal Theory

Stephen Porges began his research career in 1969 when he published his first peer-reviewed article that explored the effects that respiration and heart rate had upon attentional attunement. In 1973, he was one of the first to advance the study of heart rate variability as a measure of attention, dysregulation, and optimal performance (Porges, 1973). By the mid-1970s he was beginning to look at physiological correlates of healthy and pathological behavioral functioning. By the mid-1980s, he had become increasingly enamored with the functioning of the vagus nerve (Porges, 1985). This led him in 1995 to introduce his polyvagal theory in *Orienting in a Defensive World: Mammalian Modifications of our Evolutionary Heritage. A Polyvagal Theory*. Today, we have a much more nuanced understanding of human threat detection and response systems thanks to Porges' polyvagal theory (Porges, 1995, 2002, 2011a, 2011b, 2015, 2018, November 3, 2021).

Porges' polyvagal theory evolves older models of understanding the ANS and moves away from the view of bipolar and biphasic two systems – the sympathetic nervous system (SNS) and parasympathetic nervous system (PNS) –complementing and competing with each other to achieve homeostasis. Instead, he postulates three systems derived from splitting the PNS into two evolutionarily and operationally distinct subsystems: the dorsal vagal and the ventral vagal. Each of these subsystems is associated with a branch of the vagus nerve, and a particular reaction to a perceived threat.

### 1. The Dorsal Vagal Complex

The dorsal (or lower) part of the vagus nerve (DVC) is associated with the most ancient of defense systems (the freeze or shutdown response), which we share with reptiles and other mammals. This system acts as an involuntary brake on the SNS, managing the "feed-and-breed" system and helping the body gently return from arousal to relaxation. Anatomically, the DVC consists of a nerve pathway that connects the brain stem to the organs situated below the diaphragm, especially those associated with digestion and reproduction and the muscles that anchor these organs in place.

The DVC system first evolved in simple organisms that passively absorbed nutrients from the rich broth of dissolved organic compounds and gases found in the prehistoric ocean. Lacking organs and muscles for locomotion, these simple creatures never developed an SNS or the option to fight or flee. Instead, their defensive systems were focused entirely on preserving their energy reserves so they could recover as quickly as possible when the threat had ceased. For this reason, the DVC is sometimes referred to as the "passive defense system." The DVC system is now understood to control the third possible response to a perceived threat: freezing. We can see this survival strategy at work when we observe animals responding to danger by becoming immobilized. This is often described as the "deer-in-the-headlights" phenomenon.

Consider the case of a driver trapped in his vehicle and unable to move after a car accident. His DVC system immediately springs into action, slowing his heart rate, reducing his blood pressure, and preserving his energy resources for the key organ systems necessary for survival. If this inhibitory response is severe enough, however, the suppression of his heart and circulatory system may cause him to go into shock and lose consciousness, with potentially fatal consequences. Our driver's amygdala may also respond by creating a powerful emotional memory of the accident and its aftermath. This memory, stored below conscious awareness, might include all of the sensory impressions surrounding the accident along with the signals of biological shutdown induced by DVC activation. Consequently, whenever the memory is triggered in the future, he may re-experience some of the classic physiological and psychological manifestations of the freeze response, including such symptoms as dissociation, paralysis of thought or action, or emotional numbing and psychological disengagement.

If the stress evoking the freeze response is chronic, our driver may attempt to manage these symptoms by self-medicating (i.e., drugs and alcohol), escapism (i.e., online surfing and videogames), self-soothing (i.e., cutting), or by distancing himself from others and avoiding activities he may have previously enjoyed.

## 2. The Sympathetic Nervous System

The SNS tends to be impulsive, irrational, illogical, and reactive, which are not always bad things (Sapolsky, 2004, 2017). It's an essential system that can provide a lot of joy and satisfaction for us – an appropriately responsive SNS allows us to perform at the highest levels in various endeavors. The problem arises when it's over-utilized or compromised via trauma, resulting in chronic dysregulation when the SNS stays activated and dominant most of the day. This is known as "sympathetic nervous system dominance."

A person in SNS dominance acts in clear, congruent behaviors that align with a human being's survival mode. There is no future, no delayed gratification, no self-reflection, no self-evaluation – only *now*, in this moment. If you were to walk around a bush in the desert and be confronted by a rattlesnake, you wouldn't begin pondering whether your current career path allowed you to demonstrate all of your talents – you'd be figuring out the next moves to stay alive! And that's a completely appropriate reaction to a perceived threat, with a system that's been refined over millennia to adapt and navigate the best route for survival.

How many of you have played some kind of a sport? Think about this: if you're on a football team, would you want your quarterback to begin ruminating on the choice for dinner during the middle of a game? Probably not! They should be paying attention to the game, with an elevated SNS that's prepared to respond immediately in the event of a successful hit by the other team. At that point in time, self-evaluation and self-reflection would not be appropriate focus for your teammate.

Consider when you've tuned into the news and heard stories about individuals who made snap decisions that put themselves in grave danger, all in the name of having a good time. Perhaps you're at a party and some friends decide to jump off a roof into the pool. They do it successfully so you're up next, and your pulse is racing and your hands are sweating. You can't stop laughing, and your whole body's trembling – but you miscalculate, landing on the concrete and breaking several bones.

If you'd been sitting in the living room that morning, discussing your day, would you have agreed to that death-defying jump off a ten-foot roof? The answer would most likely be a resounding "no!" Yet in that moment, when your SNS was in full swing and the adrenaline was pumping, you made a decision that was the result of compromised neocortical functioning without access to judgment, reason, or impulse control. It seems counterintuitive that one might place themselves in a life-threatening situation *while* they're in survival mode, but it once again demonstrates how our modern-day situations are at times not conducive to our reptilian brain systems.

One more situation: a contentious discussion with a loved one. Things are getting heated, and they say something that really irritates you. Suddenly your voice is raised and you start providing them with a list of all their defects and shortcomings. You couldn't care less if it hurts their feelings (engaging in what David Schnarch, 1997, calls "normal marital sadism"). Perhaps there's a small corner of your consciousness that's whispering, "This probably isn't a good idea, you don't mean that and you definitely shouldn't say it," but you go ahead and unleash on your loved one anyway.

In the moments of that argument, you're not thinking about how it's going to be beneficial for your relationship ten years later, or the long-term consequences the disagreement may reap. You're acting in a way that would be appropriate if you were facing down a wild beast in the jungle, but one that's decidedly inappropriate for a conversation with your spouse in the home.

Human beings engage in behaviors that are SNS-driven much more often than we realize. If we want clients to benefit from what we can do for them, we need to help them to move out of this SNS mode and into one that's intentional and deliberate in word and action. If you're a doctor discussing a new medical regimen with a patient, you'd want the environment to be one of stability and safety for their compliance – if the individual is in an SNS-dominant state, they're most likely not processing much of what you have to say.

There are also mitigating or space-creating behaviors that we can fall into, and those who've suffered from trauma being especially are prone to such conduct. These behaviors create a separation between the experience of the body and the perception of the body, and we frequently see them through the lens of pathology. Humans have the ability to dissociate and create substantial emotional distance or numbness to a current state of being. If one becomes too absorbed in these instinctual and involuntary self-soothing techniques that relieve distress in the body via distraction, we see the risk for addiction, self-injury, suicidality, and other compulsive behaviors greatly increase.

## 3. The Ventral Vagal Complex

The third component of our threat response system evolved most recently and is found only in humans. The ventral vagal complex (VVC) subsystem is the second branch of the PNS, and the one that most directly reflects our status as social beings with biological imperatives to form mutually beneficial relationships. Anatomically, the VVC system connects the brain stem to the organs above the diaphragm, (i.e., the heart, lungs, et cetera) and to the muscles of the face and head. As part of the PNS, the VVC system furnishes similar capabilities for relaxing our bodies and suppressing the fight-or-flight response generated by the SNS and the freeze response generated by the DVC system. However, unlike either of these systems, it operates through the medium of face-to-face communications. For this reason, the VVC is sometimes referred to as the "social engagement system."

If the eyes are the portal to the soul, then our face is the window to the threat response system (a "safe haven" of sorts), and our voices are the music of engagement or the klaxon of rejection with those to whom we're connected. When the VVC system is dominant, we feel safe, centered, and secure. We convey this through our facial muscles by smiling and maintaining appropriate eye contact. We do the same with our tone of voice, speaking in a relaxed and rhythmic way that eschews choppy or staccato phrases. Think of a mother singing a lullaby to her baby or the sound of two lovers cooing their endearments. We hear differently too, focusing our attention on the person speaking to us and losing awareness of background noise. All of these stress reduction responses are mediated by the VVC system.

When we encounter stress, humans naturally turn to each other for comfort and support. If we see a friendly face, the VVC system activates to calm us. If we encounter someone whose face and voice communicate anxiety or distress, we may become aroused and infected by their stress.

This is the biological basis for the kind of environmentally caused stress that you would experience when engaging with someone in a distressed state. For example, recently I sat in an emergency department waiting to have my ankle x-rayed after falling during a run. I overheard a woman who had just arrived in distress speaking with the admission clerk. He says, "Are you pregnant?" she says, "Yes, of course I am pregnant" ... "I just told you, I believe I am having a miscarriage." "I need help." The woman is speaking in a rapid upset tone. She is clearly stressed and tearful. The admin clerk responds in an agitated and aggravated tone, "Don't speak to me like that, I am here trying to help!" He continues to chastise this woman, who is already weeping quietly. He looks at her but seems unable to stop his escalating response toward her.

This type of encounter is what can occur even with people trying to be helpful but engaged in an escalation driven by arousal, fear, and a fight for survival. The admin clerk likely connected with the woman's obvious distress and, instead of remaining compassionate and calm, his own reactivity became activated and his VVC disengaged while communicating with a woman in distress.

Our passive defense, social engagement, and fight-or-flight systems come online in a consistent, evolutionarily defined sequence. If we perceive danger, we look first to our fellow humans for support. If we find it, we relax. If not, our SNS takes over and we attempt to fight or flee. If we're prevented from fighting or fleeing, then our earliest evolved system takes control. This instinctual process is entirely outside of our conscious awareness and occurs almost instantaneously within a scant ten to fifteen milliseconds.

Another major player in the threat response system is the anterior cingulate cortex (ACC), found in the frontal cingulate cortex of the brain's cerebral cortex (LeDoux, 2015). The ACC operates much like a radar system does, constantly scanning the environment and searching for things that are unique to that specific person. That's what's so amazing – the ACC is only looking for what's relevant to *them*. Any two people can be in the same room having the same experience, but what they recall of it is going to be highly influenced by this system of relevancy. In other words, what's relevant to us will more likely code in our memory, and if not the physical memory, then the sensorial memory through cognition.

When the ACC perceives threat, danger, risk, adversity, or stressors the more primitive parts of the brain are activated – the SNS. In other words, it moves the individual from being able to be logical, reasonable, and rational into a primitive, reactive, survival mindset.

If the ACC is "on" for too long – it's been perceiving danger continuously due to a person's inability to perceive safety in the present context – the threat perception system becomes enhanced and expanded. The more these neural pathways are utilized, the stronger, faster, more automatic, and more efficient they become. You might think of it as a road in the mountains; the trail starts small, but over time and with enough traffic, the path widens exponentially. The hypervigilance of the ACC follows the same principle, which is detrimental to trauma survivors with histories of adversity.

Not only do the neural pathways of the ACC become better developed, but the reaction speed shortens with repeated use. With heightened sensitivity, all the body needs is the *suggestion* of a threat to jump into overdrive, so that it's fully engaged almost immediately. This leads to impulsive and reactive behavior, all led by attributions and perceptions that have been repeatedly conditioned through the process of traumagenesis.

For example, most people find flowers relatively pleasant or at least neutral, but imagine that one day you encounter a flower that caused you a tremendous allergic reaction. Your reaction required an emergency trip to the hospital, a breathing treatment, and even a painful injection.

Now, several years later, your perception of flowers is still altered. Even though it was just the one flower that caused the reaction, your brain is going to perceive flowers forevermore – and possibly even items resembling weeds or plants – with an added threat factor that never existed before. The painful learning experience really does create a binary mindset, a black-and-white view of the world that is very difficult to ignore, even when logic says otherwise.

Tens of thousands of these experiences of traumagenesis throughout a person's lifetime construct categories within our minds that are populated by painful learning. This painful learning translates to hyperattunement and hyperarousal to any other experience that remotely resembles the original traumatic event – especially the sensory components. It changes how we see the world, it influences our relationships, and it can often be to our benefit and safety. The problem arises when this causes us to repeatedly perceive threat where there is little or no danger. Constantly perceiving threat causes us to remain on high alert, resulting in physical, emotional, and relational consequences that create a myriad of health concerns.

There is considerable research pointing to chronic stress as the root cause of many diseases, psychological problems, and immune system dysfunctions. A dysregulated ANS can become self-perpetuating. Any stressful situation we encounter may provoke a full-scale fight, flight, or freeze response. Driving to work, we fly into a rage when someone cuts us off. When presented with a challenge, we find ourselves unable to act. Failing to deal effectively with minor setbacks, we become even more distressed. Our innate capabilities for intelligence, creativity, emotional connection, and considered judgment are sharply degraded to impairment. Our health and wellbeing are endangered. We live our lives on a hair trigger, ready to explode or implode at the slightest provocation.

The effects of chronic stress are wide and encompass every area of our lives. They can range from physiological symptoms like headaches, irritability, and chronic pain to habitual behaviors and belief systems that create more harm to the self and others.

However, by using the voluntary and intentional capacities of the VVC, we can begin to interrupt and regulate this threat response. This interruption and regulation, helps us to move out of the distress of the SNS and into comfort and optional functioning of the VVC. One of the most important components of good psychotherapeutic treatment for posttraumatic stress is teaching our clients skills to engage in this ability to interrupt their threat response and regulate their ANS.

The polyvagal theory is a fundamental tool that we can use in our work with clients. We can help our clients better understand why their posttraumatic nervous system is dysregulated with the model of the polyvagal theory. Secondly, it is a tool to help survivors begin to understand and embody that the emotional and physiological pain they suffer with after trauma *is not their fault*. Thirdly, it organizes clear and thorough methods for interrupting and regulating the ANS (discussed earlier in this section). Finally, and ultimately, the polyvagal theory is a roadmap to help trauma survivors to *feel safe*, something that Stephen Porges and the authors of this book agree is an essential outcome of any trauma treatment.

## Salutogenesis

Salutogenesis is a health promoting and resource/capacity-building paradigm that is based upon the work of Aaron Antonovsky (1979, 1987), a medical sociologist who coined the term in the early 1970s. Antonovsky proposed that health existed on a continuum between sick and healthy, rather than the dichotomy between disease and health central to the allopathic approach. According to salutogenesis, medical approaches should aim to optimize movement toward health for patients and not focus upon treating the sickness. In 1995, Charlton and White suggested, in their margin of resources model, that incorporating key health promoting factors, such as strengthening interpersonal resources, personal resilience building, decreasing unmet needs, and a long-term view within treatment models could greatly increase health and wellness outcomes. It is with these concepts in mind and a combined seventy years of experience applying these principles across multiple disciplines that we promote and advocate a salutogenic model and philosophy as an alternative framework for understanding and treating posttraumatic stress.

This book aims to promulgate the value of these principles and the ways in which they can be integrated and applied within treatment models for posttraumatic stress to increase effectiveness and better move them towards full recovery and good health. It is important for clients to complete treatment feeling empowered in their recovery:

to better understand their physiological and psychological processes, navigate challenges, self-regulate their arousal, and forge meaning, value, skills and resources from their experience that can help optimize their forward movement during and after treatment. In our work with trauma survivors, we have found that integrating a salutogenic approach throughout treatment has helped clients to better understand, interrupt, arrest, and extinguish the overactive physiological and cognitive threat response systems that were once necessary for survival. Helping them develop and master these regulatory skills while also helping them to understand that these skills were once necessary for their survival but are now an over-adaptation in the present, catalyzes a more compassionate and syntonic perception of themselves and their lives. This is an excellent example of how salutogenesis compares to allopathic approaches – in salutogenesis we are helping our clients remove and navigate beyond the impediments to their health instead of focusing upon treating the "disease" of PTSD. This approach not only aids recovery, but helps clients find a new way forward to a higher quality of life, with greater fulfillment, ease, and resilience.

# The Mind-Body Connection

There are several areas of the brain that have tremendous influence on our thoughts and actions following trauma. Let's look at several of these areas to see how some of these systems work in concert and how we can use this information to encourage the healing process.

## The Amygdala

The amygdala acts as an emotional control center in our brains and helps us to instantly feel certain emotions; those that we feel in ourselves and those that we perceive in others. When we feel fear, we know that the amygdala is actively engaged in the brain. The amygdala is responsible for our ability to respond rapidly to signs of danger and to activate and mobilize all resources to fight, flight, or freeze as a response to this danger. This works well with trauma survivors, but once this neural pathway is engaged in serious situations it is not always easy to turn it off or lower the stress volume. This is why individuals may experience a lack of sleep or hypervigilance long after the danger is over. The amygdala response can occur so quickly that we do not have time to confirm that our early warning signs of danger are correct. Hence, trauma survivors may respond

with anger, fear, or a startle when there is no current source of danger igniting the reaction.

## The Hippocampus

The hippocampus stores memories so that if you have a need to respond to danger in the future, you are prepared to recall triggers and prepare your mind and body for rapid response to threat. This results in the release of cortisol, the stress hormone that can interfere with memory and produce an automatic fearful response to danger signs. It is easy to see how useful this system can be when we are trying to respond quickly to true danger, but it can backfire when we are continually responding long after the danger has passed. When you store the traumatic memories of your experience, they are stored along with the strong emotions that occurred at the time as well, so anytime you experience a trigger of this memory, you may also experience strong emotions (i.e., upset, agitation, anger, fear, confusion) as well. So it is no surprise that one of the key features of PTSD is the avoidance of any triggers to the traumatic memory. However, life is full of such reminders, and working through our stories on our journeys to recovery is the best route to a better life experience.

## The Sensory Thalamus

The next thing to add to this picture is the sensory thalamus, which is responsible for gathering information and disseminating sensory input. It is postulated to be the communication gateway to the cortex, amygdala, and hippocampus. If this system is not functioning correctly, it may mobilize the amygdala to activate the body's alarm system, at times, causing us to respond to danger when no danger is present. A slower and more reflective information pathway is invoked when the sensory thalamus sends information of a noncritical nature to the cortex for analysis. The sensory cortex will assess and confirm meaning. However, by this time, the amygdala may already have set off the alarm bells of the ANS. Once this happens, we are into our reaction and may be sweating, tense, breathing quickly, and agitated before we are able to confirm that a threat has occurred.

## The Sympathetic Nervous System

The sympathetic nervous system (known as the SNS) is a part of the nervous system that is responsible for accelerating heart rate, constricting blood vessels, and raising blood pressure. The SNS, along with the parasympathetic nervous system (PNS), makes up the autonomic nervous system, the branch of the nervous system that performs involuntary functions. Once the SNS is engaged to fight, flight, or freeze, the more reflective information processing that occurs in the sensory cortex is short-circuited. So, a client might feel as if they have overreacted after a noncritical event, but while in the middle of a response (e.g., feeling angry, startled, or fearful) they will likely feel fully engaged and the response may feel entirely realistic and justified at the time. The goal is always to bring the client back to a stable base or comfort zone – re-engaging the PNS (known for its functions of rest and digestion ability) and engaging the vagus nerve to return to the inner calm steady state that is hardwired as a part of every individual's core functioning. When the SNS is engaged, all energy is moved to activate a *get-out-of-danger* impulse and away from the normal digestive functioning, the warming of fingers and toes, and the management of other bodily functions that are not critical for survival. So it makes sense that after a traumatic event, a client might describe physical symptoms such as a stomachache, poor appetite, or feelings of cold or exhaustion.

### Cortisol: The Stress Hormone

Emotional and physical strain can release a cascade of chemicals into the body and mind. Some of these chemicals, like cortisol, can have a big impact on how we function after trauma. After exposure to a disturbing event, the body and mind send signals that activate the adrenal glands, which pump out high levels of the stress hormone, cortisol.

Too much cortisol short-circuits the cells in the hippocampus, making it harder to organize the memory of the trauma or stressful experience. Memories lose their context and become fragmented. These fragments can become re-ignited whenever something reminds a client of their trauma history, resulting in another big cortisol release. Once high levels of cortisol are released, it makes it difficult to find a sense of relaxation. This is a part of the response chain that can create strong emotional reactions, even in safe circumstances, leaving an individual feeling overwhelmed, depleted, and shaken up by trauma reminders. It also reminds us as trauma professionals, that finding calm after trauma is a necessity and not a luxury item.

Please also see a video that goes into some further depth on this topic  titled "Learn About Adrenaline &

Cortisol to Help Manage Stress: Ask Dr Anna S.2.E.17," in the supplementary material, Video 4 (or see Baranowsky, 2015, April 16, https://youtu.be/rHpLoK4ZhQQ). This video is visually informative on ways that cortisol and adrenaline affect our body both normally and after trauma and is a source of encouragement about our capacity to bring our body back towards a state of greater normalcy and homeostasis after trauma.

Offering after-trauma care that addresses the impact of extreme events on our brain's functioning requires that the clinician assist the client to slow down the reactivity ignited when people are exposed to trauma reminders, setting off old emotions. It is the gap between exposure to trauma reminders and reactivity that opens the door to change. It is pausing in that gap with calm reflection that allows us to inform and reform reactivity, creating a new storage of the trauma memory associated with a more reflective and less reactive or emotionally strained response. Our goal in *Trauma Practice* is to find the route to retraining the brain along with the body, mind, and emotions.

# Traumagenesis: The Creation of Trauma

We are very grateful to our colleague Dr. Robert Rhoton (2012), who has kindly shared this section on traumagenesis. We feel strongly that this section offers a deeper insight into the root development of the trauma response. His contribution fits perfectly within the trauma practice model and we are proud to offer it as an aid to better understanding how trauma can weave itself into our world view.

Traumagenesis is a concept attempting to show that trauma as it has been traditionally understood is sometimes too narrowing and this does not give a rich understanding to what unfortunately is a relatively common experience in many lives.

The term "traumagenic" is a label for a type of environment that can create trauma-stress reactions and lead to traumagenesis, which is an origination of symptomatic behaviors and biological alterations that increase the risk of problems in physical, emotional, and psychological development. In simpler terms, the environment activates real physical, emotional, and psychological changes that become enduring characteristics in the individual.

One of the primary factors of traumagenesis is that it can occur in anyone's life, but that the young are more vulnerable to a permanent and indelible neurological as well as biological impact, changing or altering the individual at a molecular and/or genetic level. Our brains think, or create thoughts, by receiving information through our senses and then, through different forms of testing, check these against experiences that are taking place in their environment. The frequency, intensity, and duration of experiences inform the brain and body to react, without evaluation or a critical eye. We "see" pictures, "hear" sounds, and "feel" sensations, categorize and construe meaning or schemas. This journey, of course, begins before conception, not just as a fetus growing in the womb, because human beings in most circumstances receive a generational transmission of family culture, which may be free of abuse, but filled with trauma.

There are two distinct types of trauma: (1) complex (involving repetitive or continuous situations which activate the threat response system of the body), and (2) simple (involving a single and a few incidents that overwhelm the threat response system of the body). James and MacKinnon (2012) describe this as "big T" and "small T." Big T encompasses exposure to disturbing situations such as abuse, violence, catastrophe, and death, whereas small T is not life threatening but equally disturbing. The word "trauma" frequently brings to mind the plight of the veteran, or the victim of violent criminal acts, natural disasters, acts of war and terrorism, child abuse, and emotional losses. These are all possible elements that contribute to trauma on a regular basis in the lives of those that experience them. However, this is only a small portion of the entire story. This section is not intended to diminish anyone who has experienced a Criterion A "Big T Trauma." It is offered to give readers – especially clinicians – an understanding that many clients will be experiencing significant symptoms in their clinical presentation from events that DO NOT meet DSM-5 diagnostic Criterion A.

## The Biology of Traumagenesis

It seems fitting to begin a discussion of trauma creation with a brief expository on the neuroscience and biology of human beings. The brain contains a part called the anterior cingulate cortex (ACC), which is tied to many functions related to problem-solving and motivating the individual to action. Another primary function of the ACC is to warn an individual of pain. It does not appear to actually deal with the pain, but instead acts as an alarm system that activates some response to the perception that pain is imminent. The ventral part of the ACC is connected with the limbic system and involved in assessing the salience of the threat of pain (Porges, 2011b). The ACC might be thought of as the trigger or activator of the threat response system in the body, sending out the alarm that the environment is stressful, or that there is some element that is fear generating or likely to lead to the occurrence of pain. However, the ACC also serves multiple other purposes, one of which is to control and encourage social engagement or relationships. Perhaps the best way to describe this is to think about how one might feel when holding a newborn puppy or kitten – that warm flush of pleasurable feelings is initiated through the ventral vagal complex (Porges & Furman, 2011). Understanding that this polyvagal system is active in both the perception of relational connection and the fear/threat/stress reaction is the starting point for understanding trauma more broadly. –

When a child who has no language is exposed to stress, the threat response system becomes activated. The activated system triggers natural changes to the biology and neurobiology of the child, and if this activated system is distressed enough, a single or repetitive event will cause the brain and body to create preemptive reactions to avoid, reduce, or divert the distress. Now, it is impossible to go through life and not have this system activated quite frequently, so it is not generally the occasional activation, but the repeated activation that creates problems in the life of an individual. Unfortunately, repeated activation of the threat response system becomes aversive and requires the individual to adapt, and this adaptation is not based on reason or logic, but on a reactive avoidance of the contextual elements that are common when activation occurs. Sometimes this process has been labeled as "trigger," however, this description is quite reductionistic in nature. A better description might be to call the reaction a procedural adaptation (Rhoton, 2012). This does not require a highly intense activation (though it certainly could be that), but instead the much more common low-intensity activator with great frequency, duration, or both will accomplish over time the same kind of molecular changes that will occur in an intense activation.

The following exercise is designed to illustrate the automatic nature of biological and neurological adaptations. In order to be fully prepared to benefit from the exercise, think back to the last time you went hiking or were wearing a pair of new shoes or boots. Blisters are fairly natural occurrences in both of these situations. You can imagine beginning to notice discomfort as you walk along. If you are like most human beings, you will change your stride or gait without conscious evaluation – you are just perceiving pain or discomfort and automatically adjusting. This is a metaphor for what is happening with an individual in any environment that is repeatedly activating the threat response system, or threatening pain and discomfort. An audience member at a training in Tucson, AZ, who loved hiking, laughingly mentioned having had an experience with hiking in the desert where he was moderately aware of the gradual increase in pain from blisters, so he ended his trek sooner than he planned. The next morning his leg and hip muscles were all sore and he realized that they were tender because he had automatically changed how he held himself and moved to accommodate the increasing pain from his blisters.

As mentioned above, the following exercise is a useful metaphor to demonstrate the nature of automatic adaptations to perceived pain or the threat of pain. It can be used in a group setting or with individuals.

### Exercise to Demonstrate Adaptation to Painful Experience

*In a moment, I will ask you to clap your hands once, vigorously, and then we will reflect on what you experienced physically. All right, clap.*

I have them process what they experienced, the stinging in their palms, the warming of the skin, etc. After the discussion, we proceed to the next aspect of this example. I tell them I am going to ask them to clap again, this time several times, and I want them to make sure that each one is equally hard as the first one. I then have them clap with my counting out loud; I count to 15 at a nice quick pace. Then I ask them about their experience.

*How many of you noticed that after 5–6 claps you adjusted how hard you were clapping (generally about half the room admits that they had) and how many adjusted by the 10th clap, or readjusted a second time?*

While there is no conscious and linear explanation for the adaptations that occur, one of the facts of adaption seems pretty resolute: adaptations become associated with environmental patterns. Because exposure to trauma activates the body's threat response system, and repeated exposure means repeated activation of said threat response system, the adaptation or reaction to pain and discomfort evokes associated memory, emotion, and cognition – a sense of location and timing as well as behavior. So, without conscious effort or thought, the activation becomes associated with patterns of emotion, perceptions, and meaning making or attributions, cognitions or expectations associated with the activating environment, as well as body use. These patterns then become ingrained to the point of being implicit and feel instinctual when the aspects of the threat response are present in the context of the environment. The question is not *if*, but to what *degree* adaptation is in place.

In his book *Mindsight*, Daniel Siegel (2010) discusses the types of memory that are involved in the creation of trauma. Conscious memory, sometimes thought of as narrative memory, tends to be serial in nature, and reflects a more or less sequential view of experience. The other memory structure, which Siegel calls implicit memory, is tied strongly to emotionally vivid sights, sounds, smells, and physical sensations that are embedded in or associated with an environmental context. The implicit system values the retention of experience associated with loss, pain, or danger. This retention held within the implicit system is sometimes referred to as "triggers," "cues," or by what Briere and Scott (2012) label "conditioned emotional responses."

Any driver who has embarked on a road trip knows that there are road signs that convey all sorts of information to the traveler. When one leaves rural areas and approaches larger cities there seem to be more signs visible, giving more information to the driver. In some ways implicit memory can be metaphorically compared to these road signs. The experience within an environmental context that has created a conditioned emotional response can be thought of as a planted sign. The sign's purpose is to convey information to the driver. In this way, the sign becomes preemptive, warning the driver before they approach the place where the trauma actually resides. Intense or frequent negative experiences activate the threat response system, which might be compared to a large city, where there are many, many more signs. If the driver heeds the signs, then they can avoid the pain associated with the experience. If the signs are not heeded, then the threat response system again becomes activated and an additional sign or two are placed on the highway. However, most signs posted along the freeway of human experience are not conscious, well thought out, evaluated signage, but are reactionary to warn the driver away from pain.

The body's threat response system has the potential to actuate, adjust, and evolve quickly to reduce the activation of the ACC, and provide relief from the arousal that is experienced as being fearful or distressing. This brings to mind the general tenet that the human body is wired to remember threats. This threat history appears to cut across all neural processes at an earlier age than previously thought, according to Montirosso, Borgatti, and Tronick (2010).

In a workshop on the function of neurobiology in the treatment for mental health, a rather abrasive audience member asked for an example that he could relate to. He was asked how long he had worked in his current job and what kind of work he was doing on a daily basis. After describing his work and workplace, he was asked, "Who have you learned to avoid in the workplace?" With a shocked look, he began to recount a particularly disagreeable coworker. He was further asked whether he changed his navigation through the work environment to avoid this person. He began to laugh and said that just a few days earlier he had walked out of an exit near his office and gone completely around the rather large building to avoid walking past the coworker's office, which was four doors down the hallway. This may seem like a strange example, but here was someone activated by an element of his environment, who was automatically adapting when the familiar pain- and distress-related elements were present in the environment. Thus, the man's behavior was not only an adaptation but also a preemptive behavior to avoid further activation of the threat response system.

We hope this explanation illustrates how you can talk about any environment in terms of traumagenesis. Any environment that creates repeated aversive activation of the threat response system of an individual, particularly if those activations are interrupting or interfering with normal social, emotional, psychological, or spiritual development or maturity of the individual, can be perceived as being traumatic. Adaptations effectively build shields or protections from the consequences of experiences, and when those adaptations are effective, they become habituated. Habituated adaptations are implicit, and in fact can often be seen as part of the identity of the individual. Many of the adaptations that lead to addiction and an array of dysfunction within a family environment are brought into being in this manner. However, to assume that traumagenesis only occurs within a family setting is not a correct interpretation, because while it is the primary context in which most people will experience trauma, any environment that repeatedly activates the threat response system is traumagenic, be that family, employment, neighborhood, or community.

## Symptoms of Traumagenesis: Where Do Problematic Behaviors Come From?

How do the behaviors associated with traumagenesis emerge? Symptoms (see Table 5) are most often associated with preemptive adaptations that have developed over time to insulate or protect the individual from experiencing the painful familiarity of context-associated signs or triggers around the repeated activation of the threat response system. What adaptation looks like in the lives of individuals is going to be unique to the personal history of their ACC/polyvagal activations. Perhaps an illustration of this process would be helpful. Think of a family with three children, aged 5, 7, and 8, who are growing to maturity in a home that is not actively abusive physically or sexually, but is highly stressful and chaotic in nature. This is a family where name calling and put downs exist, as well as significant conflict, shouting, and angry words. Intimidation and threat are part of the active parenting structure, with few positive or even neutral interactions. Using the children in this family might be a good canvas against which to paint a picture of what can occur. Many helpers looking at traumagenesis are hoping to find a standardized set of symptoms that clearly speak to the activation history of the individual. This is problematic because the symptom development is based on individual adaptation, which is completely unique.

Using the three siblings in the foreground of our representation might help to better clarify this point. The oldest of the three, the 8-year-old, finds it difficult to handle any uncertainty, and will quit whatever activity he is engaged in if it becomes the least bit unpredictable. This makes studying and learning difficult because he spends a significant amount of time worrying about what to do when asked a question for which he lacks the answer. Additionally, he struggles with any type of confrontation with adults or peers, and when placed in a situation where it is difficult to withdraw, becomes aggressive.

The next child is a 7-year-old girl, who struggles a great deal with any emotional intensity in her environment and exhibits inconsistent or inappropriate displays of emotions, from crying inconsolably to screaming until hoarse and losing her voice. She rarely recognizes the appropriate emotional response to most engaging situations. A secondary adaptation is emotional withdrawal, shut down, or retreat. She has been known to hide in closets or under beds with her hands over her ears.

The 5-year-old boy, who is in kindergarten, has developed a great preciseness, makes lists, and engages in repetitive behaviors such as repeating out loud the instructions of his teachers several times as a way to make certain that he knows exactly what actions he is supposed to take. He does not tolerate spontaneity well and prefers not to have things occur that are not known and planned out.

Each of the adaptations shown by the children in this family are exactly right for them, because each way of being in the world is to a great extent a reaction to the road signs firmly planted to warn of danger, threat, and

**Table 5.**    Symptoms of traumagenesis

| Emotional difficulties | Cognitive difficulties | Social difficulties |
| --- | --- | --- |
| Inability to self-soothe | Extremist thinking | Poor boundaries |
| Chronic anxiety | Learning and memory problems | Seeking attention in inappropriate ways |
| Low frustration tolerance | Inability to tolerate uncertainty | Efforts to control as a response to helplessness/powerlessness |
| Fluctuating moods | Emotions interfere with thought processes | Problems with authority figures |
| Chronic fear states and phobias | Poor problem-solving | Lack of relational trust |
| Suicidality/risky behaviors and self harm | Difficulty following through to task completion | Constant demand that others prove they can be trusted |
| Hypersensitivity to minor stressors | Rigid and binary thought processes | Impulsivity |
| Intense feelings (positive or negative) can be overwhelming | | Poor conflict management |
| | | Rapid withdrawal from distressing relationships |
| | | Failure to recognize social cues |
| | | Difficulty learning from social nuances |

pain. The frustrating part for the helper becomes the need to have a set of prescriptive criteria to use to help move treatment forward, but lists of symptoms like the one included above only have a very limited capacity to be helpful. What becomes vital is understanding how the individual reacts and becomes activated, and what avenues have been developed to preempt the perception or experience of pain and distress. One can think of the warning signs as being a template or schema that houses within its structure a habituated pattern of responding to the environmental activators. These patterns have become automatic and emotionally self-reinforcing. A starting place too often in mental health and education is to look at behavior that is problematic, as if the behavior emerged through an intentional act of will. The reality is that most problem behaviors are exactly the right behaviors for the individual based on their activation history. This is not to say that these behaviors can be tolerated in schools or homes, but treating problem behaviors as intentional, character-related issues doesn't open the door to a compassionate understanding of the impact of trauma on children and families.

Another example of this automatic or habituated adaptation can be illustrated by a 9-year-old girl who had discovered a strategy that kept her physically abusive father from striking her. The girl was incredibly allergic to oleanders, and the yard of her home was surrounded by a wall of them. She discovered that being in the plants would cause her nose to run, and run heavily, so when her father's behavior began to edge toward a danger point that she recognized, she would go out into the yard and climb

into the plants. She would then blow her nose on her shirt front and wipe mucus on her arms above her hands, and the father, who was particularly repulsed by her mucus-covered arms and clothing, would order her to her room. In this way she would escape his attention for hours at a time. She also kept oleander leaves hidden in her room so that she would not recover until her father's mood had changed. While this adaptation was unpleasant and even costly to the young girl emotionally or psychologically, the benefit of the adaptation was successful protection from the traumatic activation of the threat response system.

## Traumagenesis and Relationships

Ventral vagal complex is the seat of warm positive feelings and is activated by the pleasure of normal touch, relationships, and the social engagement system.

The activated threat system includes the sympathetic nervous system and the dorsal vagus system.

These implicit-seeming adaptations that are based on repeated activations have another serious impact on the internal environment of the individual and the operations of a family. Since the system that responds to threat is so well exercised, an imbalance is created in the VVC (see Figure 5). This imbalance comes as the activity of the threat response system absorbs more and more energy, a circumstance that not only inhibits the individual from experiencing the positive ventral system activation as often as possible, but actually creates anticipatory brain potentials, where the brain learns to react with few

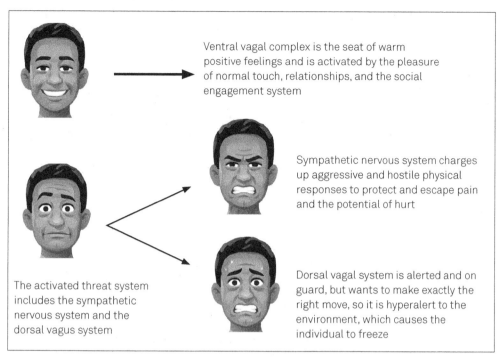

Ventral vagal complex is the seat of warm positive feelings and is activated by the pleasure of normal touch, relationships, and the social engagement system

Sympathetic nervous system charges up aggressive and hostile physical responses to protect and escape pain and the potential of hurt

The activated threat system includes the sympathetic nervous system and the dorsal vagus system

Dorsal vagal system is alerted and on guard, but wants to make exactly the right move, so it is hyperalert to the environment, which causes the individual to freeze

**Figure 5.**
Threat system activation and the consequences.

associations. This can lead to behavior that was originally attached only to the trauma contexts being generalized, to the extent that many neutral environmental contexts become activators. When this takes place, a reduction in VVC activity occurs so there is less reinforcement for relationships.

When VVC activity is reduced, interrupted, or interfered with, relationships will suffer. Either needed relationships will not develop, or those in place will be eroded, due to the lack of warm, positive associations for the individual. This is often witnessed in the adult who has grown to maturity in a traumagenic environment, struggling with or being vulnerable to difficulties forming and/or maintaining secure adult relationships. This is problematic for families, because the mature individual impaired in this way is likely to continue the life cycle of traumagenesis across generations. From the evidence provided by years of clinical work, it seems that there is a sturdy relationship between people who have grown to maturity in a traumagenic environment and poor quality or at least distressed adult relationships, increasing the likelihood of marital conflict and overly quick withdrawal from challenging intimate relationships of all varieties.

## Tri-Phasic Model

Judith Herman is a psychiatrist in the Boston area. She has worked extensively with trauma expert Bessel van der Kolk. Herman is the author of two books, *Father Daughter Incest* (1981) and *Trauma and Recovery* (1992), as well as numerous articles on the enduring effects of chronic trauma. *Trauma and Recovery* is considered a seminal work on the history and treatment of chronic Type II trauma. Herman conceives trauma recovery to proceed in three stages: safety and stabilization; remembrance and mourning, which we will now refer to as *working through trauma*; reconnection.

When writing the first edition of *Trauma Practice* in 1999, we began to closely adhere to the tri-phasic approach as a foundation for our model. We have seen increased interest in this approach and a call for research within this area of intervention with trauma survivors (Cloitre et al., 2011, 2012; Lohrasbe, 2012).

## Phase I: Safety and Stabilization

The central task of recovery is safety. Victims of chronic trauma are betrayed both by their experiences and their own bodies. Their symptoms become the source of triggers that result in retraumatization. The clinician's primary goal is to help the client regain internal and external control, thus interrupting a chronic threat response at the core of posttraumatic reactivity. This is accomplished through careful diagnosis, education, and skills development. The safety section of this book is focused on skills development to aid the trauma survivor to practice self-soothe and self-care skills to increase emotional and behavioral stabilization. In cases where the client remains in an unsafe environment, plans to establish personal and practical safety remain the focus of treatment prior to delving into the *working through trauma* phase. The overriding goal is to enable the client to make a gradual shift from "unpredictable danger to reliable safety" (Herman, 1992, p. 155), both in their environment and within themselves. Accomplishing this goal depends on the individual circumstances, as well as on the internal ability to cope with exposure to trauma memories; it may require days, weeks, or months to achieve.

## Phase II: Working Through Trauma

In the second phase of recovery, the client begins to work more deeply with exercises to process their trauma history, bringing unbearable memories to greater resolution. Because of the nature of traumatic memories, this process is rarely linear. Bits and pieces of the traumatic events emerge and can be processed. The objective is to create a space in which the client can safely work through traumatic events and begin to make sense of the devastating experiences that have shaped their life. The clinician's role is to "bear witness" to the client's experiences and help them find the fortitude to heal.

There are many excellent CBT techniques that fit well within the rubric of this stage of *working through trauma*. In addition, there are well-researched approaches such as eye movement desensitization and rreprocessing (EMDR), time-limited trauma therapy (TLTT), and traumatic incident reduction (TIR); these approaches will not be covered in this book, but they certainly fit the CBST trauma therapy framework and warrant further exploration. The book is filled with many useful approaches that have proven their worth since our first edition in 1999.

## Phase III: Reconnection

The final stage of recovery involves redefining oneself in the context of meaningful relationships and engagement in life activities. Trauma survivors gain closure on their experiences when they are able to see the things that happened to them with the knowledge that these events do not determine who they are. Trauma survivors are liberated by the conviction that, regardless of what else happens to them, they always have themselves. Many survivors are also sustained by an abiding faith in a higher power that they believe delivered them from oppressive

terror. In many instances, survivors find a "mission" through which they can continue to heal and to grow. They may even end up helping others who have similar histories of abuse and neglect. Successful resolution of the effects of trauma is a powerful testament to the indomitability of the human spirit. After Phase II of trauma practice is completed, personality that has been shaped through trauma must then be given the opportunity for new growth experiences that offer the hope of a widening circle of connections and the exploration of a broader range of interests.

# Necessary Ingredients: Treatment Codes (R, RE, CR)

We believe there are three active and necessary ingredients for the effective treatment of trauma. These include relaxation and exposure (reciprocal inhibition) and cognitive restructuring. Note, however, that none of the ingredients on its own is sufficient to accomplish the task of recovery. Each of the techniques included in this book is intended to provide at least one of these three ingredients. Because the timing of the interventions is important as well, some of the techniques are most appropriate during the *safety and stabilization* phase, while others are more appropriate to the *working through trauma* or *reconnection* phases.

We will indicate which techniques provide which of the three ingredients with the following coding system:

R = relaxation, self-soothing
RE = relaxation and exposure
CR = cognitive restructuring

We chose to include a broad variety of interventions because varying interventions work more effectively with individual clients with their unique presentations, depending on their background and/or mode of experiencing. It is by no means an exhaustive list of interventions.

The type of intervention selected for each client is left to the creative discretion of the therapist. With patient observation, symptoms and interventions can be fit to the needs of the client within each of the sessions, meeting needs more precisely to what is needed on a session by session and case by case basis. It is our hope that, with experience and an understanding of the necessary ingredients and process for trauma recovery, good therapists will be able to mix, mingle, and create interventions of their own to meet the specific needs of each client.

# Somatic, Cognition, Behavior, and Emotion/Relation

Throughout this book you will notice that sections are broken down into Somatic, Cognition, Behavior, and Emotion/Relation. In previous editions, we referenced "body" rather than "somatic" but the current use of the term "somatic" (Levine & Frederick, 1997) is a helpful redefinition of the importance of current approaches and literature supporting the need to attend to how posttraumatic symptoms profoundly implicate body or somatic systems.

We address somatic, cognition, behavior, and emotion/relation elements because we process events on many channels and sometimes it is necessary to recover both our ability to live peacefully in our bodies (e.g., psychophysiology, heart rate, breathing); our minds/cognitions (e.g., thoughts, perceptions, and beliefs); our behaviors (e.g., proactive vs. restricted); and our emotions/relations (e.g., range, depth, rationality, support level). With these elements in mind, we have made it our mission to seek out interventions that address recovery on all channels. By addressing different channels as needed, we gear our treatment to the client and thereby avoid "cookie cutter" methodology that limits our ability to truly treat the complexities that are so often common among those suffering from posttraumatic syndromes.

# Posttrauma Response

PTSD stands for posttraumatic stress disorder. In the *Diagnostic and Statistical Manual of Mental Disorders,* Fifth Edition, (DSM-5; APA, 2013), PTSD was classified as a trauma- and stressor-related disorder that can occur following a traumatic event. A psychological trauma, as opposed to a physical trauma or injury, occurs when you experience an emotionally disturbing or distressing event. Although we commonly think of trauma as a reaction to a violent event or a terrible accident, we know that individuals can also experience emotional trauma after being physically injured or diagnosed with a serious illness. During a traumatic event, you may have felt that your life, or the life of another, was in danger, and that you had no control over the outcome. Even witnessing an event in which someone died or was seriously injured can result in symptoms consistent with PTSD. It is not unusual for an individual to experience uncomfortable or upsetting memories of a traumatic event, as well as potentially strong

physical reactions. A person will likely also experience uncomfortable or distressing emotions such as anger, fear, and helplessness, as well as negative beliefs and moods. If these symptoms do not go away, or if they interfere with daily activities or enjoyment in life, it may be time for skilled trauma therapy. It is important to remember that only a qualified mental health professional can verify a diagnosis of PTSD through a series of clinical interviews and tests that determine whether the individual has experienced specific symptom responses for at least one month.

Based on DSM-5 diagnostic features, the most salient posttrauma elements result in the development of particular symptoms as a result of exposure to massive trauma in which one's personal health and well-being is threatened. One noteworthy change that occurred in DSM-5 was the move from the previous anxiety disorder classification to a re-categorization as a trauma- and stressor-related disorder. The stressor is often identified as one that may lead to one's death or injury or to that of a person close to the individual (e.g., friend, family, colleague). An important addition is the recognition of changes in mood and thoughts after trauma exposure, now included as Criterion D (Asmundson & Taylor, 2009, Solomon & Horesh, 2007). There are eight criteria that need to be met in part or whole to establish PTSD as a diagnosis. The PTSD diagnosis is based on the following criteria (APA, 2013):

A. Personal involvement in a life-or-death event that is a threat to one's personal safety or that of friends, associates, or family
B. Recurrent, intrusive mental re-experiencing of the trauma
C. Avoidance of trauma-related cues and emotional numbing
D. Negative alterations in cognitions and mood
E. Trauma-related alterations in arousal and reactivity
F. Symptoms (in criterion B, C, D, E) must be present for longer than one month
G. The symptoms must be significant enough to impair functioning of life skills (i.e., work, school, social)
H. Exclusion from diagnosis if apparent symptom disturbances are the result of medication, substance use, or illness.

Other possible diagnoses to consider might include: acute stress disorder, generalized anxiety disorder, major depressive disorder, panic disorder, adjustment disorder, dissociative disorders, dysthymia, etc.

Earlier wording of the diagnostic criteria for PTSD in the DSM-IV-TR (American Psychiatric Association, 2000) recognizes that the individual's response to a traumatic event is equal in importance to the objective evaluation of the event itself and the degree to which it might be determined to be traumatic. We remain convinced that it is essential to continue to take individual responses into account when offering after trauma care. With this in mind, we are able to begin to make sense of why some individuals become debilitated after experiencing a seemingly innocuous event, whereas others can spend long periods of time in the midst of heinous circumstances without experiencing negative effects. The essential issue here is to offer meaningful intervention that fits the needs of the individual whether they meet the diagnostic criterion in whole or part for PTSD or related disorders.

To recap, key posttrauma symptoms (see also Box 2) include:

- Recurrent, intrusive reexperiencing of the traumatic event (e.g., nightmares, flashbacks, intrusive memory replay)
- Avoidance of any trauma-related cues (e.g., places, people, or activities associated with the trauma or resulting in reminders of the trauma)
- Difficulty recalling important features of the trauma; distorted self-blame or blame of others; negative beliefs about oneself or the world; trauma-related emotions; diminished interest in significant life activities; sense of social alienation; constricted range of positive emotions

**Box 2.** Features associated with posttraumatic response

| |
|---|
| Alexithymia |
| Guilt over acts of commission or omission |
| Survival guilt |
| Suicidal/homicidal ideation/behaviors |
| Disillusionment with authority |
| Feelings of hopelessness/helplessness |
| Memory impairment and forgetfulness |
| Sadness and depression |
| Feelings of being overwhelmed |
| Loss of assumptive world |
| Behavioral reenactments |
| Self-destructive soothing behaviors |
| Somatization |
| Relationship problems |

- Anxious arousal (e.g., increase in heart rate and breathing, nervousness, fearfulness, agitation, easily ignited startle response)
- Impairment of life skills (e.g., ability to socialize, work, attend school, or manage family responsibilities)

In addition, there are two types of trauma that the traumatologist would benefit from differentiating at the beginning stage of treatment to assist in treatment planning.

**Type I trauma.** An unexpected and discrete experience that overwhelms the individual's ability to cope with the stress, fear, threat, and/or horror of the event, leading to PTSD (e.g., motor vehicle accident, natural disaster). It is possible that the trauma might be in the form of witnessing an event (secondary traumatic stress). Treatment outcome tends to be achieved more rapidly than in Type II trauma if services are offered within a reasonable period of time (months rather than years) after onset of posttraumatic symptoms.

Type I traumas are often represented by incidents such as:

- Serious accidents, including car accidents, plane crashes, and significant sporting accidents, etc.
- Natural disasters, including earthquake, fire, tornado, hurricane, and floods, etc.
- Acts of violence, such as a physical assault, mugging, or rape, that are viewed as unusual rather than a constant threat
- Terrorist attacks that are limited in scope and viewed as a one-time event

**Type II trauma.** Expected, but unavoidable, ongoing experience(s) that overwhelm the individual's ability to metabolize the event (e.g., childhood sexual abuse, combat trauma). Type II Trauma is the origin of disorders of extreme stress that can include Posttraumatic Stress Disorder, Complex Posttraumatic Stress Disorder, and/or Dissociative Disorders.

Type II traumas are expected, but unavoidable events that are sustained over a period of time, such as:

- Combat or military experiences, including blasts and the witnessing of injury or death of fellow soldiers
- Repetitive physical or sexual abuse
- Childhood abuse or incest
- Workplace harassment or bullying at school
- Terrorist attacks that come with a threat of repeated actions

# Treatment Resistance or Failure: Addressed with Integrative Approaches

For every one of the dedicated clinicians working with clients after trauma there is the added strain of the possibility of treatment resistance or failure. Certainly, the goal of the trained trauma therapist is to relieve suffering, and yet when clients are in the more chronic phases of PTSD symptoms, they can be particularly resistant to treatment, even when using approaches well-supported in the research for efficacy. Refining our approaches over time, investigating new approaches, updating our skills, reviewing client history, and uncovering treatment gaps can all help us do better work with our clients.

Friedman, Cohen, Foa, and Keane (2009) explain that:

At this time, the acknowledged reasons for treatment resistance in PTSD include those seen in other disorders (e.g., chronicity, comorbidity, poor compliance, adverse life circumstances), along with more specific, yet poorly explored, reasons (extreme or repeated traumatization, traumatization during critical developmental stages, etc.). No clear guidelines can be given to clinicians who encounter treatment resistance in their patients except to use their clinical wisdom to probe and eventually to improve their approach to the patient, to find out what might have gone wrong (too fast or too slow an exploration, incomplete mapping of current life stressors, lack of home practice, over- or underdosage of medication), and to use the variety of options...(p. 639).

In order to assist in our care, we need to look beyond traditional approaches and to the areas of treatment that are progressive and move the field forward. At times, for those who are treatment resistant and not experiencing symptom relief we need to add treatment approaches that are new to the field or innovative (i.e., biofeedback, psychotropic, plant-based medicines, yoga, massage, group support therapies, nature retreats, etc). The idea is to recognize the individual as complex who requires an approach that focuses on their unique needs. Additive care can result in a more profound resolution of symptoms allowing for progress for those who would otherwise continue to struggle with chronic, complex symptoms. As treating practitioners, we accept the need for ongoing innovation and remain open and humble in our contact with each individual we meet.

# Phase I:
# Safety and Stabilization

*Your enemy is not well or healthy or strong and is unable to think
straight or see straight because of her obsession with you ...
no longer let this poor, weak creature have the power to upset you.*

Susan Trott, *The Holy Man* (1995)

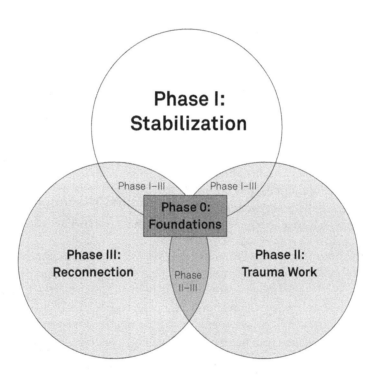

**Summary**

The effects of trauma reverberate through time and across a wide spectrum of life activities. Depending on the circumstances, these effects result in debilitating behaviors meant to alleviate anxiety that are often less than healthy and less than useful to that purpose. They may withdraw from life, use alcohol or drugs, or develop personality habits that are self-defeating. They may actually continue to place themselves in situations that are chaotic and anxiety provoking because they lack the skills and emotional stability to make better choices. They may show up on the doorstep of a therapist with every diagnosis in the DSM other than PTSD. In fact, many experienced therapists believe that almost all the symptoms they see in their practice are related to trauma in one way or another. It is important to understand that to accomplish the task of trauma symptom reduction the client must be able to create a state of relaxation. When their life is in chaos or they continue to self-soothe in less-than-useful ways, creating this state is next to impossible. Phase I defines safety and provides techniques by which the practitioner can assist their clients in creating the environment of safety necessary for trauma work. There are techniques that address the elements of somatic, cognition, behavior, and emotions/relationships essential to recovery.

# 1.  What Is Safety?

In 1996, while completing a fellowship in psychotraumatology at West Virginia University in Morgantown, Eric Gentry wrote an article on developing and maintaining safety with trauma survivors that was later published as a chapter in *Death and Trauma* (Figley et al., 1997). In this chapter, which provides a protocol for assessing and developing stabilization, Gentry attempts to define and "operationalize" the concept of safety into three levels relative to the treatment of trauma survivors. These three levels of safety are:

- Resolution of impending environmental (ambient, interpersonal, and intrapersonal) physical danger, including
  - Removal from "war zone" (e.g., domestic violence, combat, abuse)
  - Behavioral interventions to provide maximum safety
  - Addressing and resolving self-harm
- Amelioration of self-destructive thoughts and behaviors (e.g., suicidal/homicidal ideation/ behavior, eating disorders, persecutory alters/ego-states, addictions, trauma-bonding, risk-taking behaviors, isolation)
- Restructuring victim mythology into a proactive survivor identity by development and habituation of life-affirming self-care skills (e.g., daily routines, relaxation skills, grounding/containment skills, assertiveness, secure provision of basic needs, self-parenting)

One of the most difficult questions that a clinician must answer is: *What is the adequate level of safety/stability necessary to transition to Phase II:* Working Through Trauma *of treatment?* We are taught from the first days of our clinical training to "above all do no harm" (*primum non nocere*), which makes it logical to assume that the more safety and stability that we, as clinicians, can affect in the lives of our clients, the better for their treatment – right?

The answer to this question can be a double-edged sword. For example, Gentry states that early in his career as a trauma therapist he spent many therapy hours working with clients to establish safety and stability. However, upon closer inspection, he saw this delay was his own anxiety about approaching the traumatic material that actually "escalated the crises of my clients." The safety issue was as much about his own emotional safety as that of his clients. So, how safe do you have to be and how do you get there? There are no hard-and-fast rules for safety, but we will discuss various techniques to help establish safety and stabilization and discuss reference points that can be useful to help you decide which to use.

It is a commonly held hypothesis among trauma therapists that the most important tool for the effective establishment of stabilization and even treatment outcomes is the warm confidence of the clinician. A nonanxious presence, along with an unwavering optimism for the client's prognosis, is probably the most powerful intervention that you can provide toward the development of stabilization for your clients. However, you will find that destabilization and lack of safety is often precipitated by client behaviors and thoughts in response to the bombardment of intrusive symptoms (e.g., nightmares, flashbacks, psychological and physiological reactivity). A protracted period of attempting to overdevelop safety for these clients is not helpful. An approach is needed that develops the minimum ("good enough") level of safety and stabilization and then addresses and resolves the intrusive symptoms by enabling a narrative of the traumatic experience. This is often counter intuitive and almost always initially anxiety-producing for the clinician. However, the client will be much better equipped to change their self-destructive patterns (e.g., addictions, eating disorders, abusive relationships) with the intrusive symptoms resolved because they will have much more of their faculties available for intervention on their own behalf.

## Minimum Criterion Required for Transition to Phase II Treatment

Again, what is the minimal standard of safety necessary to begin Phase II of treatment? While this question has not been addressed in the literature, much less resolved, we will propose the following criteria:

*1. Resolution of impending environmental and physical danger (i.e., ambient, interpersonal, and intrapersonal).* This Level One of Safety, as previously discussed in *What is Safety*, is primary and must be successfully addressed before moving onward with treatment. Traumatic memories will not resolve if the client is in *active* danger and the clinician must use cognitive and especially behavioral strategies to assist the client in removing themselves from harm's way.

*2. Ability to distinguish between "am safe" and "feel safe."* Many trauma survivors feel as if danger lurks around every corner, at all times. In fact, the symptom cluster for arousal is mostly about this phenomenon. It is important for the clinician to confront this distortion and help the client to distinguish, objectively, between "outside danger" and "inside danger." Outside danger, or a real environmental threat, must be met with behavioral interventions designed to help the survivor remove or protect themselves

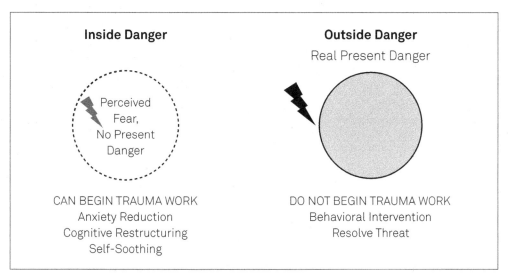

**Figure 6.**
Dealing with inside and outside danger.

from this danger. Inside danger, or the fear resultant from intrusive symptoms of past traumatic experiences, must be met with interventions designed to lower arousal and develop awareness and insight into the source (memory) of the fear (see Figure 6).

*3. Development of a battery of self-soothing, grounding, containment, and expression strategies* and *the ability to utilize them for self-rescue from intrusions.* These techniques should be taught during the early sessions prior to beginning Phase II of treatment. At a minimum, clients should be taught the following skills:
- 3-2-1 sensory grounding technique
- visualization of a "safe place"
- progressive relaxation (and/or other anxiety-reduction skills)
- development of self-soothing discipline (e.g., working out, music, art, gardening, etc.)
- containment strategy(ies)
- expression strategy(ies)

These skills are explained in detail throughout this book.

*4. Ability to practice/demonstrate self-rescue.* It is useful to ask the client to begin to narrate their traumatic experience(s), and when they begin to experience intensifying affect, the clinician should challenge them to implement the skills above to demonstrate the ability to self rescue from a full-blown flashback. This successful experience can then be utilized later in treatment to empower the client to extricate themselves from overwhelming traumatic memories. It is also a testament to the client now being empowered with *choice* to continue treatment and confront trauma memories. The metaphor of teaching a novice sailor the procedures of sailing mechanics prior to casting off so that they can assist with the management of

the boat, instead of becoming a liability during rough seas, is a useful tool for explaining this important skill.

*5. Positive prognosis and contract with client to address traumatic material.* The final important ingredient of the safety phase of treatment is negotiating the contract with the client to move forward to Phase II: *Working Through Trauma.* Remember from previous work the importance of mutual goals in the creation and maintenance of the therapeutic alliance. It is important for the clinician to harness the power of the client's willful intention to resolve the trauma memories before moving forward. An acknowledgment of the client's successful completion of the safety phase of treatment, coupled with an empowering statement of positive prognosis, will most likely be helpful here (e.g., "I have watched you develop some very good skills to keep yourself safe and stable in the face of these horrible memories. Judging from how well you have done this, I expect the same kind of success as we begin to work toward resolving these traumatic memories. What do you need before we begin to resolve these memories?").

It is not necessary that the client meet all the objective criteria before moving to Phase II; however, the clinician should be able to interpret any shortcomings to ensure that there is no danger in moving ahead with treatment. Red flags or concerns about dissociative symptoms or potential regression should alert the clinician that movement forward might be premature. Warning signs may indicate that (a) the client needs more work toward the development of stabilization skills and/or (b) the client is experiencing a dissociative regression.

What follows are a variety of techniques useful for self-soothing, grounding, containment, and self-rescue. These are not the only techniques available, merely examples. Notice that they either subtly begin to incorporate the principle of reciprocal inhibition (relaxation and exposure), or address the narrative of what occurs cognitively, or both.

For up-to-date information on training in the assessment of dissociation, regression, and chronic complex posttraumatic stress, please refer to the Traumatology Institute Training Curriculum – training programs available both online and face-to-face through http://www.psychink.com. The Traumatology Institute Course TI-202 offers a systematic assessment method for aiding clinicians in determining readiness for trauma care.

## 30-Day Video Stabilization Program for Adjunctive Online Trauma Therapy

From a therapeutic standpoint, very few of us have the opportunity to work daily with our client to keep them moving in the right direction every moment that trauma symptoms surface. As a result of increased access to online therapeutic devices, materials, and learning tools, we currently have mechanisms to guide our clients with daily instructions and strategies to keep them on track.

The 30-day video stabilization program was developed to assist clients in their daily focus on stabilization, helping them to build the foundation and hardiness required to move from stabilization into Phase II: *Working Through Trauma*. Each video focuses on a unique skill set or knowledge base with the goal of establishing a hardy sense of stabilization or capacity to harness calm along with a

commitment to required daily practice. We believe that daily practice forms a foundation that allows for improved trauma recovery.

The 30-day video stabilization program is part of the larger Trauma Treatment Online program – offering complex adjunctive therapy for clients to aid them in their recovery program. The first 10 days of the video stabilization program can be accessed at no charge on request. For details or to register, see http://www.whatisptsd.com/find-calm

# 2. Somatic

Traumatic events trigger a subsystem of the autonomic nervous system (ANS) called the sympathetic nervous system (SNS). This is a survival system that releases chemicals into the body and prepares it to fight, flee, or freeze. Although this is a normal sequence, it is an unpleasant experience characterized by fear, anxiety, and very high arousal. Remembering traumatic events can also trigger this cascade of chemicals, creating the same experience. Left unmanaged, this survival/fear response is counterproductive to the therapeutic process. There are a variety of ways to manage this sequence. This section provides body-based techniques that are useful in the management of the fear response.

## Creating a Nonanxious Presence (R – RE – CR)

**Time required:** A few minutes, but repeated often until well learned.

**Materials required:** This script

**Indications for use:** Use when the primary need is to manage the fear response. This is a self-soothing skill that can be utilized as required throughout the remainder of these techniques.

**Counterindications:** None.

This technique is adapted with permission from *A Language of the Heart: Therapy Stories That Heal* (Schultz, 2004). It is designed to help create and maintain a nonanxious presence and is one of the easiest ways to manage stress. It uses the body itself to turn off the fear response by intentionally stimulating the parasympathetic nervous system (PNS). It is an intervention that, once

learned, can be used throughout the recovery process. It is a powerful and effective way for both the client *and* the therapist to manage immediate emotional overwhelm such as fear, anger, and sadness. It combines both physiological and cognitive resources to turn off the survival response.

The first part is primarily psychoeducational for the client. When they understand the sequence of events in their brain related to the survival response, they are better able to normalize the process. In other words, they realize they are not broken when this response occurs – they are normal. And they understand there is a normal intervention they can use to manage it. However, it is a technique that needs to be practiced daily until it becomes almost second nature. Clients *and* therapists should practice it often, whether they think they need to or not. The more they practice it, the more profound the effect will be.

## Delivery of Approach

What follows is a script for explaining to clients, in simple terms, the mechanism in the brain responsible for most of their difficulties. It contains a three-step exercise that only takes a few seconds to accomplish. For it to be effective, it is useful to practice the exercise often and before they might actually need to use it. A useful practice routine will be presented after the script.

 **Script: Psychoeducation**

Our brain is layered, with different functions associated with each layer. The middle part of our brain is an old animal part that even primitive animals possess to some degree. This area is where all of our sensory information goes first. Everything we see, smell, taste, touch, and hear passes through the midbrain. This is where our emotions (sadness, fear, anger, etc.) are located. It is also where the survival routines (fight, flight, or freeze) are triggered.

Layered on top of the midbrain is the part most people imagine when they think of human brains – the part with squiggly lines running across it. This is called the neocortex. The neocortex contains functions that make us uniquely human. This is where the language areas are located, so it allows us to put words to our experiences. It is also where the logic areas are located, so it allows us to connect the dots, make sense of experiences, and attach meaning to events. In addition, it contains a function that allows us to manage our emotions.

Under normal circumstances, information comes into the midbrain, where it is quickly evaluated to determine if we are in danger. If we are not in danger, the information is sent to the neocortex, where words are added to it, sense is made of it, and it is stored for future reference as a memory. However, if we perceive danger or we are being overwhelmed by strong emotions, the midbrain triggers survival routines and begins to prepare the body for fight, flight, or freeze. This preparation is accomplished by chemical messengers that flood through the body and prepare it to either run fast, fight hard, or submit by freezing to survive. You may be familiar with some of these chemicals: they are adrenaline, noradrenaline, aldosterone, and cortisol. This preparation for survival is responsible for the experience of the adrenaline rush.

The following is a partial list of the things that happen in the body when these chemicals prepare it for survival:
1. The digestive process turns off. (There is no need to be wasting energy digesting food when you are running for your life.)
2. The immune system is depressed. (Again, immunity is a waste of energy if the goal is survival.)
3. Blood is pushed from the outer part of the body to the large muscle groups to provide them with the energy (oxygen and food) to either fight, flee, or freeze. (To accomplish this, the heart rate increases and blood pressure increases.)
4. Sugar and cholesterol enter the blood to provide energy to the muscles.

If you think for a minute, you may find these reactions familiar. This is because they all happen to relate to the symptoms of long-term stress. What we call "stress" is really just the physiological experience of the survival sequence being triggered repeatedly. In other words, if the body drops into survival mode again and again, this sequence of events leads to the symptoms of long-term stress. For instance, when the digestive system is repeatedly compromised, symptoms such as ulcers, irritable bowel syndrome, gastritis, constipation, etc. occur. When the immune system is repeatedly compromised, we end up with infectious diseases, such as colds and flu. Even cancer and ulcers are now being associated with a compromised immune system. We end up with high blood pressure, high heart rate, and high cholesterol. More recent research even suggests that a form of diabetes may also be associated with the constant release of sugar from stress.

There is, however, one more very important event that occurs when we enter survival mode. Cortisol floods through the neocortex, essentially shutting down those functions that make us uniquely human. We lose the ability to think clearly. We lose the ability to find words to express ourselves precisely. Most important, we lose the ability to manage our emotions. You have probably seen people who become enraged, turn beet red, and yell obscenities. This is the process that accounts for such things as road rage. It occurs partly because their neocortexes have begun to shut down and they do not have access to the words they need to articulate their inner experiences or communicate what they want – nor do they have access to the logic areas of their brain or the ability to manage their emotions. When we are in survival mode, it is extremely difficult to think about what is going on and choose our next response, instead of just making a knee-jerk reaction. In other words, when our neocortex is shut down, it is very difficult to be intentional.

It is a fact, however, that you cannot be stressed and relaxed at the same time. When you are in danger mode, the sympathetic nervous system (SNS) is activated. This subsystem is responsible for sending out the chemical messengers, increasing your heart rate and blood pressure, tensing your muscles, making your breathing shallower, and shutting down your digestive and immune systems. Conversely, the parasympathetic nervous system (PNS) does everything in reverse of the SNS. The PNS turns off the survival response, thereby lowering your heart rate and blood pressure, etc. Intentionally activating the PNS essentially shuts down the SNS, confirming that you cannot, in fact, be stressed and relaxed at the same time.

 **Script: Creating a Nonanxious Presence**

The following is a three-step exercise designed to help you activate your PNS. The first step will probably sound familiar because we are told to do it over and over by others when we seem upset. However, we are rarely taught Steps 2 and 3, which actually make Step 1 work.

### Step 1

To begin, take a slow deep breath. What part of you moved when you took it? If you said your chest, you are probably breathing from the top of your lungs. When you take a deep breath, your diaphragm should drop down and push your belly out of the way. This is the normal way to breathe. If you watch a baby breathe – before it has been told to hold that belly in – you will notice the belly rising and falling. When you breathe from the top of your lungs, you only move a small percentage of the air from your lungs. When you breathe into your belly, you move a vastly higher percentage of the air and, by so doing, you put more oxygen into your blood stream. The first step of the exercise is to take a single, slow, deep belly breath.

Now, before you go to Step 2, mentally go inside your body. This is a one-time internal check for tension. Start at your head and move all the way to your toes and back again. The object is to see where you are holding tension. Do not try and relax it right now, just take an inventory of where you hold it. Some people have tight shoulder or neck muscles. Some people hold tension in their chest, arms, or stomach. Some try and push their foot through the floor. Note how your body feels when you are paying attention to your tension.

Next, find the front part of your hipbones that jut out below the level of your belly button. Then, notice where your buttock bones are located (theses are sit on). If you stood up, you could imagine lines that run down the front of your body from the level of your hipbones to the level of your buttock bones. Continue the lines back to your buttock bones, then up the back to the level of your hipbones and across again to the front where you started. You have just created an imaginary box that begins just below your belly button and extends down into your lower torso. Medical professionals would call this the *pelvic floor*. Martial artists, especially those who practice a martial art called Aikido, would call this the *one-point*. It is the balance and power point of the body.

### Step 2

Now, take a deep belly breath. As you slowly exhale, intentionally relax this area called the one-point.

Relax all the muscles that begin about two inches below the belly button. Now *really* relax it! Let the muscles in the front of your torso become soft enough to touch your backbone. What did you notice? If you have successfully relaxed the one-point, you should notice that your whole body immediately relaxes, including the parts where you have been holding tension.

Now do the exercise again, slowly. This time, pay close attention to what happens inside your head when you relax your one-point. Most people report what feels like a clear spot opening. Some report it feels like tension is being released from the sides out. You should also notice that you seem more clearheaded and better able to think. It is a very simple exercise: take one deep breath and (most important) relax your one-point – the belly muscles two inches below your belly button.

This is a very stable place to be. From this position of a relaxed one-point, you are able to experience powerful emotions such as sadness, fear, anxiety, and anger without having to "do" anything. You have the ability to feel your emotions, and you can let them flow through you like water through a hose. In other words, you are in a state where you can decide (consciously intend) what you will do next.

Although it seems too simple, there are sound physiological reasons why this exercise works. Intentionally relaxing your body has one very important consequence: it stimulates the PNS, which turns off the SNS. Remember, you cannot be stressed and relaxed at the same time. When your body is relaxed, the midbrain is no longer delivering the message that you are in danger.

Did you know that zebras do not get ulcers? (see Sapolsky, 2004). Ulcers are frequently one of the symptoms humans experience from unrelenting stress. They result from a physical reaction caused by the midbrain constantly telling the body it is in danger and to prepare to survive. One of the ways it prepares the body for survival is by chemically turning off the digestive process because there is no need to be wasting energy digesting food when you are running for your life. When this occurs repeatedly, symptoms such as ulcers occur (also irritable bowel syndrome, gastritis, constipation, etc.). You would think that being chased across the savannah by a large lion would create enough stress to cause an ulcer. But, as it turns out, zebras do not get ulcers (yes, the study has been conducted!). Here is why: After zebras are finished being chased by the lion, they eat their lunch! In other words: no lion, no stress. They live in the here and now; after the lion is gone, their midbrains are no longer preparing their body to survive.

Humans, on the other hand, remember the lion that chased them yesterday and fantasize about the lion that will chase them tomorrow. In fact, many people go looking for lions to worry about because feeling like they are in danger is what they consider normal. There is never a time when their midbrain is not telling them they are in danger, and it is the physical reaction to constantly being in "danger" that results in symptoms like ulcers. Understanding this, you can now add Step 3.

## Step 3

Now that you have taken a deep breath and relaxed your belly muscles, take a moment to notice what happens inside your head and ask yourself, "Am I safe?" Right here, right now, right this second, are you safe? No lions, no stress...

This exercise is most effective when practiced often and before it is needed. The following routine has been found useful in acquiring the skill of being nonanxious. Take a business card and write on the back of it "relax your belly." Place the card where you are likely to see it throughout the day as often as 10 or 15 times (on a computer screen, in a pocket, next to your credit card). Make the agreement with yourself that every time you see the card, think of the card, or touch the card, you will do the exercise. This means you will take a moment to take a slow deep breath, let it out slowly as you relax your belly, notice what happens inside your head and ask, "Am I safe?"

Clients are likely to notice the following sequence of events. In the first couple of days, they will notice that each time they do the exercise they will find themselves relaxing more and more. This is because they are literally training their body to relax on command, which it is not used to doing. After doing the exercise 10 or 15 times a day for a week or more, they will also begin to notice something else: the body does not like being tense. When it finds a way to relax itself it will begin doing so spontaneously. They will find themselves spontaneously taking a deep breath and relaxing. And when this happens, many will notice something else. When they are experiencing a strong emotion (fear, anger, sadness) and they do the exercise, an interesting thing happens: the emotion does not disappear. However, they suddenly will not have to *do* anything about it. They will be able to watch it flow through them like water flows through a hose and they will not have to *do* anything. The neocortex will be functioning and the feeling of overwhelm will subside. This is a powerful and healing place from which to continue recovery.

## Titration Part I: Trigger List Using Braking and Acceleration (R – RE – CR)

**Time required:** One or more sessions depending on the extensiveness of the trauma.

**Materials required:** Pencil and paper (or the following chart).

**Indications for use:** Use when the primary need is to enhance physical, cognitive, and emotional coping skills in the Phase I: Safety and Stabilization of trauma recovery. The client will have been taught or can demonstrate self-soothing skills that can be utilized as required throughout the development of the trigger list in this exercise.

**Counterindications:** If client is clearly unstable, labile, actively dissociating, or dissociates during exercise.

In her excellent book, *The Body Remembers*, Rothschild (2000) encourages clinicians to teach clients how to apply the "brakes" when beginning trauma therapy. She uses the analogy of teaching a new driver to be really comfortable with the braking system in a car before accelerating. In the same manner, she finds methods for teaching clients how to brake before becoming deeply involved in trauma work. In this way, the client moderates the trauma work. A client can begin their work beyond fear after they have learned that they need not be stuck in fear forever. After an individual learns that they can touch just the surface of their experience and then return to a safe or neutral ground, they are empowered, and learn that they can master their own discomfort.

There are many ways to apply the brakes as a way of moderating the release process involved in trauma therapy. In this section, we will review many braking methods, including:

- Titration Part I: Trigger List Using Braking and Acceleration
- Progressive Relaxation
- Autogenics
- Diaphragmatic Breathing
- 3-6 Breathing
- 5-4-3-2-1 Sensory Grounding and Containment
- Postural Grounding
- Anchoring Part I: Collapsing Anchor
- NLP Anchoring Script for Safety and Confidence
- Breathe 911
- Body Scan

The idea is to be aware of many approaches because something may work for one person but not another. Layering (Baranowsky, 1997), which is taught in Phase II, is a braking and accelerating exercise that has been found to be very useful in a clinical setting as well as on a trauma/disaster site. The key with this approach is to start and stop trauma review so processing is not overly explosive or extreme for the individual.

### Delivery of Approach

There is printable handout material available for this exercise (for instructions on how to download please see the Notes on Supplementary Materials, p. 225); see Using the Tools 1 and Using the Tools 2. Here is an example of a titration of significant traumatic events that occur over a lifetime. In this example, the client reviews their life chronologically, identifying significant disturbing life experiences with short, simple descriptions in order from birth to the present.

1. **Time-Out:** Discuss time-out or stop signs with your client. This can simply be a raised hand (stop sign/time-out) to let you know a break is needed. This will indicate it is time for a temporary change of subject or pause in discussion to reclaim one's comfort.

2. **Trigger List:** Work with your client to develop a trigger list of disturbing life experiences that continue to feel unresolved, upsetting, and traumatic.

3. **Break-Down:** The trigger list is to be broken down into early childhood, middle childhood to adolescence, young adulthood, and adulthood to the present (complete sections as required by the client's age and experiences).

4. **Using Brakes:** After you have begun this list, ensure that you remind the client to stop and apply the brakes whenever things feel overwhelming. This "putting on the brakes" will give the client the opportunity to practice some self-soothing techniques and demonstrate for themselves, during the session, their ability to manage symptoms before they become overwhelming.

5. **Create Guardrails:** Ensure that the client provides one-sentence, simple descriptions (maximum 10 words) that are just enough to recall the memory without going into great detail – that will come later (e.g., I was 12 years old, in front of my family home. It was the day I walked across the street and was struck by a motorist). The first few words just give the time frame and context. The words that follow identify the traumatic memory and they are not to exceed 7-10 words.

6. **SUDS Rating:** After the list is complete, read all the memories back to the client, giving the client a chance to reflect on them and rate them based on the Subjective Units of Distress Scale (SUDS). This is a 1–10 scale where 1 represents a calm relaxed state, 5 represents discomfort but within a manageable range, and 10 is the worst feelings of distress the person can recall. Explain the SUDS scale so they can give you the number that best reflects their feelings of distress now, in this moment, when they think of that difficult moment from the past. The list is to be completed based on how the individual feels as they look back on the event now.

7. **Add Till Complete:** Allow the individual to add as many memories as they wish to each section until they feel it is complete.

8. **Identify Themes:** After the trigger list has been built, reflect again on all of the items on the list to identify any guiding principles or core beliefs that stand out or appear in various forms through significant life experiences. These may take the form of negative beliefs (e.g., I am not lovable, everyone lets me down, life is dangerous). These are the operating principles upon which a person is building their beliefs about the world around them and have a fundamental impact on how they walk on this earth.

Consider the following abbreviated trigger-list example (Table 6):

After reviewing all the items above and rating the memories, the client is asked to reflect on the themes. The list following below are the themes identified by the client based on the trigger list developed and rated above:

- I am not acceptable as I am.
- I am unlovable.
- No one will accept me once they know me.
- People are cruel.

Now it is possible to work with both the memories and the core beliefs that have been established as a result of these pivotal life experiences.

*Note:* This approach is similar to the time-line approach in the Phase II: *Working Through Trauma*, but is strictly used to capture the memory rather than to process at this stage.

**Table 6.**    Trigger-List Exercise (Multiple Events) – Example

| Life stage | Trigger list | SUDS |
|---|---|---|
| **Early childhood*** | | |
| 1. Age 10 | Teased in school yard because of weight | 8 |
| 2. Age 12 | Three young males, corner me and molest me on way home from school | 10 |
| 3. Age 12 | Parents do not want to talk about what happened after police leave the house | 10 |
| 4. Age 27 | Weight-loss doctor shames me for being unable to stay on a diet | 7 |

*Trigger-List Exercise (One Event – Multiple Hot Points) – Example*

Use this Trigger List in a graphical manner when there is one event that occurred over a long period of time with multiple "hot points" or disturbing moments related to the same event.

|  | 1 | 2 | 3 | 4 | 5 | 6 | 7 | 8 | 9 | 10 |
|---|---|---|---|---|---|---|---|---|---|---|
| Start | | | | | | | | | | |
| Driving in a snow storm | | | | X | | | | | | |
| Car cuts me off, skid but okay | | | | | | | X | | | |
| Snow starts to reduce | | | | X | | | | | | |
| Hit black ice and lose control | | | | | | | | X | | |
| Car flips in ditch | | | | | | | | | X | |
| I'm alive, not badly injured | | | | | | | X | | | |
| Ambulance & police arrive | | | | X | | | | | | |
| At hospital with internal injuries | | | | | | | | X | | |
| Family arrives for support | | | | X | | | | | | |
| Dr. good news about surgery | | | | X | | | | | | |

## USING THE TOOLS 1

**Trigger-List Exercise (Multiple Events)**

| Life stage | Trigger list | SUDS |
|---|---|---|
| **Early childhood*** | | |
| 1. | | |
| 2. | | |
| 3. | | |
| **Middle childhood to adolescence*** | | |
| 1. | | |
| 2. | | |
| 3. | | |
| **Young adulthood*** | | |
| 1. | | |
| 2. | | |
| 3. | | |
| **Adulthood to present day*** | | |
| 1. | | |
| 2. | | |
| 3. | | |

**List of themes (or core beliefs):**

1. _____

2. _____

3. _____

* Use additional pages if necessary

**USING THE TOOLS 1:**
Trigger-List Exercise (Multiple Events)

## USING THE TOOLS 2

**Trigger-List Exercise (One Event – Multiple Hot Points)**

Use this Trigger List in a graphical manner when there is one event that occurred over a long period of time with multiple "hot points" or disturbing moments related to the same event.

|  | 1 | 2 | 3 | 4 | 5 | 6 | 7 | 8 | 9 | 10 |

Start

_____

_____

_____

_____

_____

_____

_____

_____

_____

_____

_____

_____

From: Anna B. Baranowsky & J. Eric Gentry, *Trauma Practice: A Cognitive Behavioral Somatic Therapy* (4th ed.). © 2023 Hogrefe Publishing

**USING THE TOOLS 2:**
Trigger-List Exercise (One Event – Multiple Hot Points)

## Progressive Relaxation (R)

**Time required:** 5–30 minutes, depending on script.

**Materials required:** None.

**Indications for use:** Use when the primary need is to enhance physical coping skills in Phase I: afety and Stabilization of trauma recovery. Our body's nervous system is the key to healing from trauma. When we teach body calmness, we teach disengagement from hyperalert and overanxious responses of a stressed system. This is a step toward body retraining.

**Counterindications:** Actively dissociating or dissociates during exercise.

### Delivery of Approach

Ehrenreich (2001) and Bourne (2010) provide simple scripts for progressive relaxation that can be expanded with minimal effort. Begin this exercise by instructing the individual to focus on lengthening and deepening the breath. Focus on the inhalation and exhalation making the breath smooth and deep.

**Script : Progressive Relaxation**

Now tighten both fists, and tighten your forearms and biceps ... Hold the tension for five or six seconds ... Now relax the muscles. When you relax the tension, do it suddenly, as if you are turning off a light ... Concentrate on the feelings of relaxation in your arms for 15 or 20 seconds ... Now tense the muscles of your face and tense your jaw ... Hold it for five or six seconds ... Now relax and concentrate on the relaxation for 15 or 20 seconds ... Now arch your back and press out your stomach as you take a deep breath ... Hold it ... and relax ... Now tense your thighs and calves and buttocks ... Hold ... and now relax. Concentrate on the feelings of relaxation throughout your body, breathing slowly and deeply (Ehrenreich, 2001, Appendix B).

From the brief description above, the clinician can encourage tightness and relaxation throughout the body, from top to bottom or in any order they prefer. The body is progressively released and relaxed throughout.

## Autogenics (R – CR)

**Time required:** 10–20 minutes, depending on script.

**Materials required:** Script.

**Indications for use:** Use when the primary need is to enhance physical coping skills in Phase I: Safety and Stabilization of trauma recovery.

**Counterindications:** Actively dissociating or dissociates during exercise.

Autogenics is a slightly different form of self-induced relaxation than progressive relaxation. Rather than using the muscles to tighten and then release, autogenics focuses on using one's own self-talk related to the body to produce a very deep sense of relaxation. A favorite script for autogenic relaxation comes from *Mastering Chronic Pain* (Jamison, 1996). This book, though written for a different audience, provides an excellent deep-relaxation script.

Autogenics is not hypnosis per se because, as the name itself suggests, (auto) effects are produced by the individual. In fact, the script offers an ideal process for learning to use *internal* dialog to calm and soothe the internal world. The individual is in control of the process the entire time. However, autogenics *is* a very powerful technique that is capable of self-inducing a dreamlike, calm state in the individual. As you read the script to the client, take your time to inhale fully and read a line on the exhalation. This breathing-paced reading aids the clinician in sending a relaxing message to the client, further enhancing their experience. It also allows the client time to silently repeat the statement back to themselves while you inhale slowly. This technique would be counterindicated for clients who are already dissociative or for those you suspect are dissociative. In cases where the clinician or counselor does not have sufficient training with dissociative disorders, it is best to make the decision to teach the use of autogenics with caution.

### Delivery of Approach

There is printable handout material for this exercise; see Using the Tools 3. It is helpful to walk the client through the process the first time when using a script that you can later hand to them for their own use. Encourage the client to find a relaxing place and position before beginning the exercise. Although it is useful to have one's eyes closed to enhance relaxation, it is not necessary. Begin to focus on the breath. Start to soften, lengthen, and deepen the breath. Let it become the focus of attention. Recognize that relaxation is a process that occurs over time as one begins to let go of tension and tightness.

---

## USING THE TOOLS 3

### Autogenic Relaxation (R)

Ask your client to find a relaxing position.

Instruct the client to begin to focus and turn your attention toward inhalation and exhalation. Start to soften, lengthen, and deepen your breath. Let go of any tension and tightness you feel in your body.

Read the first sentence out loud to the client, instructing them to repeat each phase silently to themselves. Continue giving the client time to slowly repeat the phrase to themselves after each sentence below:

- I am beginning to notice my breath
- I am beginning to make the inhalation and exhalation slow and deep
- As I inhale slowly and deeply I am beginning to feel calm and soft
- My mind is feeling calm and quiet
- I notice a sensation of relaxation
- My right hand feels soft and light
- My left hand feels soft and light
- My right arm feels soft and light
- My left arm feels soft and light
- I notice a feeling of release in my hands, arms, shoulders, and neck
- My neck, jaw, and forehead feel soft and light
- I notice a feeling of release in my neck, jaw, and forehead
- My muscles feel comfortable and smooth
- My right foot feels soft and light
- My left foot feels soft and light
- My right calf feels soft and light
- My left calf feels soft and light
- I notice a feeling of release in my feet, calves, and thighs
- I feel completely supported by the surface I am resting on
- My body releases more and more
- My breathing is slow and deep
- I feel quiet and comfortable
- My mind is slow and calm
- My body releases more and more
- My heartbeat is slow and steady
- I can feel warmth flowing from my shoulders into my hands
- I can feel warmth flowing from my hips into my feet
- I feel deeply warm and at ease
- My mind is still and quiet
- My breathing is slower and deeper
- I feel safe and comfortable
- I feel at peace
- My breathing is slow and deep

Slowly bring your attention back to the room in which you are relaxing.
Begin to make tiny movements in your fingers and toes, ankles and wrists, legs and arms.

 **WITH AUDIO:** See Video 5 in the supplementary material of this book (or Baranowsky, 2015e, August 23, https://youtu.be/OUIJAsO3XQE) and/or Video 1 in the supplementary material (or Baranowsky, 2020, December 5, https://youtu.be/DvzwJ614frM) for guided audio versions of this exercise.

---

**USING THE TOOLS 3:**
Autogenic Relaxation (R)

---

When finished with the script, encourage the client to bring their attention back into the room in which they are relaxing. Suggest that they can bring feelings of relaxation into their regular day simply by focusing in the same manner as they have during this exercise. Close by asking the person you are working with to slowly bring their attention fully back, taking their time. It is important to inform your client that, when using the technique, they will be very relaxed. They should spend an appropriate amount of time grounding themselves to the here-and-now before attempting to stand or perform complicated tasks such as driving.

The use of autogenic relaxation in session is an excellent approach when there is a need for enhanced skills around self-soothing. This exercise can be quite instructive for the individual who has a willingness to try new approaches and remain in a self-reflective state while they are learning to relax.

## Diaphragmatic Breathing (R)

**Time required:** 5 minutes.

**Materials required:** None.

**Indications for use:** Use when the primary need is to enhance physical coping skills in Phase I: Safety and Stabilization of trauma recovery.

**Counterindications:** Any respiratory complications.

If we watch an infant sleep, we will see the rhythmical movement of deep belly breathing. This is the ideal breathing for relaxation and the nourishing of the body with the breath.

When we feel upset or anxious about something, our breathing is often the first thing to change. It is likely to become shallow, rapid, and jagged or raspy. If, on the other hand, we were to practice intentional diaphragmatic breathing, we would improve our ability to consciously regulate our breathing when we become upset.

### Delivery of Approach

**Script : Diaphragmatic Breathing**

Find a comfortable, unrestricted position in which to sit or lie. Place your hands on your belly as a guide to the breath. Begin to consciously slow and smooth out the breath. Notice the rhythm of the breath through the inhalation and exhalation. Is it smooth, deep, and full, or jagged, shallow, and slight? Now focus on bringing a deeper breath into the belly. Let a full breath be released upon exhalation. Inhale fully, not holding the breath at anytime. On the exhalation release completely and pause, counting to three after the exhalation is complete. Then inhale slowly, fully, and deeply. Continue to focus in this manner on the breath.

Placing one's clasped hands behind the neck opens the chest through the lifting and spreading of the elbows. As this occurs, breath moves much more freely, deep into the belly. This procedure is an excellent alternative (to hands on the belly) for those just learning deep breathing exercises.

At first, the individual is taught to deep-breathe in sets of five. Then this is increased to 10 inhalations and exhalations. Finally, an instruction is given to practice two times each day for 5 minutes per day. In this way, the individual is learning to relax through deep breathing.

**WITH AUDIO:** A guided audio version of this exercise can be found in the supplementary material Video 6 (or see Baranowsky, 2015b, August 23, https://youtu.be/ys3AuHFTKQg) or Video 1 (or see Baranowsky, 2020, December 5, https://youtu.be/DvzwJ614frM).

## 3-6 Breathing (R)

**Time required:** 20 minutes.

**Materials required:** This can be used in conjunction with a biofeedback system like the EmWave® Coherence System that is available through http://www.heartmath.com. This system allows the client to receive immediate feedback both before and after breath training so they can monitor their progress and see improvement as a result of training. Although biofeedback is an excellent resource, it is possible to effectively teach 3-6 Breathing without any equipment.

**Indications for use:** Use when the primary need is to enhance physical coping skills in the Safety and Stabilization stage of trauma recovery.

**Counterindications:** Any respiratory complications.

### Delivery of Approach

There is printable handout material available for this exercise; see Using the Tools 4. At the start of this exercise it is best to focus all your attention internally, and, if possible, it is preferable to begin with your eyes closed. When you are focusing on your breath, sit or lie in a relaxed position where you are comfortable and will not be disrupted. Please note that a full breath is considered an inhalation and an exhalation.

## USING THE TOOLS 4

### 3-6 Breathing (R)

1. *Noticing:* Instruct your client to "just notice the pace, depth, and movement of the breath as you take three inhalations and exhalations (three breaths). Notice if the breath is deep, shallow, smooth, or rough and how it feels moving in and out of the body." After three breaths, ask your client to report on the experience of the breath.

   *Capture Client Response*

   _____

   _____

2. *Deepening:* Instruct your client to "just notice by focusing that you can make the breath deeper, smoother, and slower. Take three breaths again, being careful not to hold your breath at anytime. When you get to the edge of a full inhalation, begin to exhale without straining the body at anytime. Bring the breath deep into the belly on the inhalation and release the breath completely on the exhalation, letting the body rest for a beat at the end of the exhalation before inhalating again. At the end of the third exhalation, let me know when you are done and what it feels like to deepen, slow, and smooth out the breath."

   *Capture Client Response*

   _____

   _____

3. *Sipping:* Now prepare your client to work with a sipping breath by instructing them to "imagine that there is a straw in your mouth and you are inhaling through that straw very slowly and smoothly. Notice that you can bring the breath deep into your belly. At the edge of the inhalation, begin to exhale through the nose. Do not hold or force the breath. Do this three-times and tell me when you are done and what this felt like."

   *Capture Client Response*

   _____

   _____

4. *Counting:* Now add another instruction (demonstrate for your client the count of three on the inhalation and six on the exhalation, – counting with your fingers so that the exhalation is twice as long as the exhalation; you will have to practice this rhythm until it is comfortable for you and easy to demonstrate). Now "following my example, begin to inhale slowly, fully, and deeply into the belly to the count of three and release slowly and completely to the count of six (counting in your own mind). Staying focused on the slow, full rhythm of inhalation and exhalation, do this five-times and tell me when you are done."

   *Capture Client Response*

   _____

   _____

5. *Biofeedback using EmWave®:* If you are using the EmWave® system or any other biofeedback system, begin this session by taking a silent 3-minute baseline of performance. After breath training, take another 3-minute reading of the performance to compare and contrast for the client. It is often amazing the progress that is achieved and can be demonstrated for the client within a short time period using this pattern of breath training.

 **WITH AUDIO:** A guided video demonstration of this exercise can be found in the supplementary material, Video 7 (or Baranowsky, 2015a, August 23, https://youtu.be/fmjoLMHPCHQ) or Video 1 (also see Baranowsky, 2020, December 5, https://youtu.be/DvzwJ614frM). Dr Baranowsky's presentation on 3-6 breathing (Baranowsky, 2010, May 11) can also be found in Video 8 in the supplementary material (or at https://youtu.be/lR0cV9vOIRM).

**USING THE TOOLS 4:**
3–6 Breathing (R)

## 5-4-3-2-1 Sensory Grounding and Containment (R)

**Time required:** 7 minutes.

**Materials required:** None.

**Indications for use:** Use when the primary need is to enhance physical and emotional coping skills in Phase I: Safety and Stabilization of trauma recovery.

**Counterindications:** None.

This technique assists the trauma survivor in developing the capacity to self-rescue from the obsessive, hypnotic, and numinous power of traumatic intrusions and flashbacks. The goal is for the survivor to break their absorbed internal attention to the traumatic images, thoughts, and feelings and instead focus on and connect with external surroundings through their senses (here and now). With this strategy the best outcome is that the accompanying fight-or-flight arousal will diminish. This technique will assist the survivor in understanding that they are perfectly safe in their present context and in understanding the value of using their sensory skills (sight, touch, smell, hearing, and taste) to ground them to this safety in the present empirical reality.

### Delivery of Approach

1. Begin by asking the client to tell part of their trauma narrative and allow them to begin to experience some affect (e.g., reddening of eyes, psychomotor agitation, constricted posture).
2. When they have begun to experience some affect (~ 5 on a SUDS), ask them, "Would you like some help out of those uncomfortable images, thoughts, and feelings?"
3. If they answer yes, ask them to describe, out loud, five objects that they can see in the room. Make certain that these are physical and not imagined objects.
4. Ask them to identify, out loud, five "real world" sounds that they can currently hear while sitting in the room (the sound can be beyond the room, just make certain that they are empirical and not from the traumatic material).
5. Hand them any item (a pen, notebook, a tissue), and ask them to thoroughly feel it and to describe, out loud, the texture of this object. Repeat this with four additional objects.
6. Return to objects that they can see and ask them to now identify four objects that they can see. Do the same with things that they can hear and feel (instead of handing items to the client, ask them to reach out, touch, and describe the texture of four objects). Repeat this until you reach one object each for sight, sound, and texture.
7. When completed, ask the client, "What happened with the traumatic material?" Most of the time your client will describe a significant lessening of negative feelings, thoughts, and images associated with the traumatic material.

*Note:* For many survivors, this technique will mark the first time that they have been able to rescue themselves from a flashback or traumatic material. It is often an experience of tremendous empowerment because it can represent the *"beginning of the end of victimization"* for the survivor. The clinician may want to allow ample opportunity to explore this process and utilize the teachable moment inherent in this process.

**WITH AUDIO:** A guided audio version of this exercise can be found in Video 9 in the supplementary material (or see Baranowsky, 2015c, August 23 https://www.youtube.com/watch?v= mwnzg4aJih4), or in Video 10 (or see (Baranowsky, 2016, April 13, https:// youtu.be/zpKOW0ylsfY).

## Postural Grounding (R)

> **Time required:** 5 minutes.
>
> **Materials required:** None.
>
> **Indications for use:** Use when the primary need is to enhance physical coping skills in Phase I: Safety and Stabilization of trauma recovery.
>
> **Counterindications:** Severe physical injury, disability, or impairment.

Postural grounding is a technique drawn from practice with clients who have dissociative symptoms. As a trauma survivor begins to experience the images and feelings associated with a flashback, they can often be observed to migrate into a constricted and fetal posture of protection. In addition, the clinician can usually notice psychomotor agitation in the form of shaking legs, tremors, fixated or scanning eyes, and shallow breathing.

### Delivery of Approach

When the client begins exhibiting these signs of reexperiencing and arousal, ask them, "Would you like some help in getting out of there [those images and feelings]?" If the client says yes, follow the script below to help them develop the capacity for self-rescue from flashbacks.

1. While the client is exhibiting the constricted and fetal posture or some other physical posture indicates a fight, flight, or freeze response, ask them, "How vulnerable to do feel right now in that posture?" You will usually get an answer like, "Very."
2. Ask them to exaggerate this posture of constriction and protection (i.e., becoming more fetal) and then to take a moment to really experience and memorize the feelings currently in the muscles of their body.
3. Next, ask them to, "stand up, turn around, and then sit back down with an *adult* posture – one that feels in con-

trol." (It is helpful for the clinician to do this with the client as a demonstration).

4. Ask them to exaggerate this posture of being in control and to really notice and memorize the feeling in the muscles of their body.

5. Ask them to articulate the difference between the two postures.

6. Ask them to shift several times between the two postures and to notice the different feelings, thoughts, and images associated with the two opposite postures.

7. Indicate to the client that they are now able to utilize this technique anytime that they feel overwhelmed by posttraumatic symptoms – especially in public places.

8. Discuss with the client opportunities where they will be able to practice this technique and make plans with them for its utility.

## Anchoring Part I: Collapsing Anchors (R)

> **Time required:** 10–20 minutes.
>
> **Materials required:** None.
>
> **Indications for use:** Use when the primary need is to enhance physical, cognitive, and emotional coping skills in Phase I: Safety and Stabilization of trauma recovery.
>
> **Counterindications:** Actively dissociating or dissociates during exercise.

### NLP Anchoring Script for Safety and Confidence

(Adapted from Bandler & Grinder, 1979; Reprint from Gentry & Baranowsky, 1998)

This exercise assists the individual to use the body (thumb, fingers, etc.) to anchor positive resource states. In doing so, the person learns to access these positive states more readily by capturing the memory in simple hand gestures. Other body parts can also be taught to be anchors for various resource states or memories.

### Delivery of Approach

 **Script: NLP Anchoring for Safety and Confidence**

*Relaxation induction.* Find a comfortable spot where you can quietly begin to relax in the knowledge that you are in a safe place where you can release any of the tensions you hold. Allow your eyes to soften and the eyelids to rest lightly on the eyes. Begin to focus on the rhythm of your breath. Pay attention to how it flows into your body and then out again. Notice that with just a bit of effort you can lengthen the inhalation, making it smooth and soft. Imagine that it is a cool stream slowly filling the lower part of your belly – filling it completely. As the breath is released, allow any tensions to flow out with the exhalation. Inhale cool soothing breath, slowly filling up the belly; notice the belly rise. Exhale completely, releasing any tensions with the breath. Allow your eyes to close completely at this time if they are not already closed. Pause before the next inhalation, allowing even more breath to release and, along with it, tensions and toxins from the body. Recognize how the body begins to feel a greater sense of relaxation just by following the inhalations and exhalations. Notice how deepening the breath enhances feelings of well-being. Be aware that you can use this breath at anytime in your day to enhance feelings of well-being, clarity, and focus. Notice that with each exhalation you feel a greater sense of inner peace and calmness. Remember that this is a tool you can use anywhere and anytime in your regular day. Allow the inhalation and exhalation to become secondary – still smooth and deep but no longer the center of your attention.

*Safety anchor.* Now search your memory for a time when you felt great feelings of safety and reassurance. You may choose to use a comforting and safe place from real-life experience or one completely based on your imagination where you feel safe, comfortable, and relaxed. Recall all the contextual cues, such as sights, smells, sounds, air temperature, texture of objects, and anything else you are aware of. Identify the "exact moment" in this situation when you felt the greatest amount of safety. Become aware of the internal dialog at that moment of safety. What was your mind saying during that time of great reassurance and security? What sensations did your body have when it felt this safety and joy and the freedom of relaxation? As this sensation reaches its height, squeeze together the thumb and forefinger on your dominant hand to anchor this experience of safety.

*Competency or confidence anchor.* Now allow your mind to recall a time in your past where you felt confident and competent. Memorize all the contextual clues such as sights, smells, sounds, temperature of the air, texture of objects, and any other contextual clues. Identify the exact moment in this situation when you felt the maximum amount of confidence and competence. Identify and experience what your mind was saying when you enjoyed these feelings of confidence and competence. What sensations did you feel in your body when you experienced that great confidence and competence? What was it like to feel that potency? As this sensation of competence and confidence reaches its height, squeeze together the thumb and middle finger on your dominant hand to anchor this experience of competence and confidence.

*Closure.* Recognize that you can utilize these anchors at anytime in your day when you feel stressed or upset. You can draw feelings of safety and confidence to enhance your access to personal resources and resiliency skills. Shortly, but not yet, you will be bringing your awareness back to this room with the knowledge that when you do you will feel fully refreshed and able to continue with the rest of your day – wiser, stronger, and more inwardly calm in the knowledge of your greater claim to inner resources. As you make your way back to this room, you can begin to have feeling in your hands and feet … arms and legs … chest and stomach. Lengthen and stretch through to your arms, hands, legs, and feet. You can begin to become more present behind your eyes. Take a deep breath and, when you are ready, open your eyes to normal waking consciousness.

 **WITH AUDIO:** A guided audio version of this exercise (Baranowsky, 2015d, August 23) can be found in the supplementary material (p. 226) Video 11 (also available at https://youtu.be/fiQJ2KXRvmQ).

## Breathe 911 (R – CR)

**Time required:** 5–20 minutes.

**Materials required:** A breath and relax app for smartphones and tablet devices (i.e., Breathe+ Simple Breath, Breethe, Calm, Headspace, HeartMath, iBreathe, Liberate, MyLife, Simply Being, etc.) Please note, there are many to choose from so familiarize yourself with a few that you can guide your clients to use.

**Indications for use:** Use when the primary need is to enhance physical, cognitive, and emotional coping skills in the Safety and Stabilization stage of trauma recovery.

**Counterindications:** Actively dissociating or dissociates during exercise.

### Breathe 911 App

This exercise assists the individual to harness calm by following steps in a breath training app with embedded cues for relaxation and safety. Breathing applications (to be used online with smart phones and tablets) are good examples of how technology can provide excellent adjunctive therapeutic support between trauma practice sessions.

In addition, current research on neuroplasticity confirms that we have the power to change the way our minds and bodies manage stress. The best route to success is massed practice, or very regular practice over a short time period. Many breath trainers are designed to help your clients engage in daily practice to harness calm and find a way to increase sensations of relaxation and comfort in both body and mind.

### Delivery of Approach

Breath trainers are designed to help individuals recapture feelings of comfort and calm anytime and anyplace. Simple breathing exercises can leave a person feeling more relaxed and at ease when facing trauma reminders or even the demands of daily life. Playing the breath trainer engages the individual in a structured approach with guided cues to slow the breath and embed corrective messages of safety. Most trainers can be set for any amount of time from (i.e., 1 to 60 minutes, depending on preference). Some have the option of embedding positive text cues or adaptive messages; some can be adjusted to go slower or faster based on the individual's pacing. Many options are available for Apple and Android devices, the list above is not exhaustive.

Practicing deep breathing daily in combination with positive messages can prove to be an excellent tool for harnessing calm in a stress moment, allowing for an increased sense of self-mastery.

**WITH AUDIO:** Please watch the guided video demonstration (Baranowsky, 2013, November 27) in Video 12 in the supplementary material (or at https://youtu.be/PyifRngs4jY).

## Body Scan (R)

> **Time required:** 10–60 minutes.
>
> **Materials required:** Script or self-guided video/audio.
>
> **Indications for use:** Use when the primary need is to reinforce feelings of comfort in the body.
>
> **Counterindications:** No counterindications – make this a completely nondemanding experience of inner self-reflection. Stop at anytime if needed.

Learning to be a patient observer of our own inner body landscape is a route to settling down the nervous system and arriving at a state of inner calm. By focusing on the body and taking the time to perform a regular self body scan or energy scan, you become the expert in what is happening within and how to tend to your inner needs.

The body needs care and attention just like a car. Tune-ups, the best fuel and maintenance are required in order for the car to perform properly, and each person is like this as well. The body scan exercise can act in a nourishing way for anyone who would like to invest in harnessing inner wisdom and calm.

### Delivery of Approach

 **Script: Body Scan**

The body scan is best performed while in a comfortable position, either lying down or sitting in a comfortable chair with the legs supported. Ensure you are warm and fully supported and that there are no distractions.

Begin by placing your hands on your belly to direct your breath deep into the body. Slowly bring the breath into the belly and then slowly release the breath three times. Imagine sensing a light entering into the top of your head illuminating every cell of your body or the internal landscape with each breath.

Starting from the top, front of your face, ears, temples, eyes, mouth, tongue, jaw. Notice if you feel any tension or tightness and with each breath exhale any discomfort you might feel. Continue to illuminate the neck and shoulders scanning for any discomfort. Exhale discomfort. Take your inner gaze to your arms, elbows, wrists, hands and fingers. Breathe in and out. Focus on the chest, ribs, belly, upper back, middle and lower back. Notice what you experience with the illuminating awareness. Is there any discomfort? Breathe in and exhale. You can even notice if there is any physical pain, emotional unease, or negative talk and you can use your breath to release this.

As you continue with your scan, energetic changes might occur within your body. Feel into this change, whether it is differences in body temperature, an image, comforting inner thought, or flash of color or light. Just continue to notice if there are any inner blocks, tension, discomfort. Breathe in and allow yourself to be present for the inner experience rather than recoiling or shutting down.

Continue to focus internally, allowing your focus to move further down the body past your lower back and belly into your legs, knees, calves, shins, feet, toes. What do you sense? Is there any residue of discomfort? Are there any energy blocks? Breathing in and exhaling fully. Allow yourself to be with the breath and focus on the body.

Stay present for the full body from top to bottom and do a final scan to ensure you have illuminated every part with light and breath, noticing everything. Accepting it all and exhaling any elements that you do not need any longer.

As you practice the body/energy scan you gain wisdom in your understanding of what is happening inside and how this might be connected with emotion, old injury, or inner blocks.

In addition to the exercise script above, there are also many great examples online of the body scan which I would encourage you to practice with.

*Here are a few of my favorite scans*

- Stop Breathe Think. (2017, September 28): *Body Scan Meditation (Tame Anxiety)* [Audio]. YouTube. https://youtu.be/QS2yDmWk0vs
- People in Pain Network (2016, July 19): *Jon Kabat Zinn Body Scan Meditation* [Audio]. YouTube. https://youtu.be/u4gZgnCy5ew
- Michael Sealey (2014, December 17): *Guided Body Scan Meditation for Mind & Body Healing.* [Audio]. YouTube. https://youtu.be/i7xGF8F28zo
- *Guided Body Scan Exercise* [Audio]. Available in Video 13 in the supplementary material (see p. 226, or Baranowsky, 2016, February 3, https://youtu.be/zYf_4tJva2M)

## Anchoring Part II: Safety (R)

> **Time required:** 10 minutes.
>
> **Materials required:** None.
>
> **Indications for use:** Use when the primary need is to enhance physical, cognitive, and emotional coping skills in Phase I: Safety and Stabilization of trauma recovery.
>
> **Counterindications:** Actively dissociating or dissociates during exercise.

# 3. Cognition

Although they are intricately connected, the brain and the mind are not the same thing. Each affects the other in ways that are only partially understood. The physical brain can overwhelm us when it perceives danger – it drops into survival mode making rational thought (cognition) and behavior difficult. Our cognitive mind (the things we think, the way we interpret reality, and the way we talk to ourselves about it) can circumvent this process. When we have good control of our thinking process, we can avert that survival routine. The use of mental images and stories, the language we use in describing ourselves and the world to ourselves (LeDoux & Pine, 2016), and the meaning we attach to events all have the power to change the fear response. This section provides cognitive techniques for managing the fear response.

There is printable handout material available for this exercise; see Using the Tools 5. This exercise is an anchoring process that enables the individual to gain access to a safety state without the use of hypnosis-type exercise.

# USING THE TOOLS 5

## Anchoring Part II: Safety I

### Safety Anchors

1. Instruct the client to identify a desired resource state (e.g., safety, courage, contentment).

   _____

   _____

2. Ask the client to identify an experience when the resource state was present.
   a. Describe context (i.e., at the cottage with the fireplace warming the room).

   _____

   _____

   b. Find the exact second that represents the resource state (i.e., place, time, objects, people present, etc.) Describe below:

   _____

   _____

   c. "Close eyes and reexperience" (10–15 seconds)

3. Make note of when the resource state was most intense. Describe below:

   _____

   _____

4. Behavioral
   a. "Close your eyes and imagine you are watching a videotape of this moment ..."
   b. "What would we see you doing ... specifically?"
   c. "What would be the look on your face?"
   d. Make note. Describe below:

   _____

   _____

5. Cognitive
   a. "Imagine that there is a tiny microphone that can listen to your thoughts at this moment ..."
   b. "What would we hear your mind say at the moment _____ (resource) is the strongest?"
   c. Make note. Describe below:

   _____

   _____

   _____

From: Anna B. Baranowsky & J. Eric Gentry, *Trauma Practice: A Cognitive Behavioral Somatic Therapy* (4th ed.). © 2023 Hogrefe Publishing

**USING THE TOOLS 5:**
Anchoring Part II: Safety I

6. Affective/Sensory
   a. "At the moment that _____ is the strongest ..."
   b. "What do you feel in your body?"
   c. "What sensations do you experience?" Describe below:

   _____

   _____

7. Establish Anchor
   a. "Close your eyes and begin to experience _____ about 15 seconds before it reaches its 'peak' intensity."
   b. Narrate context.
   c. Narrate behavioral.
   d. Narrate cognitive.
   e. Narrate affect/sensory.
   f. "Allow this experience of _____ (resource state) to intensify even more ... feel it expanding in your chest ... in your mind ..."

   _____

   _____

8. Trigger

   a. Now, squeeze together the thumb and forefinger of your dominant hand (5 seconds) ... put all of the _____ into that squeeze."

9. Return to normal consciousness

   a. Test trigger ("How much of that feeling comes back when you squeeze your thumb and forefinger together now?") _____ %

From: Anna B. Baranowsky & J. Eric Gentry, *Trauma Practice: A Cognitive Behavioral Somatic Therapy* (4th ed.). © 2023 Hogrefe Publishing

## Safe-Place Visualization (R)

**Time required:** 5–30 minutes depending on script.

**Materials required:** Script.

**Indications for use:** Use when the primary need is to enhance cognitive and emotional coping skills in Phase I: Safety and Stabilization of trauma recovery.

**Counterindications:** Actively dissociating or dissociates during exercise.

The next exercise is not hypnosis, although it is a technique that utilizes some elements that are like "hypnotherapy." It is therefore limited for use by those who have had formal training and appropriate educational background to offer that type of work. This exercise is adapted from the *Treatment Manual for Accelerated Recovery from Compassion Fatigue* (Baranowsky & Gentry, 2010, 2011a, 2011b; Gentry & Baranowsky, 1998).

### Delivery of Approach

 **WITHOUT AUDIO:**

 **Script: Previsualization**

Find a place and position where you can relax. This should be a place where you can be assured of minimal interruptions. Take the time to set the space for your maximum benefit. After you are satisfied with the environment and feel it will be one that is safe and relaxing, we will be ready to begin.

During this exercise you will have the opportunity to enjoy a sense of deep relaxation through a guided exercise. Through the exercise you will be instructed in the inner imagining of a safe place. This may be a place you have been to before or one entirely made up in your imagination.

Remember that this next exercise is a guided relaxation and imagery approach in which you remain in control while being deeply relaxed. You *can* stop at anytime if you need to, *but* we recommend that you experience the entire exercise without interruptions to enjoy the greatest benefit and insight.

Focus on creating a sense of relaxation in the muscles in the back of your eyes and notice how this relaxation can spread. Now, as your eyelids softly rest over your eyes, notice how you are able to soften your facial muscles – first those that are closest to your eyes, but then more and more as you sense a smoothing, soothing, warming sensation spread across your face. Notice this warming, soothing sensation spread gently across your forehead ... across your eyes ... through your hairline. Notice as it warms and softens the lines of your face. Just notice and let the gentle warmth calm your face. This calming sensation moves down your face ... your nose ... lips ... chin ... until your whole face becomes a numb mass of relaxation. Even the mind takes on a soothing, mellow position ... until the mind feels very quiet. Listen to the sound of my voice and any other sounds without doing anything. Let these sounds be signals to let you know that you are safe, here in this room, allowing you to pay even closer attention to the *inside* world. Simply let the sounds assure you that you are in a safe place in this room. Feeling that safety, allow yourself to relax and slowly let the soothing warmth spread through to your neck muscles, helping you to release any tensions. The warmth now moves down through your arms all the way to your fingertips. As it does you can release tension in your upper body by imagining it spilling out through the tips of your fingers and into the ground below. Allow the warmth to spread through to your chest and fill up your lungs ... relaxing your muscles, relaxing your stomach, softening the muscles of the back and warming and releasing any tensions there. Continue to pay attention to my voice. Notice any points of tension and bring the soothing warmth to those points so they too can soften and relax. Bring the warmth through to your lower back, thighs, calves, feet, and toes. Become aware now that you can release even more tension from your lower body by imagining it spilling down all the way through to the tips of your toes and spilling out and into the ground. Just let your body relax as deeply as it wants, letting your conscious mind stray where it might ... and while your body relaxes it brings a feeling of calm detachment ... and a feeling that time doesn't matter, time is not important ... you feel calm and emotionally detached.

**Script: Safe Place Imagery**

Now allow your mind to find a relaxed and soothing space – a safe place. This is a place from the past that you have been to before, or one from your imagination. Either way is okay, because it all belongs to you. Begin to develop a picture as a instant film strip would develop. Watch as the safe place develops, exposing itself to you. Notice how the lights, colors, textures that surround you are now soothing to you. Notice what is above and below you. Walk around this place, taking notice of all the sounds of relaxation ... those that are close and those that are far away. Notice the soothing fragrances in this safe place ... those that are distinct and those that seem subtle. Be aware of all the safe fragrances. Now notice the temperature and quality of the air ... reach out and touch some of the objects in this place of safety ... notice all the textures. Be aware that anything that is safe can be imported into this place by you. If anything seems unsafe or threatening, allow yourself to send it out and notice how you are able to do this. Feel and appreciate all the relaxing sounds ... assuring smells ... and the sight of safety ... feel it, appreciate it. Take it all in and memorize it so that if someone asked you to draw it at a later date you could do this in great detail... or can call it up at anytime [5–10 seconds of silence].

Also notice how you can begin to move about ... moving about with the feeling of relaxed joyfulness ... relaxed joyfulness ... this is our natural state. Remember what it feels like to be relaxed ... and joyful. Take a moment now to give yourself permission ... full permission to enjoy this state of comfort ... of relaxation ... of peace [be silent for about 10 seconds].

Slowly begin to bring your awareness back into this room, realizing that shortly but not just yet you will open your eyes. Before you do this, realize that you will feel more relaxed and better able to get on with the rest of your day. Make small movements in your fingers and toes ... make small movements in your arms and legs. Whenever you are ready, slowly begin to bring your awareness fully into this room, opening your eyes when you are ready.

 **WITH AUDIO:** Please watch the guided video demonstration (Baranowsky, 2019, April 8) in Video 14 in the supplementary material (p. 226, or at https://youtu.be/rMIAgTY_-Fc).

## Positive Self-Talk and Thought Replacement/Transformation (CR)

**Time required:** One or more sessions, continuously referring back.

**Materials required:** List of thinking errors.

**Indications for use:** Use when the primary need is to enhance cognitive coping skills in Phase I: Safety and Stabilization of trauma recovery.

**Counterindications:** Client clearly confused, labile.

This section is strongly influenced by the work developed by Dr. Albert Ellis (1961) and Dr. Aaron Beck (1967, 1976). These two individuals revolutionized our understanding of errors in thinking and how our thoughts can lead us astray. The power of our internal thoughts can shift us from relative calm to extreme distress. Harnessing our thoughts and challenging where they lead us can be the difference between unsettled internal distress and peace of mind. Intentionally learning about our automatic thoughts and challenging the roots and the power of these beliefs can offer a route to a more settled and calm state.

### Delivery of Approach

*Ten Errors of Thinking and Positive Challenges to Errors in Thinking*

There is printable handout material available for this exercise; see Using the Tools 6, Using the Tools 7, and Using the Tools 8. Assist your client by reviewing the following Ten Errors of Thinking and discussing how to transform them through positive self-talk and replacement using the Challenges to Negative Thinking presented later in this section. You can read through the items out loud with your client or have them read them out loud. Give the client time to reflect and comment on each of the Ten Errors of Thinking by asking, "Is this Error in Thinking something you recognize in yourself, and if yes, how?"

## USING THE TOOLS 6

### Ten Errors of Thinking

1. *Exaggeration or minimization.* In the case of exaggerated thinking, small errors may be viewed as major (e.g., I lost my bus ticket – I am the biggest idiot in the world!). Alternatively, in minimization we may undermine our true accomplishments or skills (e.g., "Oh yes, I did get an A on that exam but it was just a fluke").
Do you do this? If yes, how?

---

---

2. *All-or-nothing thinking.* This occurs when we fail to see things on the full spectrum of life experiences. For example, a slight inconvenience such as a meal that arrives warm instead of hot results in a declaration that dinner is ruined!
Do you do this? If yes, how?

---

---

3. *Overgeneralization.* A single occurrence is viewed as a never-ending negative pattern or prophecy of doom (e.g., a man's relationship ends and he arrives at the conclusion that all relationships he will develop in the future are doomed to failure).
Do you do this? If yes, how?

---

---

4. *Mind reading.* Here, the person believes that their interpretation of what another is thinking must be accurate without fully checking out their own version of the situation (e.g., a woman sees her friend yawning during their conversation and concludes that her friend must think she is a bore; the reality may be that the friend stayed up all night with a sick child).
Do you do this? If yes, how?

---

---

5. *Fortune-teller error.* This is an unfortunate tendency to anticipate bad outcomes and then behave as if one's prediction has already occurred (e.g., in anticipation of a job interview the person predicts that they will never get the job – then proceeds to perform poorly during the interview even though they are highly qualified).
Do you do this? If yes, how?

---

---

---

From: Anna B. Baranowsky & J. Eric Gentry, *Trauma Practice: A Cognitive Behavioral Somatic Therapy* (4th ed.). © 2023 Hogrefe Publishing

**USING THE TOOLS 6:**
Ten Errors of Thinking

6.  *Should statements.* The individual puts pressure on themselves or others to accomplish something through the utilization of guilt (e.g., "I will disappoint everyone if I don't get this new job"). Conversely, an individual may use guilt to manipulate another (e.g., "If you don't wash my car, you do not love me").
    Do you do this? If yes, how?

    _____

    _____

7.  *Labeling.* The person uses name-calling or negative labels to describe errors made by themselves or others instead of simply describing the mistake (e.g., "I'm *totally useless* for forgetting to take the muffins out of the oven in time").
    Do you do this? If yes, how?

    _____

    _____

8.  *Personalization.* Taking personal responsibility for a negative outcome that the person is not entirely responsible for (e.g., a person may say, "I lost the game" when they were playing a team sport and therefore only one player in a group).
    Do you do this? If yes, how?

    _____

    _____

9.  *Emotional reasoning.* This is the act of believing that because you feel very badly about something, everyone else must be equally devastated or disgusted by the event (e.g., "I lost my new team jacket and feel awful – I have let everyone down by my actions and they must feel devastated about this loss").
    Do you do this? If yes, how?

    _____

    _____

10. *Disqualifying the positive.* Here, positive outcomes, accomplishments, and experiences are discounted while the meaning of negative events are elevated in one's view (e.g., one negative comment is taken much more seriously than many examples of positive feedback). The constructive criticism one receives is extremely important, whereas positive feedback is quickly forgotten.
    Do you do this? If yes, how?

    _____

    _____

From: Anna B. Baranowsky & J. Eric Gentry, *Trauma Practice: A Cognitive Behavioral Somatic Therapy* (4th ed.). © 2023 Hogrefe Publishing

## USING THE TOOLS 7

### CHANGES – Positive Challenges to Errors in Thinking

In the acronym CHANGES, each letter stands for one challenge to the ten errors in thinking outlined above. There are seven items in this section to help you challenge negative thoughts and improve internal dialog. Work with your client to review all the items below and then give homework sheets "Reflection Sheet 1 and 2."

1. *C – Concretize:* Arriving at exaggerated statements of events such as "It will never get better" or "This is devastating" are the result of thinking errors like exaggerated thinking or overgeneralization. Questioning the statement of belief can bring a bit of reality back into the picture. An exaggerated statement such as those above could be challenged as follows: "Will it really never get better?" or "Is it so devastating that we should call an ambulance, police, or the Red Cross?"

2. *H – Humor:* Using humor to defuse our thinking errors can be very effective. Although we are able to laugh at comedy shows depicting events very familiar to us, when we are personally involved we become unable to see the humor. The goal in using humor is to step back, view the situation with detachment, and search for the humor in the event.

3. *A – Alternatives:* The use of alternatives broadens our currently narrow view on an event. One can challenge virtually all the errors in thinking utilizing this approach. Initially, the goal is simply to identify alternatives to the current belief. You may be unable to believe the alternative, but it starts to broaden your thoughts and that is the goal. You may think "My roommate hates me," or alternatively you may challenge this with "My roommate and I are different people and enjoy different things."

4. *N – Normal Others:* The task here is to identify others whom you admire and feel are managing their lives well. Then, when confronted with an error in your own thinking, you ask yourself "What would X say about this?" or "How would X handle this?"

5. *G – Good for Me:* Use this strategy whenever your thoughts are negative or unhelpful. For example, if I have some document to review and conclude that "I will never get this done," the challenging question would be "Is this thought helpful in achieving my goal of reviewing the document?" Of course, the answer would be no. The next question would be "What thought would help me achieve my goal?" This might be "If I put aside a little time each day this week, I will get this work completed." In this way, we find thoughts that are good for us and useful in helping us arrive at our desired outcome.

6. *E – Evidence:* Use this when you get stuck on thoughts that arrive at conclusions without sufficient evidence (e.g., "I'm going to die," in response to anxious feelings associated with a racing heartbeat). Challenge yourself with evidence-seeking questions, such as "Have you died in the past when you had these feelings?"

7. *S – So What?* Use this when thoughts are upsetting but you are not certain what error in thinking you have made. Challenge your negative thoughts or conclusions with "So what?" For example, you may be worried about an upcoming meeting and conclude, "I will make a fool of myself!" Challenge your belief by saying "So what?" If you respond with another negative thought like "It would be so embarrassing," again say "So what?" Keep challenging yourself with "So what?" until negative thoughts are exhausted.

These seven thought challenges are designed to broaden and improve your own thought patterns so as to include a more useful, nourishing, and sustainable internal dialog. Run through one or more of the challenges above whenever you have errors in thinking. Continue the process until the errors reduce or are, at the very least, exposed.

Use Reflection Sheets 1 and 2 in Using the Tools 8 to assist in externalizing negative thoughts and challenging them.

From: Anna B. Baranowsky & J. Eric Gentry, *Trauma Practice: A Cognitive Behavioral Somatic Therapy* (4th ed.). © 2023 Hogrefe Publishing

**USING THE TOOLS 7:**
CHANGES – Positive Challenges
to Errors in Thinking

## USING THE TOOLS 8

**Reflection Sheet #1**

| Date | Situation | Automatic thought | Feeling | Error type |
|---|---|---|---|---|
| **Example** 05/08/02 | Job interview | I'll blow it. They will think I'm ridiculous. | Panic, hopelessness | Fortune teller, Mind reading |
| | | | | |
| | | | | |
| | | | | |
| | | | | |
| | | | | |
| | | | | |
| | | | | |
| | | | | |
| | | | | |
| | | | | |
| | | | | |

From: Anna B. Baranowsky & J. Eric Gentry, *Trauma Practice: A Cognitive Behavioral Somatic Therapy* (4th ed.). © 2023 Hogrefe Publishing

**USING THE TOOLS 8:**
Reflection Sheet

## Reflection Sheet #2

Date: _____

| | |
|---|---|
| **Situation** | (What were you doing)? Example: Preparing for a job interview. |
| **Feelings** | (Describe and rate 1–10 where 1 = no distress to 10 = extreme distress)<br>Example: Panic, hopeless, fearful – *Rating* = 8 |
| **Trigger thoughts (images)** | (What was going through your mind just prior to the bad feelings? What other thoughts or images came up?)<br>Example: I'll blow it. They will think I'm ridiculous. |
| **How to make changes to trigger thoughts** | Concretize: "Shall we alert the Red Cross?" Humor: "How can I see the humor in this?"<br>Alternatives: "Can I see this in a more positive light or just differently?"<br>Normal others: "What would X think about this?" or "How would X handle this?"<br>Good for me: "Is this thought good for me or useful?"<br>Evidence: "Is there enough evidence for me to believe it is 100% true? How so? How not?"<br>So What: And if all else fails, "SO WHAT!" |
| **Balancing thoughts** | (Phrase a neutral or balanced statement to replace the error in thinking.)<br>(Next, rate how much you believe the new statement from 0 to 100%.)<br>Example: I will do my best at this interview and learn from my experience.<br>*Rating* = 75% |
| **Rate feeling now** | (Describe and rate 1–10, where 1 = no distress to 10 = extreme distress)<br>Example: Panic, Hopeless, Fearful<br>*Rating* = 3 |

From: Anna B. Baranowsky & J. Eric Gentry, *Trauma Practice: A Cognitive Behavioral Somatic Therapy* (4th ed.). © 2023 Hogrefe Publishing

# Flashback Journal (R – RE)

**Time required:** Approximately 10–20 minutes, continuously referring back.

**Materials required:** Journal.

**Indications for use:** Use when the primary need is to enhance cognitive and behavioral coping skills in Phase I: Safety and Stabilization of trauma recovery.

**Counterindications:** If client is overwhelmed by events and unable to self-soothe.

## Delivery of Approach

There is printable handout material available for this exercise; see Using the Tools 9. The following journal format is useful as a functional analysis of triggers and symptoms. Column labels are self-explanatory. Have the client note specific symptoms on the template. Then have them identify what was occurring at the moment that may have triggered the symptom. Next, have them identify the event with which it may be associated and make an estimated SUDS level. Have them use self-soothing skills and re-estimate their SUDS level.

You will recall from the Trigger List (Using the Tools 1 and 2) where the Subjective Units of Distress Scale (SUDS) was described in use. To recap, this is a 1–10 scale where 1 represents a calm relaxed state, 5 represents discomfort but within a manageable range, and 10 is the worst feelings of distress the person can recall. Explain the SUDS so they can give you the number that best reflects their feelings of distress now, in this moment, when they think of that difficult moment from the past. The list is to be completed based on how the individual feels as they look back on the event now.

## USING THE TOOLS 9

### Flashback Journal

| Symptom | Trigger | Memory | SUDS | Self-soothing skill(s) used | SUDS |
|---|---|---|---|---|---|
| | | | | | |
| | | | | | |
| | | | | | |
| | | | | | |
| | | | | | |
| | | | | | |
| | | | | | |
| | | | | | |
| | | | | | |
| | | | | | |
| | | | | | |

From: Anna B. Baranowsky & J. Eric Gentry, *Trauma Practice: A Cognitive Behavioral Somatic Therapy* (4th ed.). © 2023 Hogrefe Publishing

**USING THE TOOLS 9:**
Flashback Journal

## Buddha's Trick (R – CR)

> **Time required:** 5 minutes.
>
> **Materials required:** None.
>
> **Indications for use:** Use when the primary need is to enhance cognitive coping skills in the Safety and Stabilization stage of trauma recovery.
>
> **Counterindications:** If client is clearly confused, unable to concentrate, or actively dissociating.

This is an awareness technique to assist clients by improving their understanding of the necessity for processing time and the level of energy required for suppression. Most trauma practitioners recognize that people who have been exposed to traumatic events attempt to "push bad thoughts out of their minds." This approach tends to result in the unfortunate outcome of posttraumatic symptoms (i.e., intrusive thoughts, poor sleep, anxious feelings, and avoidance). By refusing to think about difficult events, we fail to establish a complete narrative, make sense of our experiences, desensitize through exposure, and recognize that we are now safe. Baer (2001) provides an excellent illustration of this technique in *The Imp of the Mind* (pp. 95–99).

When we are feeling very badly about something that has occurred or that we worry might occur, we sometimes make a strong effort to suppress our thoughts, feelings, and memories associated with the disturbing recollection. Many research studies show that this type of thought suppression does not work. In addition, it uses a large amount of energy to keep thoughts out of our mind and is therefore exhausting. It also increases the fear factor as we are hiding this thing from our thoughts, reducing our ability to review and resolve our feelings and thus making it seem even more unbearable than it is. Recall someone saying to you that something terrible has happened and then not telling you right away what it is. Your mind arrives at a conclusion that is even worse than the actual reality, in most cases.

Although the suppression of thoughts may seem to be an effective solution, this strategy can lead to an exacerbation of the very thought that one is attempting to suppress. This ironic effect is the most obvious unwanted outcome of suppression and has now been investigated empirically for more than three decades. However, the fact that suppression is an effortful process implies that, even when suppression does not lead to an ironic rebound of the unwanted thought, it puts an insidious cognitive load on the individual attempting to suppress. Moreover, whether or not suppression leads to an exacerbation of the unwanted thought, it is rarely successful, and hence adds to the individual's distress (Najmi and Wegner, 2009).

### Delivery of Approach

*Thought Exercise*

1. Instruct the individual to think of a "stone Buddha" or any other nonanxiety producing object (e.g., pink elephant, puppy dog) for 1 minute, keeping their mind as focused as possible during this time. If at anytime they lose their focus, they are to lift a finger to alert both themselves and you that they have lost their focus. Now discuss what this exercise was like, what they observed, and how much energy it took to keep their mind focused.

2. Next, instruct the individual to keep "stone Buddhas" out of their mind for a full minute. Again, they are to lift a finger every time "stone Buddha" comes into the mind. When the minute is over they are given time to reflect on the difficulty of this exercise and the amount of energy it takes to keep the mind focused.

3. Now they are asked to notice if "stone Buddhas" come to mind at a greater rate than prior to thought suppression. This is called the *rebound effect* and is also noted in a number of research studies (e.g., Abramowitz et al., 2001; Magee et al., 2012 Sayers & Sayette, 2013). Studies show that the use of suppression results in traumatic memories surfacing more often and more vigorously than prior to suppression. This is a good way to teach clients that, although they are trying to suppress traumatic memories, the use of suppression often makes it more difficult to manage trauma memory intrusions when they surface, and that suppression is simply not an effective method of managing historical trauma.

4. Explain this phenomenon to the individual so they understand the importance of reflection and resolution, as opposed to the tendency to want to suppress our negative thoughts, feelings, memories, or fears.

This is an extremely useful approach for preparing the individual for trauma review and reducing treatment resistance as the individual begins to recognize that they are continually thinking about the feared event because suppression does not work efficiently and is likely the reason for ongoing feeling of distress. This exercise is also a practical clarification as to why thought-stopping is frequently unsatisfying for individuals seeking relief of trauma-loaded thoughts.

# 4. Behavior

There is a tendency to believe that behaviors are nothing more than the end result of our body and mind working together to accomplish an end. This is seen as a one-way flow of information from inside to outside. However, the truth is that information flows both ways. How clients behave is how they will begin to see and understand themselves. If they act in unsafe ways or perform less-than-useful behaviors to manage their anxiety, they often believe that they are helpless to do anything else. In turn, if they act in ways that are more useful in keeping themselves safe and less anxious, they will come to believe they have the power to change. Many times, clients do not have the skills or experience necessary to create more useful behaviors. This section provides techniques to aid in the creation of new options.

## Rituals (R – CR)

> **Time required:** One session or more.
>
> **Materials required:** Paper and pencil/contract.
>
> **Indications for use:** Use when the primary need is to enhance behavioral coping skills in Phase I: Safety and Stabilization of trauma recovery.
>
> **Counterindications:** Depends on the ritual selected.

Ritualistic methods for safety and stabilization can vary widely. The key is to create a form of practice or ceremony that reinforces the individual's sense of reassurance, safety, or security. One meaningful ritual is to have a "marriage" ceremony with oneself. This ritual effectively strengthens the internal tie by affirming the individual's commitment for personal responsibility and fully empowers the person to act on their own best behalf. If things are not going well or goals have been set, they must look to themselves to move their lives forward in the desired direction. This takes an act of will, but it is much more likely that we will achieve our greatest hopes and dreams if we take full responsibility for these dreams. After all, who else is as fully informed of what we truly wish from life if not ourselves?

### Delivery of Approach

There is printable handout material available for this exercise; see Using the Tools 10. The ceremony is to be orchestrated in the vision of the individual. This can be completed alone or in the company of trusted counselors or friends/family. In one example, the individual chose to complete the ritual alone. Candles were lit, paint and paper were used for creative expression, a colorful silk robe was worn, and meaningful music was played. The individual wrote their wishes for the future and their commitment to themselves. They wrote a self-marriage ceremony in which they made a strong and earnest vow to "care for themselves in a manner that met their inner desires, hopes and dreams." In effect, this ceremony was a joyous occasion of personal commitment to the future and self-support. The individual concluded that if they treated themselves in this manner they would have nothing to feel disappointed about. The exercise led to an awareness that freed them up to count on themselves when needed and choose relationships where they could enjoy honest and healthy relationships.

*Examples:*

Below you will find a list of sample rituals, many of which have been described in trauma practice workshops that we offer nationally and internationally. This list offers very brief descriptions of different rituals that can be undertaken by individuals or groups. The idea is to let one's imagination open up to the possibility of a meaningful expression of self.

- Perform a ceremony alone or with others to celebrate one's earlier life and then a ceremony to celebrate a "rebirth to a new way of living" – one that allows for healthier choices and new opportunities.
- Burn a list of harmful traumatic memories.
- Collect photos of one's earlier life to use as a point of reference for moving forward in life.
- Construct a collage to make a representation of internal experiences.
- Attach objects for healing or names of survivors to helium balloons and symbolically release objects/persons to freedom along with the balloon.
- Prepare a shrine or memory collection of grief to help maintain a connection with a person who has died.
- Write a letter to a person who has died or one whom you have unfinished business with (letters do not need to be sent).
- Conduct services of thanksgiving or reconciliation.
- Maintain a journal.
- Perform positive daily affirmations.
- Videotape survival and resiliency experiences of survivors to share with future survivors.

- Construct hope quilts from squares made by survivors.
- Construct a safety collage filled with reassuring and comforting images.
- Prepare certificates of success with positive comments from others.
- Paint rocks with meaningful symbols and display them in prominent places as reminders of recovery.
- Make a self-care box filled with examples of things to do to feel good; when not feeling well, pick something out of the box.

## USING THE TOOLS 10

### Rituals

Because there are many possible safety and stabilization rituals, we offer you a place to recall and collect or imagine rituals that may be meaningful for you or your clients. Using the space available, describe rituals for which you wish to keep a record for future use.

_____

_____

_____

_____

_____

_____

_____

_____

_____

_____

_____

_____

_____

_____

_____

_____

_____

_____

_____

_____

_____

_____

From: Anna B. Baranowsky & J. Eric Gentry, _Trauma Practice: A Cognitive Behavioral Somatic Therapy_ (4th ed.). © 2023 Hogrefe Publishing

**USING THE TOOLS 10:**
Rituals

## Contract for Safety and Self-Care (R – CR)

**Time required:** One session or more.

**Materials required:** Paper/contract and pencil.

**Indications for use:** Use when the primary need is to enhance behavioral coping skills in the Safety and Stabilization stage of trauma recovery.

**Counterindications:** None.

### Delivery of Approach

There is printable handout material available for this exercise; see Using the Tools 11. Another approach is to make a concrete commitment or contract in writing to move toward healing. An example of this follows.

---

## USING THE TOOLS 11

**Contract for Safety and Self-Care**

Name: _____ Date: _____

Safety Goal Area: _____ (My goal)

I care about myself and am committed to my healing. I realize that to be well I have to make changes in my life and the way I live it. By making these changes, no matter how small, I am affirming my choice to become the person I want to be.

I want (to):

_____

_____

(My goal)

I will prove to myself that I am committed to becoming my best self by completing the following behavioral objectives (tiny achievable steps):

Self-Care:

_____

_____

Connection with Others:

_____

_____

Self-Soothing Skills Acquisition:

_____

_____

I will complete these affirmations of myself on or before: _____

Signature: _____ Date: _____

Witness: _____ Date: _____

**USING THE TOOLS 11:**
Contract for Safety and Self-Care

# Safety Net Plan (R – CR)

**Time required:** One session.

**Materials required:** Paper and pencil.

**Indications for use:** Use when the primary need is to enhance behavioral coping skills in the Safety and Stabilization stage of trauma recovery.

**Counterindications:** None.

## Delivery of Approach

There is printable handout material available for this exercise; see Using the Tools 12. A safety net plan is a personalized master plan of what you can do when you feel overwhelmed, out of control, helpless, and/or at a loss as to what you need to do to find your own safety again. Remember, it is always better to plan ahead than to have to act without a plan in a crisis.

---

## USING THE TOOLS 12

### Safety Net Plan

This document is to help you be better prepared for difficult times when they arise throughout the course of your treatment. It will help you become more self-sufficient and resilient to the daily stressors of being a survivor.

### Self-Help Capacities

You have managed many difficult situations in the past successfully and used different abilities and techniques to do so. Let us inventory some of these abilities and self-soothing techniques (activities that help you calm down) so that you can refer back to them when necessary. Remember, you might want to use one technique after the other until you find one that works.

Self-soothing techniques (e.g., talking positively with your self, taking a bath, writing, reading):

1. _____

2. _____

3. _____

Abilities used in the past to manage difficult situations: (e.g., creativity, accepting help, courage, tenacity):

1. _____

2. _____

3. _____

### Informal Support

Below, list names of friends and family members you feel free to contact when you need help. Establish that your supporters are willing to help (for your own assurance) and tell them how they can best assist you when you are in a crisis. They will not know what you do and do not need unless you tell them. Please make a check mark next to their name after you have talked with them about their willingness to help. Different people have different strengths and might be better at helping in one situation than in another.

Remember, it is the quality – not the quantity – of your supporters that counts.

| | Supporter's name | Phone numbers | Supporter's helping strengths |
|---|---|---|---|
| 1. | | | |
| 2. | | | |
| 3. | | | |

From: Anna B. Baranowsky & J. Eric Gentry, *Trauma Practice: A Cognitive Behavioral Somatic Therapy* (4th ed.). © 2023 Hogrefe Publishing

**USING THE TOOLS 12:**
Safety Net Plan

# 5. Emotion/Relation

One of the most damaging long-term effects of trauma is the way it constricts the survivor's ability to feel a full range of emotions and connect to other people. This is true whether the trauma is inflicted by another person, or experienced as an accident, or an act of nature. Fear and anxiety create such a high state of arousal that emotions are shut down. This occurs because the areas in the brain responsible for emotions are directly linked to the survival routines. If the trauma is abuse, the violation of trust makes it difficult to connect to others for fear of being harmed. Traumatic experiences can lead to intrusive fear that is overwhelming. This often results in constriction of emotion, feelings of powerlessness, and eventual withdrawal, and makes it difficult to connect to others. Learning to feel and learning to connect with others are powerful healing agents that mitigate the effects of trauma. This is a process that requires all the skills of self-soothing because the overwhelming feelings happen so quickly. This section provides techniques useful to that end.

## Transitional Objects (R)

> **Time required:** Minimal.
>
> **Materials required:** Varies.
>
> **Indications for use:** Use when the primary need is to enhance emotional coping skills in Phase I: Safety and Stabilization of trauma recovery.
>
> **Counterindications:** None.

Transitional objects are representations of supportive persons, places, things, or memories. These may take the form of soothing objects, such as a blanket that reminds the individual of safe moments in a loving care-provider's arms, a stuffed toy given by a cherished friend, or a pebble picked up at a beach while enjoying much-needed rest and relaxation.

### Delivery of Approach

A transitional object can be anything. The key is what it represents for the individual and whether they can use the object to anchor safety, security, comfort, and relaxation for themselves. One object may suffice or several may be selected collectively or individually to create a sense of grounded comfort for the individual. Objects can be identified through a visualization exercise similar to the safe place visualization exercise described earlier or simply through self-awareness by asking, "Is there something, some object that represents comfort to you?" If the individual is not able to identify anything, it may be planted through the safe place visualization by adding a suggestion of finding an object that represents safety, security, and comfort during the imaging process. In this way, the individual is able to identify an object that they can invest with meaning.

## Support Systems (R – CR)

> **Time required:** 30 minutes.
>
> **Materials required:** Paper and pencil.
>
> **Indications for use:** Use when the primary need is to enhance emotional coping skills in Phase I: Safety and Stabilization of trauma recovery.
>
> **Counterindications:** Actively dissociating or dissociates during exercise.

Research indicates that social support is a buffer against the struggles of everyday life. It becomes even more important when we face tough times and trauma. The following exercise is an imagery exercise to assist individuals in identifying social supports that can create the basis of this powerful buffer. In the following exercise, we encourage individuals to find their own "committee of comfort and support."

### Delivery of Approach

*Committee of Comfort and Support , aka "Circle of Support"*

There is printable handout material available for this exercise; see Using the Tools 13. *Invite* the client to find a comfortable position, begin to relax, close their eyes, and focus inwardly. Ask the client to imagine the safe place and safe object they visited and identified in earlier safety exercises (if they have done so - otherwise return to the safe place exercises to accomplish this first). Encourage them to recall and describe the safety object and use it to guide them right back to their safe place. Ask them to see all that they would see in their safe place, hear what they would hear, smell what they would smell, and sense or feel what they would sense or feel in their place of safety.

*Remind* your client to reclaim the feelings of safety, comfort, and reassurance associated with their safety object and place in whatever way is meaningful to them.

*Instruct* the client at this time to, "Begin to call in toward you all the people in your life who you feel would be good members of a 'Committee of Comfort and Support.' These people could be present and involved in your life right now, or helpful in the past but no longer in your life at this time for any reason. They might be imagined or ideal persons, or those who you knew and are no longer alive. These would be people who would not judge you, and who you feel completely safe with and supported by. Call them in one by one, becoming very aware of who they are, what they look like, and their names."

*Encourage* the individual to make the members of their team as concrete as possible. Remind them that, "These are the figures who you can call on when you are needing support in your everyday life … you can draw on these members for wisdom, emotional support, play time, etc. Review the members of your team and ask any members you no longer feel completely supported by and safe with

to leave. Watch as they leave the circle, urged only by a polite but firm statement that it is time for them to leave now. Once again, invite any new members in to take the places of those you have asked to leave."

*Ask* your client to lift one finger to let you know when their committee is formed.

*Now* have the individual focus inwardly again. Suggest that they imagine a member of their committee moving toward them and sharing words of support and genuine care with them. Encourage the individual to focus on establishing a positive and nourishing internal dialog.

*Inform* the client that you will be silent for 1 minute of clock time while they have this positive internal dialog.

*When* the minute is over, ask them to slowly bring their attention back into the room and open their eyes when they are ready.

*Provide* a sheet for the client to write on and instruct them to, "Write out all the names of the committee members on this sheet."

*Process* the experience. Ask the client, "What effect did this exercise have on you?"

**WITH AUDIO:** Please listen to this a guided demonstration of this exercise facilitated by Dr Baranowsky (Baranowsky & Gentry, 2015, August 23), which can be found in Video 15 in the supplementary material (also available at https://youtu.be/CcbJz4CZTbM).

## USING THE TOOLS 13

### Safe Place Imagery: My Committee of Comfort and Support

This exercise is designed to help you "fire" the "negativity committee" that creates the nonstop chatter, criticism, and self-depreciation in your mind. This exercise will help you to replace this negativity with support, comfort, and affirmation.

Write out the names of all the people from your life who have contributed to your health or esteem, and/or who you have admired. These can be real people with whom you have had relationships in the past. They can be important people from your life with whom you are no longer in contact. They can be people from public life, historical or present, that have contributed to your worth. They can be religious leaders or icons. They can be imaginary or real. There is no limit to who or how many people can comprise your committee of comfort and support. Please list your committee members on the sheet below.

Remember it is the quality – not the quantity – of persons you list that counts.

**My Committee**

| | |
|---|---|
| 1. | 11. |
| 2. | 12. |
| 3. | 13. |
| 4. | 14. |
| 5. | 15. |
| 6. | 16. |
| 7. | 17. |
| 8. | 18. |
| 9. | 19. |
| 10. | 20. |

From: Anna B. Baranowsky & J. Eric Gentry, *Trauma Practice: A Cognitive Behavioral Somatic Therapy* (4th ed.). © 2023 Hogrefe Publishing

**USING THE TOOLS 13:**
Safe Place Imagery:
My Committee of Comfort and
Support

# Drawing Icon and Envelope (Emotional Containment) (R – RE – CR)

> **Time required:** 10–30 minutes.
>
> **Materials required:** Papers, colored markers, envelope, and stapler.
>
> **Indications for use:** Use when the primary need is to enhance emotional coping skills in Phase I: Safety and Stabilization of trauma recovery.
>
> **Counterindications:** Actively dissociating or dissociates during exercise.

The capacity to contain posttraumatic images, feelings, and thoughts is a crucial skill that must be developed with a client before they can truly confront and resolve a traumatic memory from a perspective of choice. If a client is unable to set aside incomplete therapeutic work on their traumatic memories and successfully reenter normal life and its demands, then the client runs a high risk of becoming retraumatized by the work of therapy. With this in mind, it is important that the trauma therapist develop, with their clients, some effective strategies for containing these incomplete or fragmented memories, thoughts, and feelings relative to traumatic experiences.

We have found an art therapy technique to be very helpful in developing this capacity for containment. We utilize this technique often when the time of a session has nearly elapsed and the client is still deeply engrossed in the traumatic material. This method allows the client to package these difficult images, feelings, and thoughts for work in a later session.

**Home Use:** Instructing the client in the use of this method can be very helpful for the individual who is experiencing frequent disruptive flashbacks in their day-to-day life. Ask them to briefly draw an icon (less than 5 minutes) of the memory, flashback, or painful images and then put it inside an envelope and address it to their therapist's office. They should also be instructed to mail this letter as soon as possible after completing the drawing. The client should be informed that the drawing will be kept safely in their file and the therapist will address these drawings with the client at their next meeting. They will become part of the trauma treatment plan.

## Delivery of Approach

1. Using colored pencils/markers, ask the client to draw a *symbol* that represents the memory, along with its feelings, images, and thoughts. This should be only an abstract symbol, and not a drawing of the event(s). No more than 5 minutes should be allowed for this drawing.
2. When the client has completed the drawing, ask them to place it inside a manila envelope and seal the envelope.
3. Hand the client a stapler and instruct them to put as many staples in the envelope as necessary to contain this material for a time, so that it can be addressed in the future. Allow them as many staples as they wish.
4. Ask them to write the title of this memory/material on the outside of the envelope.
5. Tell the client that you will keep this envelope, along with all its negative thoughts and feelings, secure inside their case file. It will remain safely contained there until the client is ready to work again toward the resolution of this memory.
6. Inform the client that if they think of the memory in the future, they need not return to the helpless and overwhelming feelings present during the traumatic event. Instead, they can recall that this memory is safe in their therapist's office.
7. Encourage the client to utilize grounding/self-soothing strategies to regain full control before leaving the office (asking the client to count backwards from 100 by 7s is an excellent exercise to help engage neocortical functioning and reorient to the present).

# Internal Vault (Emotional Containment) (R – RE – CR)

**Time required:** 5–10 minutes.

**Materials required:** None.

**Indications for use:** Use when the primary need is to enhance emotional coping skills in Phase I: Safety and Stabilization of trauma recovery.

**Counterindications:** Actively dissociating or dissociates during exercise.

### Delivery of Approach

This technique, drawn from hypnotherapy, can be utilized in a variety of contexts. Simply, it assists the client in developing an "internal vault" into which they can place uncomfortable memories, feelings, thoughts, and other negative artifacts of trauma. This technique works well with clients who have the capacity for dissociation. One elegant strategy that includes this technique is to assist the client with visualizing a "steel vault that has a locked door" when doing the safe place visualization exercise. This allows the client to store these negative experiences temporarily between sessions and allows them to attend to the demands of their daily life without becoming overwhelmed by the traumatic memories.

Another variation of this exercise can involve creating a physical artistic representation of some of these overwhelming memories, thoughts, or feelings through pictures, colours, and/or words, and physically stapling that paper shut to be stored away in a vault, both internally and externally, so that it can be accessed at a later time when the client is ready to face them.

**WITH VIDEO:** Please watch a guided video demonstration of this exercise facilitated by Dr Baranowsky (2015, July 15), which can be found in Video 16 in the supplementary material (p. 226, or at https://youtu.be/du5MaQk-w3M).

# Positive Hope Box (R – RE – CR)

**Time required:** 5 minutes.

**Materials required:** Paper and pencil, small box.

**Indications for use:** Use when the primary need is to enhance emotional coping skills in Phase I: Safety and Stabilization of trauma recovery.

**Counterindications:** None.

### Delivery of Approach

Most of us have heard people tell of having cigar boxes into which they put their written hopes, dreams, fears, etc., and then pray for a higher power or God to "take care of it" for them. Being careful to remain sensitive to each individual's spirituality, we have utilized a variation of this technique. We ask trauma survivors to decorate a box (cigar boxes work well) with drawings and clippings from magazines that depict images of healing. With this done, we ask them to draw pictures or write words that represent all the overwhelming aspects of their trauma memories and their current life and then put these representations into the box. If they are spiritual, we suggest that they allow their higher power to intervene on their behalf in these areas. If this is not appropriate for the client, we ask them to pick one or two of these areas to bring each week to work on in therapy and to build a ritual that indicates completion (for the individual) when one of these areas has been successfully resolved.

**WITH VIDEO:** Please watch a guided video demonstration of this exercise facilitated by Dr Baranowsky (2015, July 8), which can be found in Video 17 in the supplementary material (or at https://youtu.be/1zbudRJ5muU).

## Make Peace with Your Sleep (R – CR)

> **Time required:** 5 to 25 minutes depending on protocol used below.
>
> **Materials required:** Pen or pencil, timer, and the form we have provided on the following pages.
>
> **Indications for use:** Use when the primary need is to improve sleep quality, re-build good sleep hygiene habits after trauma, or reduce impact/likelihood of trauma induced nightmares.
>
> **Counterindications:** Always reflect on your inner state and notice if you need a break from the exercise to find your inner calm.

Research indicates that trauma has been increasingly identified as a potential precursor to clinical insomnia (Sinha, 2016). Sleep quality disruption is one of many ways that trauma can have a significant and prolonged impact on health and well-being, and this is largely because of the ways in which trauma can sensitize the central nervous system to become more hyper-aroused. However, there are ways to mitigate this, improve sleep quality, and regulate the body's sleeping patterns again after trauma.

An excellent article by Havens et al. (2019) outlines this research and has informed some of the exercise guidelines below. This exercise is intended to help remove barriers that may be disrupting restorative sleep after trauma.

### Delivery of Approach

**WITHOUT AUDIO:** The exercise in Using the Tools 14 provides basic steps for sleep hygiene as well as exercises to assist the client in remaining calm when not able to sleep.

**WITH AUDIO:** Please watch the video demonstration in Video 18 in the supplementary material (see p. 227, or Baranowsky, 2015a, September 9, https://youtu.be/ 5HjzyLMsygM), or listen to a more in-depth guided audio facilitation in Video 19 (or Baranowsky, 2015b, September 9, https://youtu.be/n9BRRCdj0s4).

## USING THE TOOLS 14

### Make Peace With Your Sleep

1. **Sleep hygiene basics steps checklist**

   ☐ Remove television/laptop/smartphones/tablets from the bedroom – no bright screen 1 hour prior to sleep

   ☐ Regulate your sleep/wake schedule – this will be difficult to start – same time to sleep and same time to wake daily

   ☐ No caffeine after 1 pm

   ☐ No heavy meals 3 hours before bedtime

   ☐ Exercise daily

   ☐ If something is bothering you, write out your thoughts during the day well-before you go to bed

   ☐ Ensure the bedroom is dark, quiet, and comfortable

   ☐ A cool room is easier to sleep in

2. **Cannot fall asleep, stay asleep or get back to sleep**

   ☐ If you waken and cannot fall asleep, work on deep breathing or relaxation exercises (Watch sleep exercise "Improve sleep, relax deeply and embed positive messages" in Video 20 in the supplementary material or Baranowsky, 2015, April 12, https://youtu.be/ZQmfCEtzvEE)

   ☐ If after 15–20 minutes of this you cannot fall asleep, get out of bed and do some rewriting the ending exercises (see outline below) for dreams or for anxious worries or fear

   ☐ Then go back to bed for more deep breathing and relaxation

3. **Having nightmares**

   ☐ Write out the dream content/or anxious feelings and rewrite the ending to a positive outcome ... then try to return to sleep. (Haven et al., 2019)

   ☐ Work on any of the deep breathing / relaxation exercises that you have found to be helpful in the daily practice/or the video exercise links found for stabilization throughout this book.

   ☐ If you can focus on your breathing and remind yourself that you are safe and able to harness calm, it will help the body/mind find some rest even if you are unable to sleep

4. **Practice Whenever needed**

   ☐ Keep a copy of the sleep practice by your bed as a reminder

   ☐ Practice whenever you need to recapture feelings of comfort or calm

From: Anna B. Baranowsky & J. Eric Gentry, *Trauma Practice: A Cognitive Behavioral Somatic Therapy* (4th ed.). © 2023 Hogrefe Publishing

**USING THE TOOLS 14:**
Make Peace With Your Sleep

# Relaxed Breathing Guided Meditation (R)

| | |
|---|---|
| **Time required:** 5 minutes. |
| **Materials required:** None. |
| **Indications for use:** Use when the primary need is to enhance physical coping skills in Phase I: Safety and Stabilization of trauma recovery. |
| **Counterindications:** Deficits related to the respiratory system or nasal airway. |

Relaxed breathing is a helpful breathing exercise that is designed to help settle the nervous system and find a sense of calm in the storm that is trauma recovery.

## Delivery of Approach

 **WITHOUT AUDIO:** Below is a script that can be utilized to facilitate the Relaxed Breathing Guided Meditation exercise:

> ### Script: Relaxed Breathing Guided Meditation
>
> Find a quiet and comfortable place where you can sit or lie down without being disturbed. Allow yourself to focus attention within, letting go of anything related to the past or future.
>
> Notice how the breath moves in and out of the body without changing anything. Allow the breath to slow down. Inhale, allowing the breath to be nourishing to the body. Release, letting go of tension and tightness in the body.
>
> Notice your inside world. Allow yourself to feel whatever you feel inside your body, without any judgement.
>
> Inhale, allowing the breath to move slowly and smoothly into the belly. Exhale, letting the breath fully release. Enjoy the release.
>
> Pay attention to the sensation of breath. Bear witness to the sensation of the breath, moving in and out of the body without any struggle. Focus on the simple sensation of the breath entering and leaving the body. Let any thoughts you might have come and go. Gently concentrate in a relaxed manner with minimal effort.
>
> Notice that the mind can slow down and settle. Feel yourself release tension and stress in the body. Allow yourself to release more and more with every exhalation.
>
> Allow the body and mind to relax, as the breath slows down. Let yourself notice, how focusing on relaxation can lay a foundation of calm. Recognize that you are increasing your self-awareness, as well as the wisdom of your body.

**WITH AUDIO:** Please watch a guided facilitation of this exercise as part of the Trauma Recovery Online Program in Video 21 in the supplementary material (p. 227, or Baranowsky, 2015, September 24, https://youtu.be/XxoLhLvdscw).

# Phase II:
# Working Through Trauma

*In the words of Ingrid Collins, a British consulting psychologist,*
*When you give patients time and attention, they can relax into healing."*

Carl Honore, *In Praise of Slow* (2004)

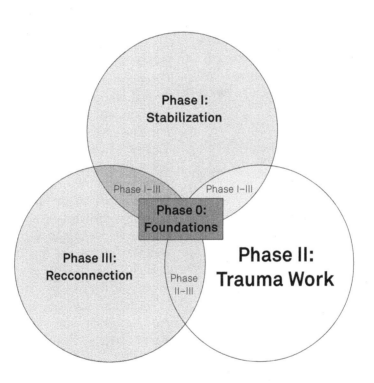

### Summary

In this section, we cover *Working Through Trauma*, moving into the core of the trauma practice work that allows the client to process and work through unresolved traumatic memories. As mentioned previously, we believe there are three active and necessary ingredients for the effective treatment of trauma. These include relaxation, exposure (reciprocal inhibition), and cognitive restructuring. From the physiological perspective, this can be understood as facilitating the natural process of the neocortex without triggering the survival routines that shut down processing and might potentially result in retraumatization. In each of the techniques that follow, notice how this could be happening. In addition, each exercise utilizes one or more of the ingredients (i.e., relaxation, exposure, or cognitive restructuring).

Much of the work in this section can be linked back to the Trigger List developed in Phase I: *Safety and Stabilization*. Progress can also be checked by reflecting on changes in the trigger list SUDS ratings (see Using the Tools 1). It is not unusual to see a SUDS reduction when one significant trauma memory is resolved. Returning to the Trigger List gives us a map to review progress over time. Remember, now that you are moving into Phase II: *Working Through Trauma* of this work you will need to ensure that your client is emotionally, physiologically, and cognitively prepared to move forward into this phase. It is important that the transition from Phase I to Phase II is managed with caution to ensure readiness in the individual to face trauma history. These steps have been outlined in the first edition of *Trauma Practice* (Gentry & Schmidt, 1999; Baranowsky, Gentry & Schultz, 2005) and are discussed as part of the four active ingredients in this book (see section The Four Active Ingredients in Phase 0).

Start by reviewing the five essential criteria required to signal client readiness to move to Phase II: *Working Through Trauma*:
1. Resolve danger
2. Distinguish "am safe" vs. "feel safe"
3. Develop self-soothe and self-rescue skills
4. Practice-demo self-rescue
5. Negotiate contract and informed consent

# 1.  Somatic

The physiological key to successful recovery is relaxation. The goal is to have the event fully processed by the neocortex. As anxiety levels go up, processing goes down due to the mechanisms previously discussed. Teaching clients to be aware of their own anxiety levels and providing them with tools to titrate and lower their anxiety will facilitate this process. The techniques discussed in this section will provide a variety of methods to accomplish that task.

## Titration Part II: Braking and Acceleration (RE)

Braking and acceleration is a necessary skill when conducting trauma work. This enables the client to begin their work with the knowledge that they can stop whenever needed. In Titration Part I: Braking and Acceleration we began to look at initial skills through the lens of *safety and stabilization*. Now we begin to look at useful methods that can be implemented during the core of traumatic memory processing. In this way, clients can begin their processing with the assurance that they can always put the brakes on. They can maintain some control over their experience and decide how fast or slow they will progress.

In braking and acceleration, the central requirement is lowering the volume on feelings of distress. Any activity that achieves this can likely be modified to assist clients. This may include humor, breathing, talking about a favorite activity or person, imagining safety, or holding a transitional object, among other activities. Some of these methods have already been covered in this text and some new ones will be added in the subsequent sections.

After trauma processing begins, we need to have a series of approaches to suggest when things get too hot. Sometimes nothing seems to work and we must drop all techniques and simply provide a safe and reassuring holding environment for the client's grief and discomfort. Alternatively, we might suggest an imagined barrier between the person and their traumatic memories or cycle through any or all of the approaches we have utilized successfully in the past.

The following three exercises are braking and acceleration tools that have been used successfully for many years. Other excellent suggestions can be found in Rothschild (2000) and van der Kolk (2015).

## Layering (RE – CR)
(Baranowsky, 1997)

**Time required:** One or more sessions.

**Materials required:** Paper and pencil for therapist.

**Indications for use:** Use when the primary need is to enhance physical, cognitive, and emotional coping skills in Phase II: Working Through Trauma of trauma recovery.

**Counterindications:** Actively dissociating or dissociates during exercise; respiratory ailments.

This approach draws on techniques that the client will have already begun to utilize through the earlier stages of trauma therapy. Deep breathing is a central component to this approach. The client needs to be familiar with and competent in the use of a deep breathing method prior to utilizing layering. It is possible to teach deep breathing in the same session prior to introducing the layering approach. The individual is informed of the entire procedure prior to commencing. This exercise can be used when a client arrives for sessions with a heightened sense of distress over a recent or current event that is related to, but not necessarily a direct memory of, the traumatic event. Over time, after clients become skilled at layering, they can use this approach on their own as a mastery technique for managing feelings of distress. A layering – charting form is also included for the clinician's use.

*Note:* For clients who are unable to utilize deep breathing, this can be substituted with Comfort in One Part exercise, especially when using the exercise of focusing on Comfort on Palms of Your Hands described in that exercise.

### Delivery of Approach

There is printable handout material available for this exercise; see Using the Tools 15. This exercise is begun with the Ericksonian approach commonly referred to as the YES SET (I. Bilash, personal communication with master hypnotherapist, February 19, 1997).

To establish the YES SET, recognize the individual's distress, then state the obvious to achieve consent. A good statement to begin with is, "I see you are feeling upset about X (the identified trauma or concern). I know you want to be able to handle this in the best way possible."

You will generally get consent or a "yes" in response to this statement.

The next statement is, "I would like us to work to together to achieve your goal, is that okay?"

Again, you will likely receive a "yes." Now we move toward a description of the exercise and will again await consent.

You can start your description of layering as follows:

"We have shown you some type of breathing exercise to practice at this point that we hope has been useful. Because it has helped you in the past, we can use this approach to give you a sense of mastery over your own feeling of discomfort related to X. In this exercise, we speak about the disturbing event and then work on the deep breathing. In this way, you will be able to take breaks from telling your story, thus keeping the feelings from overwhelming you while still having the opportunity to speak about what has occurred."

1. Identify the source of discomfort or disturbing memory. Rate it on a 1-to-10 SUDS scale.
2. Remind the client of the deep breathing approach. Have them practice with three to five deep inhalations and exhalations or focus on the Comfort in One Part exercise. Encourage them to follow the directions as described in the deep breathing exercise found in this text.
3. Tell them about layering and how the exercise will progress.
4. Ask them to begin by telling you what has occurred or what keeps their memory disturbing. Request that they keep their expression descriptive but succinct as possible to begin with. Tell them that you may interrupt them when you notice their breathing beginning to change.
5. As they begin describing the event, keep an eye on their breathing. Ask them to stop their description when you recognize a noteworthy change in their breathing (it will become shallow and rapid or labored).
6. Now have them focus inwardly and begin five deep inhalations and exhalations in the prescribed manner. After the fifth exhalation, have the individual focus outwardly again. Take a SUDS rating based on how they feel now. If the SUDS is higher than 5, ask them to take five more deep breaths; if it is 5 or lower, ask them to tell you more about the event that is causing them discomfort.
7. Follow Steps 4 through 6 until the SUDS rating has been consistently reduced to below 5 while the client describes the entire event.

**WITH AUDIO:** Please listen to this a guided demonstration of this exercise facilitated by Dr Baranowsky (2014b, August 25), which can be found in Video 22 in the supplementary material (p. 227, or at https://youtu.be/qWCLQbF6A50).

---

**USING THE TOOLS 15**

Layering (Baranowsky, 1997)

A Mastery Approach to Disturbing Physical and Emotional Sensations

| Target Event | SUDS |
|---|---|
| | |
| **Emotional Reaction** | |
| | |
| **Thought** – What is it that makes this event so upsetting? | |
| | |
| **Outcome** – What happened? | |
| | |
| **DEEP BREATHING** (5 times) (or Comfort in One Part) | |
| **Target Event** (Further description) | |
| | |
| **DEEP BREATHING** (5 times) | |
| **Cognition** (What thoughts go along with this experience?) | |
| | |
| **DEEP BREATHING** (5 times) | |
| **Emotion** (What feelings do you have about this event?) | |
| | |
| **DEEP BREATHING** (5 times) | |
| **Body Sensation** (What feelings of discomfort do you have in your body?) | |
| | |
| **DEEP BREATHING** (5 times) | |
| **Emotion** (What feelings do you have about this event?) | |
| | |
| **DEEP BREATHING** (5 times) | |
| **Emotion** (What feelings do you have about this event?) | |

**Alternatives** (Refer to Comfort in One Part or Positive Self-Talk/Thought Replacement exercises in this book.) Continue with this process until SUDS rating is below 5 for the identified event prior to ending the exercise. If this is not achieved, then end with a safety and stabilization grounding exercise for closure.

**USING THE TOOLS 15:**
Layering (Baranowsky, 1997)

## Comfort in One Part (RE)

**Time required:** 10 minutes.

**Materials required:** None.

**Indications for use:** Use when the primary need is to enhance physical coping skills in Phase II: Working Through Trauma of trauma recovery.

**Counterindications:** None.

This exercise assists the individual in using bodily-felt sensations to retrain the body to a new state of comfort or relaxation. After they have achieved this state, they will be able to retain calmness, even if it is in only one small part, while facing difficult memories. In this way, they will be able to reassure and soothe themselves through the maintenance of comfort in one part while bravely forging ahead in the resolution of past experiences.

## Delivery of Approach

This approach was initially introduced in Erickson's work (Erickson & Rossi, 1989) and later revisited by Dolan (1991, p. 26). The individual is taught to deeply and completely relax one part of their body (this can be a part of their choosing). First, general relaxation can be achieved through inductions described earlier in this text (Anchoring, Deep Breathing, or Safe Place Imagery). After the individual is deeply relaxed, they are instructed to select a part of their body that is prepared to completely release all tension and relax. They are encouraged to let this part feel a complete sense of ease, calmness, and a soft and deep contentment. Allow them time to fully feel that sense of comfort and to let it soak into that body part. After they give you a cue (lifted finger) that they have fully enjoyed this experience, ask them to return their attention slowly to the room in which they are seated.

The client is now prepared to retain comfort in one part while agreeing to proceed with traumatic memory processing. During the processing or telling of the story, they are instructed to monitor the body part that retains comfort. The body part becoming aroused out of comfort is the signal to take a break and find comfort again.

*Comfort on the Palms of the Hands.* A good approach to begin with is to have the individual focus on the center of the palms of their hands. Instruct the client to imagine warm sun beaming into the center of the palms of their upturned hands. Encourage sensory feelings of warmth and relaxation soothing and smoothing out the sensation of release in the center of the palms of the hands. Allow the individual to imagine the warmth spreading and easing any discomforts they may have.

Please view a guided audio recording (Baranowsky, 2014a, August 25) of this exercise available in the supplementary material, Video 23 (p. 227, or at https://youtu.be/_g1gUcjY28I).

## Timed Reflection (R – RE – CR)

> **Time required:** 15–30 minutes.
>
> **Materials required:** Template.
>
> **Indications for use:** Use when the primary need is to enhance ability to tolerate strong emotions and sensations that have been triggered difficult interactions, triggers, or circumstances.
>
> **Counterindications:** Inability to engage relaxation or harness calm.

Containing emotion is at times less effective then learning how to show up for oneself in a soft and meaningful way. I like to think about being very friendly and accepting with emotions as a starting point for this exercise. In allowing for a deep sense of acceptance with whatever surfaces we create a holding place that allows for space and integration of one's own internal truth, whether that is anger, hurt, sorrow, or sadness. In contrast, resistance creates a battle ground and restriction that increases tension and discomfort. Emotional acceptance can be the starting point of understanding and may result in creating a new relationship with oneself, where emotions can be guides to personal truth and growth. Timed reflection can lead to increased ability to self-soothe combined with the capacity to lean into the places of personal suffering with empathy. This perspective can assist in lowering the internal negative dialog while witnessing the truth of one's own history, fears, and struggles. Being gentle with oneself while witnessing the internal experience can change old internal patterns/negative beliefs and reactions, and the dynamic of feeling unsupported, unheard, and unloved. There is nothing as powerful as being compassionate with oneself and this is a great exercise for growing this skill.

This expressive strategy should only be used when (a) the client is adept at self-soothing strategies in order to ground and contain this energy or (b) the client has articulated the desire to work with the expression of this negative effect.

The goal of this work is to develop a safe, controlled expression and resolution of negative feelings and not to trigger a full-blown abreaction. This exercise should begin and end with the client applying Phase I stabilization strategies as needed.

The main outcome is a deepening capacity to attend to one's emotional inner world. After all, emotions are our own inner wisdom system and need to be treated like a gift, if we are truly to grow.

## Delivery of Approach

1. Identify a theme/emotion/struggle that the individual is prepared to sit with or attend to.
2. Take a SUDS level (0–10). Look for SUDS ratings that are at least 6 or higher so you have sufficient content to work with.
3. Provide the client with details of the exercise – including the need to use a timer for 1-minute reflections – to add a writing portion or talking portion. Once there is consent you can begin with timed reflection rounds.

4. The client will need to close their eyes and focus inwardly for the 1-minute reflection. The goal is to pay attention, notice, observe in a nonjudgmental way to whatever surfaces (i.e., sorrow, worry, grief, fear, etc.)

5. Encourage the individual to simply notice and lean in toward the feeling in a friendly and accepting way, just noticing the internal experience.

6. After each timed round of 1-minte, ask what they noticed without any judgment. Encourage continued focus on the internal lived experience (i.e., heaviness in their heart, belly tension, deep core sadness, etc.) Continue to focus on the emotion and body sensation rather than any stories or specific past trauma.

7. Continue with another round of timed reflection once again helping to guide the individual into noticing what is happening deeply within themselves without judgment. Although the individual may notice internal negative talk or stories, it is important to refocus on the inner emotion or body sensation (inner lived experience).

8. As soon as the timer goes off, instruct the individual to open their eyes and either write out what they noticed – or speak about what they noticed. You can try both options and see what suits your client best. If they write, ask them to read what they wrote or for permission to read it out loud for them.

9. Whatever content surfaced simply refocus again on another round of timed reflection, following the instructions above.

10. The primary goal of this exercise is to provide a safe and stable environment with guardrails (one minute maximum) and witnessing (within the therapeutic relationship) of the inner content. With this structure the hopeful outcome is that an increased personal tolerance will develop over time – allowing for greater self-acceptance of the internal messaging and less self-judgment.

11. At the end of a series of 8–10 rounds, stop the client. Take a SUDS level. Ask the client to discuss with you what has happened and describe that experience.

12. Continue as needed

## Timeline Approach (RE – CR)

(Gentry, personal communication, 2002)

> **Time required:** 20–30 minutes.
>
> **Materials required:** Paper and pencil.
>
> **Indications for use:** Use when the primary need is to enhance physical, cognitive, and emotional coping skills in Phase II: Working Through Trauma of trauma recovery.
>
> **Counterindications:** Actively dissociating or dissociates during exercise.

What follows is an approach that incorporates much that is useful in the techniques of braking and acceleration, self-soothing, systematic desensitization, looped tape scripting, cognitive restructuring, and reciprocal inhibition. Recall from a cognitive-behavioral perspective that reciprocal inhibition (relaxation with exposure to memories of a traumatic event) and cognitive restructuring helps mitigate the negative sequelae of traumatic stress. While there are a number of available techniques with more or less research to support them to address posttraumatic stress difficulties, the manner in which you accomplish reciprocal inhibition and cognitive restructuring is limited only by your creativity.

### Delivery of Approach

This approach is grounded in the notion of reciprocal inhibition and cognitive restructuring with a self-controlled start/stop element. It may be done in a group setting or in individual therapy. This technique is, of course, done after safety and stabilization has been successfully attained and the client has adequate skills for self-soothing, including the ability to relax using exercises, self-talk, breathing, etc. In this exercise, the therapist will act as a witness and monitor the distress level of the client. In a group setting, a partner can fill this role.

*Step 1*

1. Identify the specific traumatic event to be processed.

2. Have the client take an A4 sheet of paper, turn it the long way and draw a timeline in the middle like the following:

[_____]
Beginning                                          End

3. Have the client relax completely and ask them to view the event from a distance. Without actually fully entering the memory, have them start at the beginning of the event and separate it into time segments. This is similar to the Trigger List exercise earlier. They may separate it into as many segments as needed.

4. Then have them draw a line up from the timeline on their paper to indicate each segment in the order it occurs and label it with a word to help remind them of which segment it is.
5. Have them make the height of each line reflect SUDS level (from 1 to 10) associated with the segment.

Now have them relax. They have just created a symbolic representation of the traumatic event. They may begin to process this at anytime they have relaxed and their SUDS level is at 0 or 1, or they may wish to leave it and come back later. When they choose to begin, proceed as follows:

*Step 2*

1. Starting at the beginning, have them narrate the events of the first segment of the timeline.
2. Monitor their SUDS level. If it begins to rise too quickly and the client feels overwhelmed, they may wish to break that segment into smaller segments. If SUDS levels rise and the client does not feel overwhelmed, have them continue to narrate that segment and that segment only.
3. Stop at the end of the segment.

4. Have the person begin a self-soothe exercise. As they relax, ask them to discuss whatever comes to mind with you.
5. When their SUDS level has reached 0 or 1, they may choose to continue, or may choose to wait. If they choose to wait, they may leave the representation of the event with you, and you will explain to them that you are capable of keeping it until they are ready to finish. They do not have to take the event home with them. If they choose to proceed, repeat Steps 1 through 5 of the second set of steps for the next segment on the timeline.

By the time they have finished, they will have worked their way completely through a traumatic memory, creating a narrative of the event that includes insights gained from the process. And they have done so without being overwhelmed by emotion. To further facilitate the processing of the event, it would be helpful for you to then retell the story back to them as accurately as possible. The client should continuously practice self-soothing exercises while this is being done. In a group setting this can be accomplished by having it read to the group by their partner.

## Biofeedback (R – RE – CR)

**Time required:** Varies.

**Materials required:** Varies.

**Indications for use:** Use when the primary need is to enhance physical coping skills in Phase II: Working Through Trauma of trauma recovery.

**Counterindications:** Actively dissociating or dissociates during exercise.

### Delivery of Approach

Biofeedback is simply any technique that provides the client with regular and ongoing feedback on one or more of their physiological responses to imaginal and/or *in vivo* stimuli. This can be as simple as monitoring (or helping the client to self-monitor) their respiration rate to as sophisticated as watching positron emission tomography (PET) scans. The most common techniques used are computer-aided monitoring of blood pressure, respiration, heart rate, skin temperature, and skin electrical conductivity (electrogalvanic skin response [EGR]). These monitoring techniques are used in conjunction with relaxation

strategies to help the client memorize thoughts and behaviors that produce visible lowering of anxiety responses (e.g., elevation of skin temperature in the hands, lowered heart rate, lowered respiration, lowered EGR). The EmWave® product, available at http://www.heartmath.com, is an excellent example of a biofeedback system that is well researched, easy to operate, and efficient in providing a feedback system for client use. Clinicians can set up the system in the office and train the individual on the system, and then use the biofeedback to monitor change while initiating an exposure exercise. This will enable the client to focus on their trauma memory while monitoring their heart rate and breathing. They can stop trauma exposure to relax, thereby improving the feedback from the system, and then resume the exposure exercise.

This technique has a specific application in trauma treatment by allowing the client to have ongoing awareness of their arousal level while they are accessing and confronting trauma memories. This feedback stimulates the client to activate a relaxation response, therefore invoking reciprocal inhibition while renegotiating and resolving trauma memories.

## Hands Over Heart Space (R – CR)

**Time required:** 5–10 minutes.

**Materials required:** None. Or use of video below.

**Indications for use:** Use when the primary need is to enhance emotional coping skills in the Working through Trauma stage of trauma recovery.

**Counterindications:** The Palms/Hands Over Heart Space exercise is a simple but deep stress release exercise that can help lower stress, anxiety and lighten internal negative self-talk. A client may begin by expressing strong emotions over a current event/ trigger from the past or intrusive trauma memory.

### Delivery of Approach

The following are some cues and instructions that can be used to help guide an individual through the hands over heart space practice. It is best for the practitioner to demonstrate each step prior to beginning the exercise and to explain that they will not need to remember any steps as this will be guided:

Guide the individual to focus their attention on the sensation in the palms of their hands. They will then use two fingers to draw very slow and soft circles around their palm, three times, while feeling the sensations that arise. Then switch and do the same with the other hand.

Then, instruct them to place hand over hand with palms facing each other, and allow them to rest on their lap in a comfortable position for a few moments, allowing themself to feel the sensation and warmth, from the left palm to the right, and vice versa.

Next, they will place hand over hand again, but this time with the top hand facing the back of the other hand rather than the palm, and then place both hands over their heart space, with the palm of the bottom hand facing towards the heart. With eyes closed, ask them to feel the sensations from the palms of your hands transferring to the heart space, softly inhaling and exhaling.

As they do that, and keeping hands over the heart space, the next step is imagining themself being able to take all of their inner awareness and attention and externalize it to the other corner of the room, or a distant corner away from them. Imagining from that distant place, being able to turn themself around and gaze at themself from that distant corner, as they see themselves with hands over heart, resting quietly with their eyes closed.

Then, guide them to inhale and exhale, allowing the individual to remain in an observer position of this resting place, and finally bringing themself back inside of their body, landing fully, hand over hand over heart space, bringing their hands back down to open neutral position on their lap, opening up their eyes, and checking in with how they feel.

Repeat this entire process another three times or more, to help turn down the volume of stress and mental chatter.

**WITH AUDIO:** A guided video demonstration of this exercise facilitated by Dr Baranowsky (2018, July 17) can be found in Video 24 in the supplementary material (see p. 227, or at https://youtu.be/Ah46XMY1YpA).

## Paced Breathing (R – RE – CR)

**Time required:** 10–30 minutes.

**Materials required:** Pen or pencil, paper.

**Indications for use:** This exercise is excellent to use for individuals struggling with a current issue, difficult thoughts that they want to share with others, or upsetting details that they need to practice speaking about, and should be utilized after diaphragmatic breathing and 3-6 breathing.

**Counterindications:** Paced breathing is an exercise that combines some written narrative work for your client about their difficult experience, with a breathing exercise that will help lessen the anxiety or stress response that would usually accompany that story. Through paced breathing, the client can gain a sense of empowerment in their ability to better regulate their nervous system in times in which they are safe, but perhaps don't feel safe when speaking about or re-visiting their past traumatic experience.

Paced breathing is excellent for anyone who is struggling with a current issue, difficult thoughts one wants to share with others, or upsetting details one needs to practice speaking about (i.e., like a client of mine, who managed to testify in court using this exercise, or our other client, who used this approach to enable her to speak at a close friend's funeral).

### Delivery of Approach

1. Have the individual begin by identifying something that they wish to speak about but recognize the difficulty they have in sharing this story or expressing their experience or perspective. In brief, what is it they want to share?
2. What makes it difficult for them to express this?
3. Have them spend 10 minutes (use a timer) to write out the event (or details to share) in as much detail as possible, as if they will be reading it to an audience.
4. After 10 minutes of writing, ask them, "Is there anything else that needs to be said about the event?" If yes, spend another 10 minutes (timed) adding more detail.
5. Continue adding increments of 10 minutes until they have written all that needs to be expressed about the event.
6. Add paced breathing to the exercise. Practicing the 3-6 Breathing exercise creates a good foundation for paced breathing. They can use the 3-6 breathing or follow the next set of instructions below:
   a. Have them take a slow deep inhalation until they can feel the belly, chest, and back body fill with air. Do not over work the inhalation. At the edge of a full deep inhalation, begin to exhale. On the exhalation, have your client read the story that they prepared in Step 3 until the exhalation is complete. Pause for a moment to let the body and mind rest.
   b. Then have them take another full deep breath – not rushing either the inhalation or exhalation, and have them continue the story (while only speaking on the exhalation).
   c. Now work with paced breathing (or 3-6 Breathing) to read through the story out loud. Follow the instructions above.
   d. They can do this repeatedly until they notice a lightening of their mood or an evident lowering of anxiety. If you cannot achieve a lowering of anxious feelings or reduction in emotional upset, then move on to a self-relaxation exercise to settle the participant back down to the state of inner calm for which we are all hardwired.

**WITH AUDIO:** A guided audio version of this exercise can be found in the supplementary material, Video 25 (p. 227, or see Baranowsky, 2014c, August 25, https://youtu.be/VDasBQQxqNE).

# 2. Cognition

The following section describes a number of techniques that address the cognitive coping skills of traumatized individuals. Trauma survivors are likely to present with any number of cognitive distortions about themselves and the world in which they live, created as a way to make sense of their world and to be safe. These distortions often result in significantly problematic behaviors. The recovery of clients from traumatic events includes not only the processing of the events themselves, but also identifying and restructuring the beliefs that have proven to be less than useful in managing their lives. It is also important to remember that trauma, and particularly stress, have a negative impact on one's ability to think, for reasons discussed earlier. Clients who are actively dissociating and/or are clearly experiencing ongoing, unmanaged stress in their lives may have difficulty performing these techniques because they will have difficulty thinking clearly. Stress issues and dissociation should be addressed first to achieve optimum outcome.

## Downward Arrow Technique (RE – CR)

> **Time required:** 5–30 minutes.
>
> **Materials required:** None.
>
> **Indications for use:** Use when the primary need is to enhance cognitive coping skills in Phase II: Working Through Trauma of trauma recovery.
>
> **Counterindications:** Client appears confused, stressed, and/or actively dissociating, or dissociates during exercise.

This approach, initially introduced by Burns (1980), is particularly useful when working with intrusive thoughts that inhibit recovery. The following illustration exhibits how to apply this approach when intrusive negative thoughts overwhelm individuals. In many cases, the greatest source of distress is linked to the notion that one must not have negative or intrusive thoughts, which leaves the individual with an additional internal battle. It is necessary to shift the battle to a challenge of beliefs to lessen the impact of the intrusive material.

### Delivery of Approach

*Example*

Polly is a 36-year-old woman who has negative intrusive thoughts related to an experience of childhood sexual abuse when she was 6 years old.

**Automatic thoughts related to a traumatic or disturbing event:** What happened to me is my fault.

**Challenging statement:** And if that were true, what would it mean? (This statement or some variation is repeated until fundamental or core beliefs are revealed.)

**Automatic thoughts:** I was a very bad girl.

**Challenging statement:** And if you were a "bad girl," what makes that thought upsetting to you?

**Automatic thoughts:** Everyone would know I am dirty and disgusting.

**Challenging statement:** If you were "dirty and disgusting," what then? What is the meaning of this to you?

**Automatic thoughts:** People would hate me and I need to feel loved.

We continue to process downward until the individual feels some lightening of the impact of their negative thought or hits a core belief at the source of their grief.

**Core Belief:** I am not lovable.

Once the client has revealed their core beliefs you can now focus on the following:

**Do you wish to keep this belief?:** The client will likely say, "No," or, "I don't know how to change." As this point, explain the following: it is possible to "install" a positive alternative to the internal core belief.

**Identify the opposite to the core belief:** (You can aid the client in identifying this. Remember, the goal is to find the opposite, not to ensure that the client believes the opposite in this moment. That will come in time.) I am lovable. I am good enough.

Initially, we can expect that the opposite to the core belief will lead the client to feel some discomfort, but just as it is true that exposure to disturbing events combined with relaxation leads to extinction of discomfort, it is also true that exposure to the positive combined with relaxation can lead to a calm, comfortable, and integrated response.

The goal now becomes exposure to the new positive alternative belief. Instruct your client to listen or repeat the new positive alternative until the SUDS rating when reflecting on this new belief is a 5 or lower.

---

## Cognitive Continuum (CR)

> **Time required:** 5–30 minutes.
>
> **Materials required:** None.
>
> **Indications for use:** Use when the primary need is to enhance cognitive coping skills in Phase II: Working Through Trauma of trauma recovery.
>
> **Counterindications:** Client clearly confused, unmanaged stress, actively dissociating, or dissociates during exercise.

Baer (2001, p. 102) and Wenzel, (2012) recommend the use of a cognitive continuum to further challenge negative beliefs about oneself. This is an especially useful technique when an individual arrives at a rigidly held negative belief that has a traumatic basis. For example, Polly, the same woman discussed above who had experiences of early childhood sexual abuse, arrives at the negative conclusion that she is "extremely bad" and "despised by others" for her involvement in the abuse.

This approach is also useful when dealing with clients who make pronouncements of themselves that are harsh generalizations and not based on reality.

For example, a client declares that she is a "terrible mother." One would think that a blanket statement like this might be based on something quite significant, but when the woman is questioned, she admits to the following:

1. She makes meals for her children daily.
2. She takes them to school and picks them up.
3. She never hits them and rarely raises her voice.
4. She reads to them at bedtime.
5. She finds interesting activities for them to engage in after school and during weekends.
6. She regularly brings them to socialize with family and friends.

So what did this woman do? *She forgot to pack her child's lunch and the teacher called her about it.*

When she was speaking about the forgotten lunch it was with such utter self-contempt that there was absolutely no space for all the good things that she does every day in parenting her children.

## Delivery of Approach

There is printable handout material available for this exercise; see Using the Tools 16. This is an exercise to aid people to gain perspective on their behaviors and better respond to their own normal shortcomings.

We begin to catalog a range of truly bad things that occur daily in our society. Start with the following question: What things might go on a list of truly bad behaviors?

### Example 1

You will see checkmarks to the right of the item signifying, to perception of best to worst, the item ranked for the individual (we are not endorsing a ranking, only recognizing a given client's ranking):

|  | 0 (best) | 50 (neutral or ok) | 100 (worst) |
|---|---|---|---|
| 1. Being a serial killer |  |  | ✗ |
| 2. Molesting a child |  |  | ✗ |
| 3. Hitting a pedestrian with a car |  |  | ✗ |
| 4. Punching a spouse |  |  | ✗ |
| 5. Drinking and driving |  |  | ✗ |

We also need to develop a list of good or neutral behaviors. What kinds of things might go on a list of good or neutral behaviors?

### Example 2

You will see checkmarks to the right of the item signifying to perception of best to worst the item ranked for the individual (we are not endorsing a ranking only recognizing a given client's ranking):

|  | 0 (best) | 50 (neutral or ok) | 100 (worst) |
|---|---|---|---|
| 1. Feeding the cat |  | ✗ |  |
| 2. Buying a loved one a gift for no reason |  | ✗ |  |
| 3. Sharing a laugh with a friend | ✗ |  |  |
| 4. Discovering a cure for cancer | ✗ |  |  |

Now we ask the client to rate all these items from 0 to 100 using the following rating scale:

0 = best ever behavior
50 = neutral or okay behavior
100 = worst or most despicable behavior

After all the items are listed and rated, the client is then asked to add their own item. In our example, the client adds "I forgot to pack my child's lunch" to the list. Suddenly her conclusion that "I am a terrible mother" changed to "I guess I just got busy that morning and forgot. It was a good thing that the teacher called so she should make sure my child got her lunch."

## USING THE TOOLS 16

**Cognitive Continuum**

Negative declaration (write out the negative statement or belief below):

_____

_____

List your good qualities related to this situation:

_____

_____

Give examples of truly bad behaviors or occurrences:

| 0 (best) | 50 (neutral or ok) | 100 (worst) |
|----------|--------------------|-------------|

_____

_____

_____

_____

Give examples of good or neutral behaviors:

| 0 (best) | 50 (neutral or ok) | 100 (worst) |
|----------|--------------------|-------------|

_____

_____

_____

_____

Now add and rate the negative declaration:

| 0 (best) | 50 (neutral or ok) | 100 (worst) |
|----------|--------------------|-------------|

_____

_____

_____

_____

_____

**USING THE TOOLS 16:**
Cognitive Continuum

## Calculating True Danger (CR)

| | |
|---|---|
| **Time required:** 10–30 minutes. | |
| **Materials required:** Paper and pencil. | |
| **Indications for use:** Use when the primary need is to enhance cognitive coping skills in Phase II: Working Through Trauma of trauma recovery. | |
| **Counterindications:** Client clearly confused, unmanaged stress, actively dissociating, or dissociates during exercise. | |

Baer (2001, p. 102) suggests another technique for challenging negative cognitive beliefs. This is useful when feelings of safety are compromised – a common occurrence among trauma survivors. Use this exercise only when you are assured that the true probability of an event will be much less likely than it is perceived by the client. For example, Sheldon believes that if he takes a much-needed vacation to a destination where he must fly, his flight will certainly crash and he will die.

This is a good example to work with because we know that globally more than 3 million people fly daily on commercial aircraft. In 1998, the world's airlines carried approximately 1.3 billion passengers on 18 million flights worldwide while suffering only 10 fatal accidents. The risk of being involved in a commercial aircraft accident resulted in one fatality per 3 million passengers that year. To put this in perspective, you would have to fly once every day for more than 8200 years to accumulate 3 million flights. Flying by commercial airliner is believed to be 22 times safer than driving your own car.

In cases where there is a real imminent and personal danger, we would not use this exercise of calculating true danger.

### Delivery of Approach

*Example*

First, Sheldon is given the opportunity to estimate the probability that his flight will crash (he believes the probability of this event is 25%). The next step is for Sheldon to work with the therapist to identity each step required for the feared outcome to occur. After all events leading up to "dying in a plane crash" are identified, each are again given a rating based on an assumed "chance of this event occurring." Then a "cumulative chance of all events" is calculated (see Table 7). Given our example of Sheldon's fear of dying in a plane crash, let us identify events and calculate the true probability of danger. Despite Sheldon's deep fear, he assesses the following events and still arrives at a very low percentage of probability using the exercise above. In this case, Sheldon's own estimate produces a chance of danger at the remarkably low 0.0000001%. This is a vast contrast to his pre-existing perceived fear of dying in a plane crash of 25% probability. This is a good example of how we can assist our clients in challenging their own notions of actual versus perceived fears.

**Table 7.**    Calculating the true probability of danger (adapted from Baer, 2001, p. 102)

| Event | Chance of this event occurring | Cumulative chance of all events |
|---|---|---|
| 1. Sheldon must select a flight with some mechanical or other problem that will lead to a crash. | 1 / 1000 | 1 / 1000 |
| 2. The error or problem will not be noticed before takeoff | 1 / 10 | 1 / 10,000 |
| 3. The pilot, staff, or passengers will not be able to correct the problem while in air | 1 / 10 | 1 / 100,000 |
| 4. There will be a crash landing | 1 / 10 | 1 / 1,000,000 |
| 5. Sheldon will not survive the crash | 1 / 10 | 1 / 10,000,000 |

# Looped Tape Scripting (RE – CR)

**Time required:** 10–60 minutes.

**Materials required:** Paper and pencil.

**Indications for use:** Use when the primary need is to enhance cognitive and emotional coping skills in Phase II: Working Through Trauma of trauma recovery.

**Counterindications:** Client clearly confused, unmanaged stress, actively dissociating, or dissociates during exercise.

This is a particularly challenging exercise. However, if we have built in all of the precautions with our clients as suggested in this book, they will likely be prepared to proceed with some reassurances. Looped Tape Scripting is an approach based on exposure therapy and habituation to the feared memory or thoughts. This requires the clinician to be skilled in handling disturbing clinical material and be able to stay calmly present for the client during the entire session.

Habituation occurs over time, when we are exposed to situations, memories, thoughts, or occurrences that may have caused distress or discomfort initially but become commonplace over time and no longer create the same level of distress. This requires practice and tolerance for initial discomfort. Research consistently shows improvement over time through the use of this exposure technique. Most of us can understand the notion of habituation when we recall times where we were initially annoyed or disturbed by something that over time we completely forgot about (i.e., a fear of the dark, a noise in our car, the sound of airplanes or traffic when we move into a new apartment, a distracting open-concept work environment, etc.). Remarkably, it also works the same way with much more disturbing material.

*Note:* Looped Tape Scripting can also be used to install positive cognitive or new core beliefs, such as those identified in the Downward Arrow technique.

## Delivery of Approach

There is printable handout material available for this exercise; see Using the Tools 17. In this exercise, the individual is asked to identify a memory or a perceived fear/threat that they are prepared to work on with the goal of resolution at this time. Recall the Trigger List developed earlier in this book during Titration Part I: Trigger List Using Braking and Acceleration. The Trigger List can provide the basis for selecting an event. When an event is selected, ask the individual to give it a SUDS rating from 1 to 10.

Now the individual is asked to write out the worst parts of the event or anticipated fear in great detail. Using this document, the individual is now encouraged to speak into a tape recorder or video camera. The entire script is read repeatedly until 30 minutes of recording is completed. The recorded document is now watched or listened to during the clinical session at least once. The individual's homework is to watch or listen to the script for an hour each day until the tape no longer results in a heightened SUDS rating. In this way, the individual achieves habituation to the feared past event.

The time required for habituation is different for each individual and clinicians need to have great tolerance for individual differences in processing time.

## USING THE TOOLS 17

**Looped Tape Scripting – Installing the Positive**

Memory or Fear                                                    SUDS = _____

_____

_____

_____

_____

An alternative method is to itemize positive self-statements that the client is not yet comfortable with and use this list to work with the exposure method outlined in the Delivery of Approach for Looped Tape Scripting.

**Example:**

The positive exposure list below provides a challenge to the individual to integrate new, more adaptive self-talk utilizing a Loop Tape Script exercise.
I am loveable.
I am wonderful.
I am brilliant.
I am successful.
I am exciting.
I am interesting.
I am fun.
I am attractive.

Read through the above list above once and then give it a SUDS rating.
SUDS = _____

Work with deep breathing, Comfort in One Part, or any other self-soothe exercise.

Read through the list again working with the self-soothe method of choice.

Rate the SUDS again:
SUDS = _____

Continue with the exercise above until the SUDS rating is 5 or below.

From: Anna B. Baranowsky & J. Eric Gentry, *Trauma Practice: A Cognitive Behavioral Somatic Therapy* (4th ed.). © 2023 Hogrefe Publishing

**USING THE TOOLS 17:**
Looped Tape Scripting –
Installing the Positive

## Cognitive Processing Therapy (RE – CR)

> **Time required:** One to several sessions.
>
> **Materials required:** Paper and pencil.
>
> **Indications for use:** Use when the primary need is to enhance cognitive coping skills in Phase II: Working Through Trauma stage of trauma recovery.
>
> **Counterindications:** Client clearly confused, unmanaged stress, actively dissociating, or dissociates during exercise.

### Delivery of Approach

There is printable handout material available for this exercise; see Using the Tools 18. This approach was developed expressly to treat rape victims and incorporates both techniques of cognitive therapy and exposure therapy. In using the techniques of cognitive therapy, the clinician works to assist the survivor in confronting and restructuring the problematic cognitions that result from their traumatic experiences, especially self-blame (Resick & Schnicke, 1992, 1993; Nixon et al., 2016; Asmundson et al., 2019). Building upon the work of McCann and Pearlman (1990), this approach also asks the survivor to address overgeneralized and often distorted beliefs about trust, power/ control, self-esteem, and intimacy. A recent meta-analytic review (Asmundson et al., 2019) has demonstrated and showed cognitive processing therapy to be an effective treatment for PTSD with long term benefits across a variety of outcomes. Exposure therapy techniques are utilized by asking the client to write a detailed account of their traumatic experience(s) and read it back to the therapist as well as other willing witnesses. This intervention assists individuals in achieving a loosening of affect, which, in turn, often helps the survivor navigate through "stuck points" that they have heretofore been unable to either recall and/or move through.

## USING THE TOOLS 18

**Cognitive Processing Therapy**

Follow the steps below:

1. Identify the unresolved memory, concern, or situation:

   _____

   _____

2. For 1 minute, remain in quiet reflection, letting your thoughts run with no judgment on the content. This should be a timed minute ending when a buzzer goes off.

   _____

   _____

3. Now take as much time as needed to write out the details of your thoughts during your 1-minute reflection, leaving out nothing (add paper if needed).

   _____

   _____

   _____

   _____

   _____

   _____

   _____

   _____

   _____

   _____

   _____

4. Repeat steps 2–3 until the SUDS ratings are 5 or less.

   _____

   _____

From: Anna B. Baranowsky & J. Eric Gentry, *Trauma Practice: A Cognitive Behavioral Somatic Therapy* (4th ed.). © 2023 Hogrefe Publishing

**USING THE TOOLS 18:**
Cognitive Processing Therapy

## Story-Book Approach (RE – CR)
(Gentry, personal communication, 2002)

> **Time required:** 10–30 minutes
>
> **Materials required:** Paper, colored markers.
>
> **Indications for use:** Use when the primary need is to enhance cognitive coping skills in Phase II: Working Through Trauma of trauma recovery.
>
> **Counterindications:** Client clearly confused, unmanaged stress, actively dissociating, or dissociates during exercise.

### Delivery of Approach

Another technique that utilizes reciprocal inhibition and cognitive restructuring is the Story-Book Approach. Have your client identify the event on which they would like to work. Divide the event into at least four segments from beginning to end, timewise. (This may be used in conjunction with the timeline created in the previous technique Timeline Approach or done separately.) Then take a sheet of paper and draw each segment. This can be done in comic-strip format or any other style the client chooses. Have the client practice continuous self-soothing while they complete the drawing and monitor their reactions to remind them. When the drawing is finished, have them tell the narrative using the pictures as a guide. Then retell the story back to them as accurately as possible. In a group setting, the drawing can be shown to the group and the narrative told by a partner.

## Written Narrative Approach (RE – CR)
(Gentry, personal communication, 2002)

> **Time required:** 10–30 minutes.
>
> **Materials required:** Paper and pencil.
>
> **Indications for use:** Use when the primary need is to enhance cognitive coping skills in Phase II: Working Through Trauma of trauma recovery.
>
> **Counterindications:** Client clearly confused, unmanaged stress, actively dissociating, or dissociates during exercise.

### Delivery of Approach

Here is another technique that utilizes reciprocal inhibition and cognitive restructuring. Have your client write out the context of what occurred in as much detail as they care to include. As before, have them self-soothe as they are writing their story. After they have written about what happened, have them write down what they think they have lost as a result of the events. Finally, have them write what they think they might have gained as a result of what happened. They may then read it to you and/or have it read back to them.

## Corrective Messages from Old Storylines (CR)

> **Time required:** 30–50 minutes.
>
> **Materials required:** Paper and pencil.
>
> **Indications for use:** Use when the primary need is to enhance cognitive coping skills in Phase II: Working Through Trauma of trauma recovery.
>
> **Counterindications:** Client clearly confused, unmanaged stress, actively dissociating, or dissociates during exercise.

### Delivery of Approach

There is printable handout material available for this exercise; see Using the Tools 19. Sometimes what we say to ourselves is absolutely untrue, misguided, and damaging. This exercise focuses on challenging old storylines or belief systems and replacing them with new corrective messages. In order to be successful at guiding a client through this approach, we absolutely must find the core of an incorrect message. We need to start with understanding what we are trying to capture as well as how to capture the core of an incorrect old storyline.

The way our mind works is that it gathers information and then makes a core statement which we carry forward, possibly to help guide and protect us in life. Now, this can be wonderful if we remain in an unchanging world where something that was dangerous remains dangerous and we need to continue to memorize and protect ourselves from that threat. However, in many situations some old perceived threat is no longer real, and yet we can continue to behave as if we are at risk, leaving us in a reactive mode that may prove detrimental in all sorts of ways.

Here is a hypothetical example that you can share with your clients to help them understand how to find their own storylines.

Julia grows up in a family where she is chronically neglected as a child, exposed to drugs and alcohol, and mistreated by a man with short, spiky hair who was providing her mother with drugs. She concludes that she is unworthy of kindness, always needs to be on guard, and that men with spiky short hair are always dangerous.

She manages to get herself through university with intelligence and great effort on her part along with a cheering section made up of friends. She is the first in her family to achieve a university education and she does not use drugs or drink alcohol. She finally feels like she is a success at something.

Unfortunately, she carries a strong belief that despite her accomplishments she is unworthy of kindness and remains constantly on guard – keeping those she does not know well at a distance.

She is offered a great job in her field of choice. Yes, her boss (a nice man with unfortunately spiky hair) is now the focus of her strong emotional reactions. She is engaged in an internal battle for growth. What this really means is that she will continue to feel distressed unless she is able to challenge and win the battle of her internal message that she is "unworthy of kind treatment and men with spiky hair are dangerous."

Remember, sometimes what we say to ourselves is absolutely untrue, misguided, and damaging ... what Julia is saying to herself is exactly this type of lie.

In therapy, we would encourage Julia to follow the steps I will outline for you right now.

A powerful option is to write out the story in third person rather than from the personal perspective. Research suggests that this re-phrasing, "Julia was treated very badly by a man with spiky hair when she was a child" rather than, "I was treated very badly by a man ..." allows for perspective and reduces the feelings of immediate threat (Andersson & Conley, 2013).

## USING THE TOOLS 19

### Corrective Messages from Old Storylines

Follow the steps below:

1. Identify the incorrect statement that you are ready to challenge today right now – in Julia's work she chose, "I am unworthy of kind treatment and men with spiky hair are dangerous."

   _____

   _____

2. Now identify a corrective statement – here Julia worked out, "I am safe at work and my boss Ben is a nice man with spiky hair – I am worthy and ready to embrace kind treatment."

   _____

   _____

3. Now she begins to implant the corrective statement, "I am safe at work and my boss Ben is a nice man with spiky hair – I am worthy and ready to embrace kind treatment." Now identify your corrective positive statement.

   _____

   _____

4. Can you imagine what Julia might say to herself the first 3–4 times she tries to implant the corrective statement? If you thought that she might suffer, struggle, feel anxious and upset, you would be correct. Initially, she doesn't believe it and instead feels like a fraud, and judges herself unfairly. This is the reaction phase and this is normal and fine. Outline below the reactions you have when you initially try to install the positive corrective statement.

   _____

   _____

5. Now stick with it and continue to repeat the corrective phrase 10 times at a sitting 3 times each day. Remember what I mentioned earlier about how remarkable Julia is in her ability to persevere? Well, we can all do this, especially if the task is bite sized. Write out what you notice after you persevere by the third sitting each day.

   _____

   _____

6. Julia notices that her reactions are no longer as powerful over time – either to the corrective statement or to her own feelings of being unworthy or at risk with men with spiky hair. She is surprised that simply by challenging an old belief with a challenging corrective statement she is able to unglue herself from the old storyline she has carried for so long. What do you notice after practicing regularly for a week?

   _____

   _____

   _____

From: Anna B. Baranowsky & J. Eric Gentry, *Trauma Practice: A Cognitive Behavioral Somatic Therapy* (4th ed.). © 2023 Hogrefe Publishing

**USING THE TOOLS 19:**
Corrective Messages from Old Storylines

7. We are all vulnerable to carrying negative fear-based stories, personal lies, or untruths. They usually come from a place where we are trying to protect ourselves so the beliefs become powerfully wired in our brains. Remember, since we are being wired for survival this is a good thing. Yet, we need to recognize that some beliefs limit us and we can challenge them so they are not as sticky and hardwired. When we free ourselves up from the "immediate go to negative fear-based beliefs" this allows us to live the lives we are meant to live. What do you notice when you free yourself up from old fearful beliefs?

_____

_____

8. So the challenge for you today is to find an old storyline that is no longer useful for you and to follow the same steps that Julia followed until the new corrective message is more powerful than the old storyline.

From: Anna B. Baranowsky & J. Eric Gentry, *Trauma Practice: A Cognitive Behavioral Somatic Therapy* (4th ed.). © 2023 Hogrefe Publishing

## Traumagram Exercise (RE – CR)

**Time required:** 30–60 minutes or more depending on complexity of history and knowledge of generational family events

**Materials required:** Paper, pen/pencil or computer generated

**Indications for use:** Used to delve deeper into one's history and identify significant family of origin events. An excellent tool for better understanding and integrating the events that may have shaped a person through the generations.

**Counterindications:** Do not attempt until the later stage of Phase I, following established practice of stabilization skills and ability to demonstrate capacity to harness calm on demand.

The Traumagram Exercise is a powerful tool that can help to visually illustrate and map out generational trauma that might otherwise undermine personal healing. As opposed to a genogram, which is used extensively in family systems therapy to highlight relationships between family members along with significant events that have taken place within the family (the system), a traumagram is focused on traumatic events that have occurred throughout the generations. In resolving trauma, it can be very helpful to recognize that trauma can and often does go through the generations.

There is increasing evidence that generational trauma may impact the current or future generations.

For an interesting video on this topic, watch Dr. Baranowsky discuss the impact of inherited family trauma with Mark Wolynn (Baranowsky, 2017, July 19), author of *It Didn't Start With You: How Inherited Family Trauma Shapes Who We Are and How to End the Cycle*, which is available in the supplementary material, Video 3 (or at https://youtu.be/WzQ5FM3hCgo).

The Traumagram is a good choice as a transition exercise for individuals moving into Phase II of trauma practice. Clients should have established some grounding and containment skills and practices. Once the individual can demonstrate these skills and can stabilize emotionally and physiologically, the Traumagram can be a liberating exercise where one recognizes that our physiology and emotions can be shaped even prior to our birth.

There is an increasing interest in research on trauma and stress being transferred through the generations. For more on this topic, please review the section on Epigenetics in this book. In addition, you will also find more on Epigenetics as well as a "how to" on applying this exercise in this video *Traumagram and Epigenetics: The Healing Power of the Traumagram* (Baranowsky, 2017, July 26) available in the supplementary material, Video 26 (p. 227, or at https://youtu.be/TQUOjoAODAo).

### Delivery of Approach

1. Begin by reviewing the example below of Charlie's written (Table 8) and visual traumagram (Figure 7). This will help to outline what is needed to begin to build the elements.
2. These templates will aid in building a traumagram from scratch using the examples. However, remember everyone has a unique traumagram so the framework provided is for example only. There is no right or wrong traumagram.
3. Client instructions:

**Script: Traumagram Exercise**

a. Begin by filling out a *traumagram* list for your family. Base this on the knowledge you have or gather information from conversations with family or friends. Focus on any traumas that may have occurred during the past several generations including accidents, violence, war, health trauma, etc. Try to go back several generations (to your grandparents or even great grandparents).

b. Try to simplify your language providing, one-sentence, simple descriptions of no more than ten words. This should include a timeline (i.e., age, year, general time frame) and a context (i.e., in the kitchen, in Afghanistan, etc.). Write just enough to document the trauma experienced by each close family member.

c. Complete the sections as required by year of occurrence or age at the time of the event. These can all be approximate. In the traumagram, we are framing events rather than reviewing an entire story of an event. We are not looking to capture the whole story or all of the worst details but rather to capture a snapshot in order to gain insight into family patterns.

d. Begin your list. Be sure to remind yourself to stop in order to pace your exposure and intensity whenever things feel over-whelming. This pacing gives you the opportunity to practice managing your symptoms with the self-soothing techniques you have learned. This helps you gain confidence in your ability to manage your symptoms, if they become evoked.

e. Add as many family incidents as you wish to each section until you feel your family traumagram list is complete and we can begin your traumagram graphic.

f. Using the symbol system below, prepare your traumagram showing the type of relationship each member has with each other.

g. On the following pages, you will see an example of Charlie's family traumagram (both the list and the graphical representation) along with legends specific to his relationships and the incidents that helped shape his family dynamics. The traumagram has been simplified and does not include all family members (i.e., aunts, uncles, siblings, and offspring). For your own traumagram, we encourage you to add all the people in your family.

h. You will notice that in the sample, we do not have exact dates for births or deaths, etc. A general age or timeframe is enough for this exercise. However, it is important to note what has occurred to each member of the family and to recognize the conflicts and behavioral patterns in a visual form as shown below. Now you can follow the steps to create your own family traumagram.

**Table 8.**   Example of a traumagram list for Charlie's family

| | | | |
|---|---|---|---|
| Mother | Age 8: Mother severely injured and nearly died as a result of an accident | Mom has always been supportive but is always overly cautious with me and everyone in the family. She argues a lot with my sister about this. | I see that my Mom is stressed and I try to keep her from worrying. I get angry with my sister for arguing. |
| Father | Age 14: became disabled as the result of a stroke during a surgical procedure; was forced to learn how to walk and talk again. | Dad is always careful and moves slowly. Everyone seems to be concerned about his health. He is a kind man. | I'm always concerned that Dad will get sick again. It scares me still. |
| Grandmother | 1940: Grandma was in London during the bombing blitz. She still cries when she remembers it. | Mom and Grandma argue especially when Grandma gets upset. Grandma is really nice but can be difficult when she gets upset. | I tend to leave the room when Mom and Grandma argue or when she is upset. Maybe avoidance keeps me from getting close to others. |
| Sister | Age 22: admitted to the family that her marriage was ending and her husband was abusive. | Seeing as her troubled marriage has been a source of conflict with everyone in the family, we were all relieved when she ended it. | I feel uncertain about my choices in relationships. |

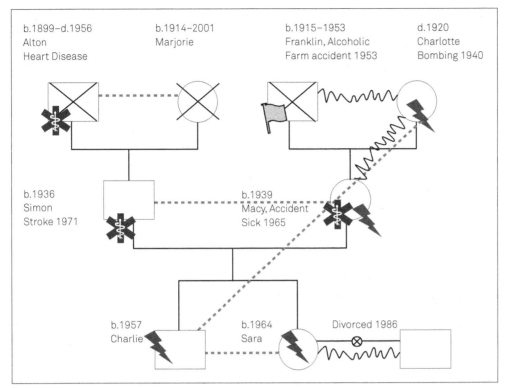

**Figure 7.**
Example of a traumagram graphic for Charlie's family.

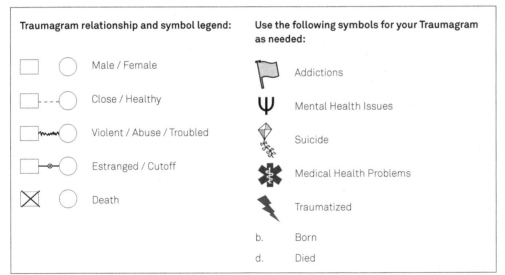

**Figure 8.**
Legends used in Charlie's family traumagram.

# 3. Behavior

The most obvious indicator of successful treatment for trauma is the ability to translate this new learning into behavior. Is the client more relaxed? Are they better able to interact with others socially? Have they decreased self-defeating behaviors and less-than-useful self-soothing behaviors? Our clients have often spent a lifetime per-forming behaviors used to adapt to difficult circumstances and do not always have a repertoire of more useful be-haviors. Also, performing new behaviors is anxiety pro-voking in itself, because individuals attempting the new behaviors cannot predict the outcome. The techniques that follow are useful in generating new behaviors and provide practice for individuals to gain comfort and re-duce anxiety before using new skills in their daily life.

# Behavior Change Rehearsal Exercise (RE – CR)

**Time required:** 10–30 minutes.

**Materials required:** None.

**Indications for use:** Use when the primary need is to enhance behavioral coping skills in the Working Through Trauma stage of trauma recovery.

**Counterindications:** Client clearly confused, unmanaged stress, actively dissociating, or dissociates during exercise.

This approach has been based on Grinder and Bandler's (1981) New Behavior Generator exercise. The technique is offered as a procedure to utilize the imagination as a process for eventually freeing actual behavior in more desirable directions. The steps that follow incorporate several techniques introduced earlier (i.e., Anchoring Safety Part I & II and Safe Place Visualization). This technique can be used in Stress Inoculation Training as the imaginary rehearsal component that is integral to that approach.

## Delivery of Approach

1. Identify the response or behavior the individual is dissatisfied with (e.g., cannot say no to overwork).
2. Identify all the payoffs to the current manner of handling this type of situation (e.g., everyone likes me; no one laughs at me).
3. Identify the disadvantages to maintaining the current behavior (e.g., exhaustion; I feel others take advantage of me).
4. Which weighs more or has greater appeal: the payoffs for staying the same or the disadvantages? Do you want to stay the same or is it too painful to stay the same?
5. What alternative positive behavior could you substitute for the current behaviors?
6. Set up an ideomotor signal for yes and no (e.g., yes = thumbs-up; no = thumbs-down).
7. Determine which type of grounding to relaxation or safety you wish to use for this exercise (e.g., Diaphragmatic Breathing, Autogenics, Progressive Relaxation, Safe Place Visualization, Sensory Grounding and Containment, etc.). Prepare the individual for this induction.

8. Once grounded in safety, ask the individual to do the following:

 **Script: Behavior Change Rehearsal**

a. Imagine that part of you remains in safety while another part of you acts as an observer and steps away from safety.
b. Recall a past experience that left you feeling dissatisfied with your behavior.
c. Once you can recall this memory, show me a thumbs-up to let me know you have the memory. *[Say "good" when you see thumbs-up.]*
d. Imagine you are going to watch a videotape of this memory. You have control to start or stop the tape as you wish.
e. Rewind the experience to just before the unpleasantness. Show me a thumbs-up when you are at the beginning of the tape.
f. Play it all the way through to the end. Watch yourself behave in the manner that you wish to change. Remember you are an observer still grounded in safety.
g. Now recall what new behavior you would like to replace for the old response. Give me a thumbs-up to let me know you have recalled the new behavior.
h. Good. Now watch and listen to yourself as you replace the old response with the new, desired behavior. Watch as you are able to handle this situation that in the past would have given you difficulty. Play the video all the way through to the end, watching the new behavior in the old situation.
i. Show me a thumbs-up when you are done. Good.
j. Having observed this new behavior in the old situation, was it completely satisfactory to you? Show me a thumbs-up if you were completely satisfied and a thumbs-down if not.

9. If the answer to 8j is yes, go through the script above imagining a future imagined scenario similar to the actual memory. Have the person imagine one that might have caused difficulty in the past but which they wish to practice this new behavior on.
10. If the answer to 8j is no, replay the same script until they are satisfied with their rehearsed imagined behavior. After they are satisfied, follow Step 9.

## Skills Building Methods (CR)
(Foa, Keane, & Friedman, 2000; Foa, Keane, Friedman, & Cohen, 2009)

---

**Time required:** 10–30 minutes.

**Materials required:** Paper and pencil.

**Indications for use:** Use when the primary need is to enhance cognitive coping skills in Phase II: Working Through Trauma of trauma recovery.

**Counterindications:** Client clearly confused, unmanaged stress, actively dissociating, or dissociates during exercise.

---

### Delivery of Approach

This treatment method is designed and recommended for severely and/or retraumatized women (Foa, Keane, & Friedman, 2000; Foa, Keane, Friedman, & Cohen, 2009). Cloitre (1998) offers the acronym STAIR (Skills Training in Affect and Interpersonal Regulation/Prolonged Exposure). In this model, clients are guided through skills training and development in three distinct areas:

- Identifying and labeling feeling states (especially feelings of threat)
- Tolerating distress and modulating negative affect
- Effectively negotiating difficult interpersonal relationships requiring assertiveness and self-regulation

There is more comprehensive training for the STAIR approach. The image below outlines some of the key elements.

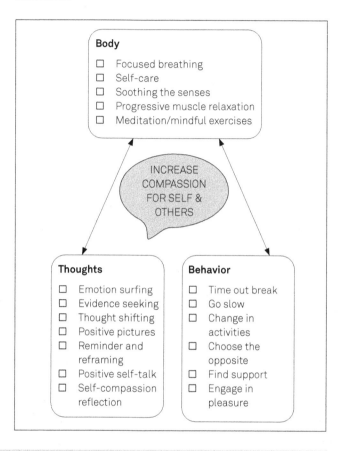

## Imaginal and In Vivo Exposure (RE)

---

**Time required:** One or more sessions.

**Materials required:** Varies.

**Indications for use:** Use when the primary need is to enhance behavioral and cognitive coping skills in Phase II: Working Through Trauma of trauma recovery.

**Counterindications:** Client unable to self-soothe, actively dissociating, or dissociates during exercise. This exercise requires a significant level of stability and self-soothing ability.

---

Imaginal and *in vivo* (live) exposures rely on a willingness to expose oneself directly to the actual feared person, place, thing, or event. Following trauma, individuals may become extremely distressed when returning to the scene of the trauma or the item associated with the trauma. Un-

fortunately, it is possible and even common that traumatic memories and feared triggers become generalized to other areas of our lives. For example, if an individual is in a motor vehicle accident, they may fear entering a car and even fear trains, planes, boats, buses, and all other modes of transportation. Repeated exposure to anxiety-arousing stimuli without danger supposedly provides a corrective learning experience. It is our belief that simply exposing a client to the imagined or actual stimuli until resolution of anxiety occurs is potentially retraumatizing and we believe that relaxation is a necessary ingredient for resolution. A method such as Systematic Desensitization (presented shortly) titrates the exposure and provides the client with the experience of self-management of the anxiety. Nevertheless, Imaginal and *In Vivo* Exposures are sometimes quick and effective ways to address the traumatic event.

## Delivery of Approach

1. Identify the feared person, place, thing, or event.
2. Provide a SUDS rating (1-10) that indicates the degree of distress associated with this stimulus.
3. Self-soothe until the current SUDS rating is below 3.
4. Either imagine the event or stimulus, or recreate the event or stimulus as closely as possible in real life (*in vivo*) to begin the exposure.

Exposure is continued until the SUDS rating drops below 50% of the original rating. Ratings are taken at regular intervals, approximately every 5-10 minutes. When the SUDS rating has dropped to below 50%, the therapist may assist the client in further lowering their current SUDS level to 3 or less. It is very important to allow the client time to discuss and process their experience of the exposure. When the individual demonstrates adequate self-soothing and self-rescue abilities, they may be given homework to complete the exposure task daily until SUDS levels continue to remain low during exposure.

*Example:*

It is best to start with a list of gradually increasing activities leading to the most feared thing. For someone who has been in a motor vehicle accident, you might generate a list similar to the one below:

|   |   | SUDS |
|---|---|------|
| 1 | Look at pictures of cars | 5 |
| 2 | Go to a parking lot | 5 |
| 3 | Touch a car's driver's seat | 6 |
| 4 | Sit in a passenger's seat | 7 |
| 5 | Sit in the driver's seat | 8 |
| 6 | Be a passenger in a moving vehicle | 8 |
| 7 | Be the driver in a moving vehicle | 9 |

The goal for each of these gradual steps, whether imaginal or *in vivo, is to expose the client to each step, lowering the SUDS to a manageable level before moving on to the next step and eventually extinguishing the list.*

## Stress Inoculation Training (RE – CR)

> **Time required:** 8–14 sessions.
>
> **Materials required:** Varies.
>
> **Indications for use:** Use when the primary need is to enhance physical, cognitive, behavioral, and emotional coping skills in Phase II: Working Through Trauma of trauma recovery.
>
> **Counterindications:** Actively dissociating or dissociates during exercise. Client must have ability to self-soothe.

This classical cognitive behavioral treatment approach to posttraumatic recovery was developed and first presented by Meichenbaum in 1987 (Meichenbaum, 1994, 2012). There is considerable research expressing the efficacy of this approach (Kashani et al., 2015; Jackson et al., 2019, VA/DoD Clinical Practice Guideline Working Group, 2017). It is a well-accepted protocol in the field of trauma treatment. Stress inoculation training (SIT) teaches individuals coping skills and practice opportunities to enhance their mastery over disturbing stress responses. SIT generally consists of 8-14 sessions and can be applied in groups or among individuals.

This treatment approach is broken into three phases (the outline below is adapted from Meichenbaum, 1994):
• Phase 1: Conceptualization
• Phase 2: Skills acquisition, consolidation, and rehearsal
• Phase 3: Application training

### Phase 1: Conceptualization

In this phase, the individual is informed of the treatment format and provided with psychoeducational training to better understand their symptoms and reactions. It is at this stage that the client works collaboratively with the therapist to identify positive coping strategies.

### Phase 2: Skills Acquisition, Consolidation, and Rehearsal

In Phase 2, the clinician draws heavily from materials reviewed earlier in this text. This is the most complex and time-intensive part of the book. The core focus is cognitive, behavioral, and physiological (body) skills acquisition to moderate or manage feelings of stress, anxiety, fear, guilt, and anger. The individual is encouraged to make it their goal to change:
1. the stressful environment or situation whenever possible;
2. one's perception or "meaning" of the situation; or
3. emotional reactions evoked by the situation or recollections of disturbing occurrences.

Strategies for moderating or managing disturbing or stressful situations include:

1. Leave the situation
2. Change the situation
3. Accept the situation as it stands and achieve satisfaction or support in other areas of one's life
4. Reframe the situation differently or develop new interpretations

The goals and strategies listed above can be traversed through the utilization of many coping skills. It is during this phase that skills are taught and practiced. Skills covered include: "direct-action and problem-focused coping and emotional-regulative palliative coping" (Meichenbaum, 1994, p. 394).

The coping skills taught in this section include relaxation exercises, positive self-talk or challenges to negative thinking, problem-solving, distraction, etc. After skills are in place, individuals are taught to prepare, confront, and cope with disturbing events and feelings. When the event is over, they are encouraged to reflect on the effectiveness of the coping strategy and either reinforce it or select another approach to stress management.

**Phase 3: Application Training**

Imaginary rehearsal, role-playing, and *in vivo* graduated exposure are applied in this phase. Relapse prevention through follow-up sessions is an integral part of SIT.

**Delivery of Approach**

There is printable handout material available for this exercise; see Using the Tools 20 and Using the Tools 21. The clinician can utilize the following steps to help the client complete the SIT. After one or two trainings, the client will be able to initiate and complete this exercise without the aid of the clinician.

## USING THE TOOLS 20

**SIT Phase Oriented – Task Checklist**

**Phase 1: Conceptualization**

1. This is the interview stage. Identify stressors and types of occurrences that are demanding for the individual.
2. Request narrative accounts of stressors and coping strategies. Identify available strengths and resources.
3. Deconstruct disturbing reactions as they relate to distressing incidents. Recognize automatic responses and coping resources. Assess the utility of each.
4. Clarify the difference between the things you can change and those you cannot.
5. Begin the process of goal setting. Focus on achievable and specific tasks.
6. Achieve self-awareness of stress reactions and early warning signs (i.e., emotional, behavioral, physical, cognitive, relational). Using this awareness assist the individual to closely self-monitor.
7. Recognize coping deficits and identify for future training efforts.
8. Normalize stress response, reinforce the positive strengths utilized, and begin to bring meaning into one's perception of experiences.
9. Reassure that everyone responds to stress in a unique manner and there is no "right way."

**Phase 2: Skills Acquisition and Rehearsal**

1. Provide skills training that fit the individual's or group's needs.
   a. Identify what works for the individual and how to reinforce this strength.
   b. Introduce problem-focused instrumental coping skills. Problems are broken into subcomponents that can be addressed individually. Appropriate skills are taught to manage a given problem.
   c. Begin solution-focused problem-solving activities that include recognizing desired change and rating alternative solutions. Introduce behavioral coping activities for in session and in vivo practice.
   d. Introduce emotionally focused palliative coping skills. These are essential when situations are beyond one's control and not likely to change. Helpful exercises include: relaxation, cognitive reframing, humor, and self-care.
   e. Encourage the use of social supports and introduce appropriate social skills development when required.
   f. A wide spectrum of skills development is required for long-term recovery or management of distress. Encourage a broad picture of coping resources.

2. Integrate a skills rehearsal component.
   a. Use imaginary and behavioral rehearsal activities to better prepare the individual for real-life use of new skills.
   b. Provide a demonstration (live or videotaped) of "coping modeling" (Meichenbaum, 1994, p. 397). The coping model displays both initial discomfort or distress and then resourceful coping strategies. Allow for discussion and rehearsal after the demonstration.
   c. Challenge negative self-defeating internal dialog and reinforce positive adaptive self-talk.
   d. Make a commitment to future resourcefulness and resiliency efforts.
   e. Identify blocks to adaptive coping.

**Phase 3: Application, Relapse Prevention, and Follow-Through**

1. Application of adaptive coping skills:
   a. Utilize early stress warning signs to cue individual to access new coping skills in response to stress.
   b. Increase imagery exposure exercise to include more stressful and disturbing material.
   c. Integrate graded exposure techniques and in vivo exercises.
   d. Rehearse coping responses as a relapse prevention technique. Recognize trigger situations or occurrences and rehearse positive coping skills to stressful and automatic reactions.
   e. Involve the individual in recognizing the utility of any given exercise through direct questioning of where, how, and why skills will be used.
   f. Teach the individual to take "credit" for new skills development and utilization through "attribution retraining." Review successful and unsuccessful attempts to use new skills.

**USING THE TOOLS 20:**
SIT Phase Oriented – Task Checklist

2. Maintain new skills and then generalize to more situations.
   a. Spread out timing of sessions to include "booster and follow-up sessions" (Meichenbaum, 1994, p. 398).
   b. Involve family, friends, and other care providers in the ongoing success of the individual.
   c. Offer a coaching opportunity to the client so they can teach what they have learned. This is best attempted with group models.
   d. Make life changes where possible and encourage a sense of self-control through the establishment of "escape routes" where necessary.
   e. Reinforce a realistic attitude where there is recognition that life can be stressful at times, and they will not handle every occurrence in an ideal manner. These times can simply be opportunities for learning and a chance to gain new skills. In this way, the individual can learn over time and not feel guilt or shame for perceived failures or setbacks.

From: Anna B. Baranowsky & J. Eric Gentry, *Trauma Practice: A Cognitive Behavioral Somatic Therapy* (4th ed.). © 2023 Hogrefe Publishing

## USING THE TOOLS 21

### SIT Book Developer

The purpose of this exercise is to integrate teaching from this book by recognizing what approaches you can utilize to achieve each of the tasks required in this SIT Book Developer. Use the contents of this book as a resource and write the name of the approach you choose for each task required. See the SIT Checklist above for further details and explanations.

*Note:* There are additional tasks required during a full SIT found in the checklist.

**Phase 1: Conceptualization**

Identify your target group or individual:

_____

_____

Recognize automatic responses and how they are damaging or useful. Normalize stress responses and reinforce the positive.

_____

_____

**Phase 2: Skills Acquisition and Rehearsal**

Provide appropriate skills training for your individual or group.

_____

_____

Integrate a skills rehearsal component.

_____

_____

**Phase 3: Application, Relapse Prevention, and Follow-Through**

Encourage the use of specific coping skills.

_____

_____

Maintain new skills and generalize these to additional situations.

_____

_____

_____

From: Anna B. Baranowsky & J. Eric Gentry, *Trauma Practice: A Cognitive Behavioral Somatic Therapy* (4th ed.). © 2023 Hogrefe Publishing

**USING THE TOOLS 21:**
SIT Book Developer

## Systematic Desensitization (RE)

> **Time required:** One to several sessions.
>
> **Materials required:** Paper and pencil for therapist.
>
> **Indications for use:** Use when the primary need is to enhance behavioral coping skills in Phase II: Working Through Trauma of trauma recovery.
>
> **Counterindications:** Actively dissociating or dissociates during exercise. Client must clearly have the ability to self-soothe and self-rescue.

Developed in 1969 by Joseph Wolpe, this technique is the basis for most behavioral treatments for anxiety and traumatic stress (Wolpe, 1969). Drawing upon the principles of reciprocal inhibition, Wolpe combined a hierarchy of negative associations connected to a triggering event or object with relaxation strategies. He theorized that, as the client was able to develop the relaxation response at each level of the hierarchy, they would then be able to accommodate a move to the next higher level of anxiety-producing stimuli. Systematic desensitization is said to be complete when the feelings of anxiety are extinguished with *in vivo* exposure to the original anxiety-producing situation or object.

### Delivery of Approach

*Example*

A client feels overwhelming anxiety when confronted with returning to work as a bank teller after a robbery.

1. Develop a hierarchy of real and imagined situations in which he would feel increasing levels of anxiety due to demands placed upon him in the work context.

   SUDS = 10   Serving customers from the same section where the robbery occurred

   SUDS = 8   Working at a bank station

   SUDS = 6   Entering the bank

   SUDS = 4   Parking at the bank

   SUDS = 2   Driving past the bank

2. Learn and master a set of self-soothing and anxiety-reduction behaviors and practices that the client can use to lessen arousal when confronted with anxiety-producing stimuli.

   a. Progressive Relaxation

   b. Safe-Place Visualization

   c. Diaphragmatic Breathing

   d. Positive Self-Talk

3. The clinician then leads the client through an imaginal exposure of the hierarchy created above, beginning with the situation with the lowest SUDS level. After the client has demonstrated the ability to successfully lower their anxiety at the lowest level of exposure, the clinician guides them to the next level of anxiety-producing stimuli. This continues, often over several sessions, until the client has demonstrated the ability to remain calm when confronting the highest level of anxiety-producing stimuli.

4. The clinician then assists the client in seeking out *in vivo* situations that are similar to those above, during which they can practice relaxation while confronting situations that previously provoked anxiety.

## IATP Narrative Exposure Therapy (CR)

> **Time required:** A previous session with a 15–30-minute set-up and a second 50-minute session or the full process can be completed in a 90-minute session.
>
> **Materials required:** Handouts for Graphic Timeline (GTL) Written Narrative and Pictorial Narrative, paper and pencil for therapist.
>
> **Indications for use:** Use when the primary need is to enhance behavioral coping skills in Phase II: Working Through Trauma of trauma recovery.
>
> **Counterindications:** Actively dissociating or dissociates during exercise. Client must clearly have the ability to self-soothe and self-rescue.

This unique treatment procedure developed by Gentry (2012) for the International Association of Trauma Professionals (IATP) synthesizes several cognitive-behavioral techniques that have generated robust evidence for their effectiveness with trauma survivors. This method contains elements of cognitive processing therapy, eye-movement desensitization and reprocessing, prolonged exposure, traumatic incident reduction, and time-limited treatment for trauma and dissociation. It is a highly structured process designed to help survivors quickly and effectively confront and desensitize the painful intrusive and anxiety symptoms associated with PTSD. It is a simple, quick, and easy-to-utilize framework that allows trauma survivor clients to achieve immediate resolution of their trauma memories through constructing and sharing narratives of these experiences. It is a nonabreactive method that minimizes the discomfort and fear associated with many exposure methods, and has been utilized by hundreds of trauma therapists globally to help their clients heal from their traumatic pasts.

IATP narrative exposure therapy (NET) utilizes five separate narrative procedures (i.e., the survivor sequences and then shares the micro-experiences that occurred during a trauma) – Graphic Timeline Narrative, Written Narrative, Pictorial Narrative, Verbal Narrative, and Recursive Narrative. This five-narrative process is conducted in a single session that requires an additional 15–30-minute set-up in a previous session or a 90-minute session, during which all processes can be completed. When a survivor completes these five processes, they will have successfully confronted and navigated through their memories of the traumatic event: the memories from which they have most likely been avoiding since the time of the trauma. This is a gentle, thorough, and rapid procedure for helping survivors gain immediate mastery for processing a traumatic memory. It is also an effective treatment for trauma phobia, which is sometimes more difficult to treat than the trauma itself.

The primary reason the IATP NET method works well is that it requires both the client and the therapist to understand and be skilled in self-regulation (see Phase I exercises in this book). The ability of the client to monitor and regulate their level of arousal is required and one of the primary tasks of the therapist during an IATP NET session is to monitor the survivor's arousal level, not allowing the autonomic nervous system to become dysregulated during the session. This is done conjunctively with facilitating the completion of each of the five narrative processes. In essence, the session is an hour-long exposure to the traumatic material – by constructing and sharing narratives – while maintaining a relaxed body. This reciprocal inhibition process is an active ingredient in all evidence-based trauma treatments. However, no other treatment dedicates as much time, effort, and as many resources to give survivors the ability to recognize when their nervous system is overcharged and then provides them with the necessary tools to master the skills of self-regulation than does IATP NET. IATP NET requires that each survivor, prior to engaging in this treatment protocol, has completed the following: (a) understands how their nervous system – including brain functioning – reacts to perceived threats; (b) develops an appreciation for the constant confrontation of perceived threats in the their lives (and how this threat matrix is elevated for trauma

survivors); (c) demonstrates the ability to keep their body regulated and relaxed when confronting perceived threats, both imaginal and *in vivo*; and (d) successfully completes the Phase I: *Safety and Stabilization* of treatment. With this criterion met, the survivor is now ready to confront their traumatic memories without becoming overwhelmed or re-traumatized. Successfully developing this knowledge and skill set is at the core of IATP NET and, when done correctly, allows the clinician to be confident in their ability to help survivors confront, navigate through, and desensitize trauma memories with minimal pain, fear, and resistance.

## Delivery of Approach

### Preparation

There is printable handout material available for this exercise; see Using the Tools 22. Before beginning the IATP NET protocol with a client, they must have completed the Phase I: *Safety and Stabilization of trauma treatment. There are many components to this phase of treatment – too many to enumerate here. However, the following tasks must be completed before moving forward with the IATP NET:*

- Survivor is in no immediate physical danger in the present or near future
- Survivor has stable living arrangements and is able to complete activities of daily living
- Survivor understands rudimentary processes of the autonomic nervous system
  - SNS vs. PNS; SNS activation in context of perceived threat
  - Diminished functioning with SNS dominance
  - Trauma = increased perceived threat = increased autonomic dysregulation
  - Stress = SNS dominance
  - ANS is regulated when the body is relaxed
- Survivor learns and demonstrates competency in self-regulation (i.e., ability to keep body relaxed while confronting perceived threat both *in vivo* and imaginal)
- A "good enough" therapeutic relationship has been established and is continuing to be enhanced through a feedback-informed process
- Survivor understands current distress experienced from historical trauma is the eruption of nonverbal memories encoded during the time of the trauma
- Survivor further understands that to resolve these intrusive and hyperarousal symptoms they will need to confront the past trauma and have enlisted the therapist to assist them with this work (as contrasted with therapist coercing the client to address traumatic material)

Once these conditions have been satisfied in the early sessions of the treatment trajectory (generally 4–6 sessions), the survivor is ready to transition to Phase II: *Working Through Trauma* of treatment and begin the IATP NET process.

### Graphic Timeline (GTL)

This model requires 30 minutes of preparation in a previous session to set up properly. As soon as your client has determined that they are ready to confront and resolve a trauma memory, then you should schedule this work for a subsequent session. During the final 30 minutes of the preparatory session, you will need to instruct your client on the procedure for creating a graphic timeline (GTL). Demonstrating this process with a mildly traumatic experience from your own life is an excellent way to teach this process. The important components of the GTL are the two endpoints (i.e., beginning and end). You will need to instruct and coach your client to make certain that they have solidly identified and recorded the beginning and end points of the trauma you will be working on within the next session. A good way to help your client identify the beginning point is to ask: *When was the first moment during this experience that you perceived threat? When did your arousal start to increase?* You should assist your client with inserting a vertical line on the left-hand side of the GTL that will represent the beginning.

Figure 9 is a graphic timeline with the beginning and end points of a motor vehicle accident one of the authors survived in 2004. The beginning point of this trauma for them was seeing, out of the corner of their eye, a small black Nissan coupe careening at an acute angle towards their vehicle. This startled the author and was the first moment that they perceived threat during this experience. Therefore, it becomes the beginning point of this trauma.

The figure also shows an endpoint (i.e., "EMT = OK"). The trauma part of this experience resolved for the author when the emergency team had taken their vital signs and reported that everything was normal. Even though they were taken to the hospital and had a couple of stitches as well as a CAT scan, the next 11 hours were not part of the trauma. These experiences were tedious and uncomfortable, but the fear and terror had resolved when the paramedics informed the author there were no significant injuries.

In this preparatory session we want to help our clients to circumscribe the trauma for narration to its essential micro-events. Sometimes clients start this process wanting to desensitize a memory that has multiple episodes (e.g., childhood sexual abuse). When these experiences are volunteered, I suggest working with one single episode somewhere in the middle of distress level when compared with the other memories of this trauma. I suggest approaching the more distressing episodes once the client has developed sufficient mastery of the process by working through one or two of the less anxiety-producing memories.

Some effective coaching statements to assist you and your client in identifying the endpoint are: *When was the first time during this experience that you knew you were not going to die? When did the intensity of this experience begin to diminish? When did you come back to yourself? When did you realize that this experience was not about you?* It is important that your client leave your office having a firm understanding and an articulated decision of the beginning and end of their trauma. These two endpoints provide the structure and containment for all that follows.

Contract with your client to complete the GTL by identifying all the significant micro-events of the trauma with vertical lines perpendicular to the horizontal timeline (see Figure 8). For micro-events that have a negative valence in the present, these lines will begin at the horizontal and will run downward toward –10. The lower the line goes, the more distressing this micro-event feels to the client in the present. Positive-feeling micro-events will begin at the horizontal and move upward toward +10.

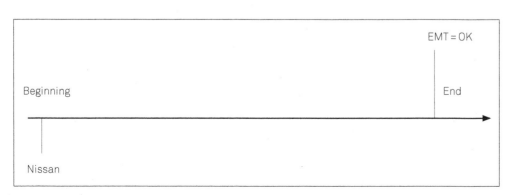

**Figure 9.**
Example of graphic timeline with endpoints.

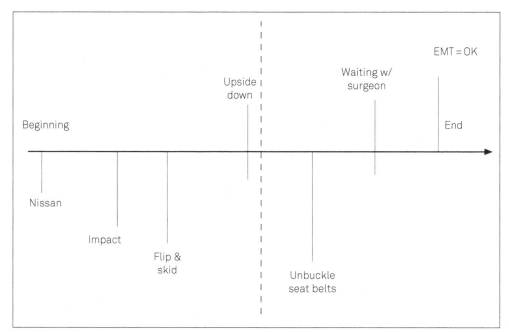

**Figure 10.**
Example of graphic timeline with micro-events and divider.

Offer your client the choice of coming in an hour before their scheduled appointment and completing the GTL in the waiting room just prior to meeting with you. If this is not possible, request that the client complete the GTL the evening before the scheduled session. The survivor should be cautioned not to begin working on the GTL until the 24-hour window before the next session. You do not want them to become overwhelmed with the traumatic material for several days before they see you. This can have significant negative effects on the outcome of your work to help your client confront, navigate through, and desensitize their trauma memory(ies). The template for the GTL can be found in Using the Tools 22.

This next session is highly structured in order to help the client navigate through their traumatic memories without becoming overwhelmed. This is achieved by monitoring your client's energy level throughout the session and intervening to help the client lessen arousal by softening muscles anytime you identify signs of dysregulation.

It is most effective to adopt an attitude of benign authority when facilitating this session; while you are preserving your warmth and empathy, you are also giving clear and unambiguous directions to your client throughout the session. The structure and pace of the day's session are as important as the content, so take a few moments before your client arrives to center yourself. Review your client's file and prepare yourself for this challenging session by relaxing your body and aligning with your intention.

Once your client has arrived in your office on the day of the intended desensitization and reprocessing session, begin immediately with the question, "Were you able to complete your GTL?" (This is one of the few sessions that the authors do not review the Subjective Units of Distress Scale with their clients at the beginning of the session).

If the client answers "yes," and produces the completed GTL worksheet, then move on to the Written Narrative exercise. If they were not able to complete the GTL worksheet - for any reason - this may be interpreted as a nonverbal communication that they are not ready to address the traumatic material. They have used behavioral language to indicate that they need a little more help. For the clients who do not show up with a completed GTL, ask them: "Do you still wish to work through this memory?" If they answer affirmatively, utilize the remainder of the session to coach them through constructing a GTL of the traumatic memory they've chosen to address. This usually takes 20-40 minutes. Once the GTL is completed, seal it in an envelope (see Drawing Icon and Envelope [Emotional Containment]) to hold for your client until their next appointment. At the start of the following session, open the envelope with your client and then continue to the next narrative procedure. If the client says they no longer wish to address and resolve the memory, thoroughly discuss the decision-making process they used to arrive at this choice. If, after this discussion, the client still chooses not to address the memory it is important to then collaboratively renegotiate treatment goals and agenda.

*Written Narrative*

Upon the client's arrival in your office, begin the scheduled work immediately. Do not allow yourself to become embroiled in preamble discussion, which often manifests due to both the client and therapist's anxiety about addressing the traumatic material. Every moment of this 50-minute session is vital so it is important to be intentional and optimize time management from the very beginning.

Once again, act in a benignly authoritative manner throughout the session. Foster a sense of warmth and connection with your client while being directive and unambiguous when introducing and managing the therapeutic tasks.

The first direction of the session is to ask the client to find the "geographic middle" of their timeline and draw a vertical dotted line bisecting the line into two equidistant halves.

With this accomplished, provide the client with instructions for the completion of the Written Narrative. Begin by providing your client with a clipboard that has on it the template for the Written Narrative (see Using the Tools 22). Then say something like the following:

*Start at the beginning of the GTL and write the story to the middle line, using as much detail as possible. Take 5 minutes to write a narrative of the events from the beginning to the middle. It is extremely important that you keep your body relaxed while you are doing this writing. If you allow your muscles to clench and remain constricted, you are potentially retraumatizing yourself. Conversely, as you keep your muscles relaxed you are healing this trauma right here and now.*

About every 90 seconds while the client is writing the therapist can prompt the client to remain relaxed ("keep your body relaxed" or "soften your muscles"). The therapist should not interrupt the client's writing unless the client begins to show signs of dysregulation (e.g., bouncing leg, fidgeting, tremors, etc.). If the therapist sees the survivor exhibit outward signs of sympathetic activation, the first step should be a nonverbal audible deep breath. Most clients will respond to this cue by relaxing their bodies and, with intention, decrease their arousal level. However, for those clients who do not respond to the nonverbal cueing, a direct intervention from the therapist is required (i.e., "Jennifer, notice your body right now and go ahead and soften your muscles... excellent... now continue writing.")

NOTE: This protocol works well to both resolve traumatic stress and lessen the phobic relationship most survivors have with their trauma history. What makes this procedure such an effective and safe way for survivors to process their trauma is the therapist's ability to assist their clients in maintaining a regulated autonomic nervous system throughout the session. Helping clients remain relaxed while confronting the nonverbal and affective elements of their trauma history creates for them a pathway to desensitize and resolve trauma memories with minimal discomfort and maximal mastery. When a client is able to retain this regulation while confronting their trauma, they complete the session knowing they have the capacity to address additional trauma successfully. This knowledge will significantly lessen the survivor's aversion to working through their traumatic history. For these reasons, it is imperative that the therapist develop the capacity to monitor their client's motor functioning for any signs of dysregulation and be prepared to intervene and help the survivor reestablish a relaxed body while confronting the traumatic material.

At the conclusion of the 5-minute period, the therapist should say, "Put your pen down and look at me." It is important to maintain fidelity to the time constraints of this session, so you will have enough time to complete the important debriefing process with the client at the end of the session. Allowing a client to go beyond the circumscribed time frame for each exercise will compromise the integrity of the protocol, potentially derailing the effectiveness of this procedure. However, if the client completes the exercise before the conclusion of the allotted time, simply move on to the next task of the session.

When this procedure was initially developed in 2004, the Written Narrative component was a 10-minute exercise, and clients were asked to write the entire narrative of the traumatic experience in that time frame. Many survivors became overwhelmed during this 10-minute time frame, compromising their ability to sustain exposure to the traumatic material while remaining relaxed. The protocol was then changed, separating the Written Narrative into two five-minute components, lessening the dose of exposure for the client. A 2–3-minute intermission was placed in between the two segments, allowing for a brief period of time for the therapist to coach the client through a short relaxation protocol (Hands-behind-the-head diaphragmatic breathing works well here). Upon completion of the intermission, say to your client: "Now, pick up your pen and complete writing the story from the mid-point to the end."

After five minutes of writing, during which the therapist remains vigilant for any autonomic dysregulation and provides cues for continued relaxation, the same

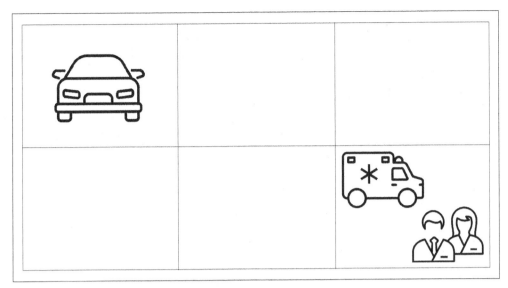

**Figure 11.**
Example of Pictorial Narrative with beginning and endpoints.

concluding direction as from the first writing exercise is given: "Put your pen down and look at me."

*Pictorial Narrative*

At this time (about 15 minutes into the session), the survivor has completed two narratives – the GTL and the Written Narrative. The client is not likely feeling better as a result of completing these narratives, but instead may be feeling worse. There is little, if any, relief in the *construction of narratives but in order for the survivor to obtain the relief that comes with the sharing of their traumatic material, it is necessary for them to, with your help and support, construct these thorough and succinct narratives.*

The next treatment activity in the IATP NET session is yet another narrative construction, albeit probably the most important one. With the completion of the Written Narrative, have a template for the Pictorial Narrative (see

Using the Tools 22) ready to give to your client. As soon as the client completes the previous exercise, slide the template onto your client's clipboard.

Then instruct the client to take the next 10 minutes to complete the Pictorial Narrative by drawing six pictures that tell the story they have just written. The same instructions for the GTL apply to this narrative – clients should first draw the micro-event that began this traumatic experience (i.e., the first time that the client perceived threat) in the upper left box. Follow this with a drawing portraying the end of the traumatic experience (i.e., the first time the client became aware that they were going to survive this experience) in the lower right-hand box of the template (see Figure 11).

When finished drawing the beginning and the endpoint, the client is to then complete the middle four drawings, creating a sequential six-picture narrative of the trauma (see Figure 12). Reassure your client that this is

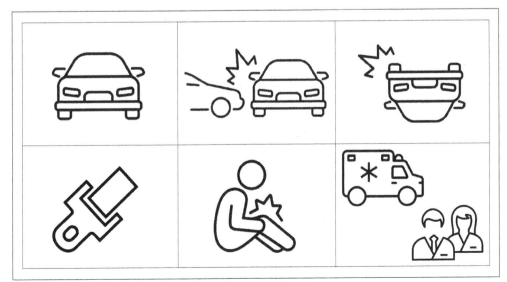

**Figure 12.**
Example of completed Pictorial Narrative.

therapy and not art class! They can draw stick people, stick houses, stick dogs, and stick cars. The quality of the drawings is not important, but the process of drawing visual representations is extremely important. The drawing process will likely elicit nonverbal memories of the trauma more readily than verbal methods. Remind your client to maintain a relaxed body while they are completing the drawings. If your client completes the drawings in less than 10 minutes, move forward to the verbal narrative portion of the session.

### Verbal Narrative

The Verbal Narrative is the centerpiece of the IATP NET Method. It is, in essence, an opportunity for your client to tell and to hear the story of their traumatic memory, as well as to be heard, probably for the very first time. It utilizes the Pictorial Narrative as a storyboard, allowing your client to share their trauma narrative in an object-mitigated way. They can point to the pictures while telling you about the trauma without having to bear the weight of looking at you during this difficult time. Completing these activities will be challenging enough for most survivors, and using pictures to help them navigate through the telling of their story makes it a little easier for them.

Once the client has completed the Pictorial Narrative, the therapist asks, "May I approach you?" With permission granted, the therapist moves to the side of the survivor (never directly in front) and says: "Using your pictures, would you please tell me the story... please remember to keep your body relaxed." While listening, remain warm, empathetic, and most of all, quiet! There is no need to ask clarifying questions, summarize, or paraphrase. Simply listen in a relaxed and resonant way until your client has completed the narrative. The only interruption to your client's Verbal Narrative would be if you notice any display of heightening anxiety (e.g., jumping leg, fidgeting in seat, wringing of hands, etc.). If you do notice your client becoming anxious, the first intervention should be nonverbal using an audible and exaggerated sigh. Most clients, if you have been diligent with the *Safety and Stabilization* phase of treatment, will recognize this cue and immediately reestablish a state of relaxation. However, if after this intervention your client is still exhibiting signs of dysregulation, say your clients name and then clearly remind your client to relax their body ("Jennifer, I am noticing your energy level seems to be increasing; take a second and get your body relaxed before continuing... excellent!").

It is common, during the Verbal Narrative, to see your clients beginning to come back to themselves. They frequently become brighter, more present, and less anxious or agitated as they complete this part of the session. Research has demonstrated that clients get little if any relief from constructing trauma narratives (i.e., journaling). However, they do experience significant lessening of trauma-related symptoms after sharing their narratives. This process of sharing within a safe relationship, such as therapy, is the most potent form of relief presently available for treating PTSD. Sharing narratives as a method of completing reciprocal inhibition (i.e., exposure + relaxation) is at the core of most effective treatments for PTSD.

### Recursive Narrative

This fifth and last narrative process is frequently the most impactful for the survivor. It involves a retelling of the survivor's narrative by the therapist, using third person perspective and language. As soon as the survivor has completed the verbal narrative say something like, "*Thank you. It was an honor to receive that.*" Follow immediately by asking, "*May I see your pictures?*" Then take the pictures from the survivor and turn them around so that the survivor can see the pictures. After this, begin the narrative by saying, "*When _____ (survivor's name) was __ years old they had the experience of _____ (name trauma)."* The therapist invites the survivor to correct any mistakes, add any omissions, or to insert any additional details that may be omitted. The therapist continues the story, using the pictures as a storyboard, until the narrative is complete.*

Once again, during the Recursive Narrative, monitor the client's energy level and body language, intervening if the client exhibits a spike in arousal. As before, this can most often be accomplished by simply taking an exaggeratedly deep breath with an audible exhale. Most clients will respond to this cue by relaxing the tension in their bodies.

### Session Closure

Utilize the few minutes remaining at the conclusion of the session to process how your client experienced the session and what insights they developed throughout the process. Inform the client that they may have some intrusive thoughts or feelings relating to today's work for the next 24–48 hours. Let them know that this is normal. Assure the survivor they will begin to experience a significant lessening of the symptoms associated with this memory during the next week. Survivors should be encouraged to utilize their support networks, engage in healthy activities (eating right, exercise, sleep), and journal their thoughts over the next week. It is important to be sure your client has regained full utility of their neocortical functioning before leaving the office (one procedure helpful in accomplishing this is having the survivor count backwards from 100 by 7s).

## USING THE TOOLS 22

### IATP NET Checklist

#### Preparation

☐ Client is safe
☐ Client can determine difference between "being safe" and "feeling safe"
☐ Client can self-regulate/keep body relaxed when confronted with memories of the trauma
☐ Client has menu of skills for relaxation, containment, grounding, and expression
☐ Client has been instructed in the procedure for constructing a GTL Line of their trauma (15–30 min)

#### Session

☐ Client presents with completed GTL
☐ Client completes vertical line bisecting GTL
☐ Written Narrative Part 1 (5 min)
☐ Intermission (Diaphragmatic Breathing)
☐ Written Narrative Part 2 (5 min)
☐ Pictorial Narrative (10 min)
☐ Verbal Narrative (10 min)
☐ Recursive Narrative (5–7 min)
☐ Closure (5–10 min)
☐ Client maintains relaxed body throughout session

#### IATP NET Handouts

1. Graphic Timeline Template (GTL)
2. Written Narrative Template
3. Pictorial Narrative Template

**USING THE TOOLS 22:**
IATP NET Checklist

**Graphic Timeline**

+10 Positive

Beginning                                                                                    End

−10 Negative

From: Anna B. Baranowsky & J. Eric Gentry, *Trauma Practice: A Cognitive Behavioral Somatic Therapy* (4th ed.). © 2023 Hogrefe Publishing

## Written Narrative

First Half

_____

_____

_____

_____

_____

_____

_____

_____

_____

_____

_____

_____

_____

Second Half

_____

_____

_____

_____

_____

_____

_____

_____

_____

_____

_____

_____

_____

From: Anna B. Baranowsky & J. Eric Gentry, *Trauma Practice: A Cognitive Behavioral Somatic Therapy* (4th ed.). © 2023 Hogrefe Publishing

## Pictorial Narrative

# 4. Emotion/Relation

Survivors of traumatic events have often spent a lifetime struggling with strong emotions and people pleasing to avoid any conflict. This diminishes skilled coping with emotions and less than satisfying relationships. The following techniques focus on skills for navigating strong emotions as well as engaging in more satisfying human relations.

## Learning to Be Sad (CR)

> **Time required:** One to several sessions.
>
> **Materials required:** None.
>
> **Indications for use:** When one needs to feel sad.
>
> **Counterindications:** Inability to actively self-soothe.

This exercise is adapted with permission from *A Language of the Heart Workbook* (Schultz, 2005, 2016). It is especially useful when used in conjunction with the Creating a Nonanxious Presence technique. As in that technique, the first part is primarily psychoeducational, giving clients a different understanding of the meaning of sadness. It is not a replacement for trauma reduction techniques and, in fact, relates more to the everyday feelings we all must process. However, it is a very powerful technique that has the ability to elicit unprocessed and sometimes unremembered trauma and the feelings associated with it. Therefore, this technique should be done during sessions the first few times to ensure the client has the self-soothing abilities to manage this unprocessed trauma and hold it for processing in session.

### Delivery of Approach

There is printable handout material available for this exercise; see Using the Tools 23. Clients quickly recognize that their fear of sadness is one of the biggest blocks to their doing the work necessary for recovery. As they proceed in recovery, they begin reflecting on things they have managed to push outside of their consciousness for a long while. They actually begin to feel the sadness, dejection, disappointment, aloneness, or abandonment from these past experiences. And this is what they should do about that: nothing! That, however, requires a bit of explaining. Dr. Schultz uses the following script when preparing clients for this technique.

## USING THE TOOLS 23

### Sadness Script

What we have been doing all along when we become sad is "something." We have been taught since we were children that it was not okay to be sad. We were called a "baby" and told to "grow up," or to "get over it," to "quit your crying," or (my favorite), "quit your crying or I'll give you something to cry about." This leads us to find ways to "stuff" away or shut down our sadness. We deny, cover up, run, distract ourselves, get busy, drink, work, play, get angry, whatever it takes to stuff it. And the problem with stuffing our sadness is that it does not go away. It piles up. Soon the pile is so big we're afraid if we ever touch it, it will come roaring out and never stop. It will flood us, drown us, or leave us dead or dying. And so, we shut it down.

The truth about sadness is that although it feels as if we will die or be overwhelmed by it, we actually will not. But we have to learn how to be sad – how to be sad without becoming reactive, doing something to "stuff" our sadness. Why, you ask, would someone want to do that? Because sadness is a normal, natural emotion. Sadness is about loss: loss of childhood, loss of innocence, loss of love, loss of relationship, loss of control, etc. Sadness has a unique ability to change a painful experience of loss into information about what is useful, important, and valuable or about what is not useful, not important, and not valuable in the choosing of our own behaviors. If we allow ourselves to feel our sadness all the way to the end of it (and there is a beginning, a middle, and an end), it will change the experience into information, and we will be better able to choose our own behaviors to avoid unnecessary harm to ourselves and others. In other words, sadness has the ability to change pain into wisdom. If we stop our sadness from running its course, we just manage to restuff it and never really learn the lessons.

We have this story that we tell ourselves. It is "our" story, about our life. It contains all of the experiences we have that we can think about that define us and tell us who we are. We tell others some of the story, but mostly it is a personal story. When we have painful experiences that we cannot think about because they are too painful and we have not grieved them, the experiences never have an opportunity to take their place in our stories. They never have an opportunity to inform us what is useful, important, and valuable or not useful, not important, and not valuable about what we experienced. Therefore, these experiences cannot provide us direction as we choose our own behaviors. When we allow ourselves to feel sadness all the way to the end, these experiences get to take their rightful place in our stories and we become wiser.

Consequently, the question is, "How do you treat yourself when you are sad?" Is this difficult to answer? If you have children (even imaginary ones), you might ask, "How do I treat my children when they are sad?" As it turns out, one of the best things we can do for our children is teach them how to be sad. Here is how: mostly by doing nothing! Of course, we make sure they are safe and loved, but then we should do nothing. We should just hold them. We should be kind and patient. We should not try to distract them from their sadness, tell them it is okay, tell them it is not important, give them an ice cream cone, or tell them to quit crying. We should just be with them. We might reassure them that they are loved. We might acknowledge their sadness and suggest that sometimes the world is a sad place. We might tell them we will be sad with them while they are sad because sometimes we are sad, too. Often, when this happens, children begin to open up about what they are feeling. They will tell you amazing little details about what they are worried about or what they have been sad about in the past. And this is what you should do: nothing. It is important to simply acknowledge this information. Do not try to fix it. Do not tell them it is nothing to worry about. Just acknowledge it. Your job is to be a witness. If you do not react to their sadness by shutting it down, when they are finished being sad they will usually get up and go play.

And this is how you learn to be sad with yourself: be kind and patient – with yourself. Do not listen to those words in the back of your head that say "grow up," "get over it," etc. Just be sad – without reacting to distract yourself. With permission, you may sob. Your tears may fall. Your nose may run. And this may last a day, a week, a month, or more. You may have weird thoughts and odd memories come up. If you are lucky enough to have a significant other who will hold you, ask them to not try to do anything to fix it. Just allow yourself to be sad. Eventually, you will come to the end of it. When you do, you will know it. You will feel strangely empty and light – as if a 5-ton weight had been lifted from your shoulders – and also sad. Oddly, you will also feel happy.

From: Anna B. Baranowsky & J. Eric Gentry, *Trauma Practice: A Cognitive Behavioral Somatic Therapy* (4th ed.). © 2023 Hogrefe Publishing

**USING THE TOOLS 23:**
Sadness Script

Have you ever tried to sit on a beach ball in a swimming pool, trying to keep the beach ball completely under water? It takes lots of concentration and energy to struggle with the ball, and it always seems to find its way back to the surface. Eventually you get tired of the game but the beach ball does not. Keeping your sadness from coming up into your consciousness requires tremendous concentration and energy; yet, like the beach ball, it seems to find its way to the surface much too often.

What if you let the air out of your beach ball of sadness? Then you could spend that energy doing something you really wanted to do – like feeling good about yourself.

This does not mean you will never be sad again. Sadness is a constantly recurring emotion. In fact, a friend of mine thinks we may be sad as often as 10 or 15 times per day. We usually work harder, play harder, watch more television, drink more, or eat more to distract ourselves. However, when you learn to be sad when it is time to be sad, you then can get on with your life without carrying the burden of that huge bag of sadness and have more energy left over to do the things you really want to do. As you learn to be sad without reacting, you realize how often old sadness and fear from your past has dictated your behaviors.

This technique is somewhat unusual because you are being asked to allow yourself to feel things you have possibly pushed out of your awareness for a long time. If you experienced significant traumatic events in your childhood that are unresolved through personal work and/or therapy, this exercise has the potential of eliciting very strong emotions. Monitor yourself. Feeling completely overwhelmed is a good indication that you need to work on self-soothing skills. Talk with your therapist about how to more effectively accomplish that.

**The Sadness Exercise**

For this exercise, you are asked to make an agreement with yourself to do nothing other than sit and be curious. You may stop anytime you wish, especially if you are feeling overwhelmed. However, while you are doing the exercise, you should not do anything to avoid the feelings other than a self-soothing technique such as Creating a Nonanxious Presence. You should also make an agreement with yourself to not make any decisions about the information you think about. In other words, you may come to conclusions and think you need to go fix something right away. I suggest that you wait before you make any big decisions. When information comes up, just sit with it and let it process. Most of the things that arise will be old stuff. So just let it come up and witness it. Allow yourself to feel the perhaps long forgotten sadness associated with it. This exercise is not meant to affix blame or point fingers. It is a process by which you finally assimilate your past experiences and allow yourself to move forward.

To begin, find a comfortable place to sit where you will not be interrupted for an hour or two. This is very important. Schedule a specific amount of time to do this exercise. Make an agreement with yourself that you will do this exercise for exactly 1 hour or exactly 2 hours. You may even want to set a timer. Try to hold fairly exactly to this time frame. You will have plenty of time to do this exercise again. Do not imagine that you will get completely to the bottom of things in one sitting. Scheduling a specific amount of time and not exceeding it is a way for you to control what may, at first, seem overwhelming. This does not have to overwhelm you. It will, however, be emotional. Also, make sure to plan an additional hour after the exercise to relax. You will probably need a little additional relaxation time when you have finished.

Take some time to relax and breathe. Try to feel your connection to the earth. Give yourself permission to think about whatever comes up and feel whatever emotions arise with those thoughts. Make an agreement with yourself that your intent is to just witness what you have inside, not to "do" anything about it. Your goal is to begin to review your life and identify those experiences that left you feeling bad about yourself or sad. You may want to start by walking through your life year by year from earliest memories to more recent memories. Another possibility is to pick a movie you found especially difficult to watch because it made you emotional. Notice, especially, those areas where you might initially think you were just angry. Underneath the anger is, invariably, sadness. Make a space inside yourself for all of the emotions that might arise. Try not to reject any thought or emotion that comes up. Welcome these thoughts and emotions as information about how you came to think about yourself the way you do and how you came to behave to protect your heart.

From: Anna B. Baranowsky & J. Eric Gentry, *Trauma Practice: A Cognitive Behavioral Somatic Therapy* (4th ed.). © 2023 Hogrefe Publishing

This is not necessarily a pleasant experience at first. It sometimes may feel like a roller coaster out of control. Emotions will well up and come flooding out. Eventually, you may find yourself tearful or even sobbing. This is very important: do not judge yourself. If you are tearful, it does not mean that you are broken, bad, weak, stupid, or a baby. The stuff that is coming up is the stuff you have been hiding from your whole life. Be kind and gentle with yourself. Insist that you think of yourself with respect and dignity.

The best thing you can do when these emotions arise is keep your belly soft. Do a self-soothing technique such as Creating a Nonanxious Presence again and again. Breathe slowly and deeply and relax your belly. Keep your neocortex functioning. Remember where you are (in the here and now) at all times. Check that you are safe. Allow yourself the right to be as sad as you need to be. Do not expect that you will solve all of your problems. Just relax and let whatever comes up come up.

The next step is very important. At the end of your allotted time, stop the exercise. Do not let it extend beyond your agreed-upon allotted time. You will always have time to come back and do it again. Take some time to fully ground yourself to the here and now. Take several slow, deep breaths. Open your eyes, if they are closed, and look around you. Relax your belly. Congratulate yourself for the courageous work you just accomplished. You will probably be somewhat to very tired. This is because you have just done some very difficult work. Take the next hour or so to relax. Treat yourself. Take a nap or a walk or try a nice bath or shower. Do whatever you like to just wind down. Do not, however, drink alcohol or caffeine or turn on the television. Allow yourself to decompress as slowly and naturally as possible.

Notice the language you are using with yourself. Did you immediately drop back into the old habit of scolding yourself for being weak? It is not true. Relax your belly. Remember, you gave yourself permission to do this. Some people report this to be a very difficult exercise because they are not used to letting go. Not only are they telling themselves that it is not okay, they are reminding themselves of what their friends and loved ones would say if they heard or saw them. This would be a very good time to work on your self-validation. This is your opportunity to let the air out of the beach ball. Your friends and loved ones may not understand that, so how can they have an opinion about what you are doing? You do not have to please them to accomplish this goal. In fact, take this as your first opportunity to be healthy for your own sake rather than someone else's.

Come back to this exercise as often as you like. You may find that you spontaneously begin to process sad information. Good! The object is to keep it flowing through you like water through a hose. You will find that once you give yourself permission to be sad, it will happen more often. However, now when it happens, it will not be nearly so painful and objectionable. We are sad every day – sometimes very sad, sometimes a little sad. Do not stuff it. Learn what it has to teach you.

There is only one follow-up question. Ask yourself, "What did I learn about that is important?" The insights you will get from doing the exercise will come for a significant amount of time after you have done it. You will have "aha!" experiences that seem to just pop into your mind that will help you understand significant pieces of your past and the pasts of those around you. Remain curious and keep your belly soft.

From: Anna B. Baranowsky & J. Eric Gentry, *Trauma Practice: A Cognitive Behavioral Somatic Therapy* (4th ed.). © 2023 Hogrefe Publishing

## Assertiveness Training (CR)

> **Time required:** One to several sessions.
>
> **Materials required:** None.
>
> **Indications for use:** Use when the primary need is to enhance cognitive and emotional coping skills in Phase II: Working Through Trauma of trauma recovery.
>
> **Counterindications:** Inability to actively self-soothe.

There are some basic principles of Assertiveness Training that are covered in most books. Primarily, individuals are assisted in achieving a sense of their rights and an ability to clearly state their wants, needs, and desires. Individuals are encouraged to move from "suffering in silence" to identifying unsatisfying situations or those that clearly violate our basic rights. With this knowledge, individuals are empowered to respond in a new and more personally gratifying manner to meet their own needs.

### Delivery of Approach

Common tips include:
- Clearly state what you want, need, or prefer.
- Use "I" statements to declare negative emotions and dissatisfaction.
- Receive compliments simply with "thank you." Self-depreciating statements and other qualifiers are not required.
- Pose questions to tradition or authority when you are not satisfied with just going along.
- Share personal experiences, opinions, and feelings with confidence. Your viewpoint counts.
- Resolve frustrations and minor irritations before they escalate into major catastrophes and explosions of anger.
- Say no when you mean no. Saying yes will lead to feelings of resentment.
- Look at your own family of origin to identify where your submissive tendency developed.

There are many excellent resources on Assertiveness Training, including items found easily on the internet through any search engine. Try https://www.mentalhelp.net for a starting point.

Practicing each of the tips above can assist clients in taking "assertiveness" from the clinician's office to their personal life.

## Thematic Map and Release (CR – RE – R)

Developed by Dr. Anna Baranowsky for the trauma practice approach

> **Time required:** 40–90 minutes.
>
> **Materials required:** Scripts & TMR Templates.
>
> **Indications for use:** Use when the primary need is to enhance cognitive and emotional coping skills in Phase II: Working through Trauma of trauma recovery.
>
> **Counter indications:** Inability to actively self-soothe.

We gain access to trauma stories that our clients share by asking the right questions and establishing a sense of therapeutic alliance or trust so that the individual feels able to share in session. However, at times we cannot seem to get access to the root of the distress, even when we have worked on the trauma memories or multiple previously unresolved critical incidents. Pulling back the layers we often find that, as a result of life experiences, we develop belief systems or themes that we carry along with us that are very hard to shake. The DSM-V diagnostic criterion for PTSD - negative alterations of cognition and mood - capture this well and reinforce need to address how beliefs are shaped and embedded after trauma. The Thematic Map & Release exercise was developed to better access how trauma shapes negative and rigid beliefs.

If we are unable to learn to become a compassionate observer of this content, we may forever remain disturbed by beliefs that no longer serve us in life.

In this section, you will find a scripted approach to access the theme as well as to guide the client through a step-by-step approach for learning to sit with and work through belief systems borne out of a trauma history. Rather than addressing any single trauma, the focus here is to identify the conclusions or themes that we carry with us. A theme may be many things (i.e., Nobody loves me; I am a bad person; I am always in danger, etc.)

### Delivery of Approach

TMR is designed to help clients get unstuck from negative beliefs. Even after resolving traumatic memories individuals can suffer from limiting beliefs that can keep them stuck for a lifetime. Using the powerful TMR approach you can identify and work through negative thoughts and cognitions.

When working with a client you will need to use the TMR scripts and template (Using the Tools 24). This is a more complex intervention and it requires time to explain to the client and gain permission prior to beginning. TMR often takes a full 40–90 minutes and should be started at the beginning of the session. It is often useful to set this up by capturing the theme and explaining the approach in the previous meeting. You will also need to demonstrate some of the activities prior to beginning to familiarize the individual with the steps. In addition, providing some understanding of the mechanisms behind the intervention may aid in client buy-in.

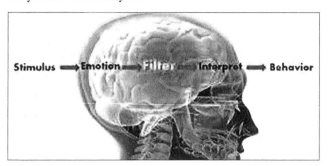

Stimulus ➡ Emotion ➡ Filter ➡ Interpret ➡ Behavior

 **Script: Introduction to TMR**

- In this exercise we will focus on the emotionally driven thematic result of traumatic or difficult life events rather than on a specific trauma.
- The best way to identify what to focus on is to reflect on either the thematic results of a trigger list that we have worked on or a core belief or a negative conclusion that troubles you (i.e., I am never safe, etc.)
- I will walk you through each step of this exercise and you will not need to remember the sequence.
- You might have noticed that when you think about something you might look up or down to right or left. You might notice other people doing this as well. For the purposes of this exercise, we will assume that in doing so we are accessing or gathering some type of information (i.e., past memory, anticipated fear, anxious feelings, hopes, thoughts). We will call those attempts to access information by looking in various directions as "focus points." *[For more information, see section Research-Based Assumptions About Eye Movements.]*
- In this approach we will deliberately try to access different types of information by engaging your focus on various points – being open and willing to allow whatever surfaces without judgment or suppression when pointing our gaze on that focus point.
- You will be instructed to gaze at a number of different focus points in a pre-established pattern *[show template with focus points to explain]*.
- During the gazing strategy your job is to just let anything associated with the theme we identify as your starting point … then let your mind become aware of emotions, thoughts, and body sensations associated with that focus point. You will hold the focus point for 30–60 seconds and then close your eyes.
- The next step is to let emotions, thoughts, and body sensations surface with your eyes closed and when asked, express what you are aware of when holding that focus point.
- Finally, we will work on the release portion of the exercise before moving onto the next focus point in the sequence.

## Script: Imagery Preparation

- The release portion of this exercise will require you to use your mind to open up your imagination
- I will explain how the imagination release exercise works before we start – if you would like to proceed, please let me know and you can choose your preferred imagery focus (either sand or light). *[See Sand Imagery and Light Imagery description below:]*
- You can choose the type of imagery to use throughout the exercise. *[There are two examples below, but I have also used "breeze" "leaves", etc.]*
- Would you like to proceed, or do you have any other questions? *[If yes, proceed or respond to questions as needed before proceeding or selecting a different approach, if the client does not consent.]*
- Is it ok to try out the imagery portion of this exercise? *[If yes, begin with preferred imagery below.]*

### Sand Imagery

You may have been to a place where there is a sandy beach or you can imagine the feeling of warm sand in your hands even if you have not been to a beach on a warm day ... can you try that now? It is easier to picture this if you have your eyes closed/or your eyes can be focused downward and gently unfocused, if you prefer ... is that ok? [if yes, begin].

Continue focusing inside and use your mind to open up your imagination ... start by holding your hands open resting lightly on your lap ... picture that you have a hand full of warm sand. The sand is warming the center of the palms of your hands. The sensation of warmth and heaviness is deeply soothing on your hands ... it moves through to your fingertips and upward toward your arms and shoulders. It feels soothing and warming. Picture that the sand is slowly spilling between your fingers down and away from you.

Now imagine that you are an empty vessel ... again, focus inwardly and let your imagination help you with this. Picture that warm soothing sand is filling up slowly from the top of your head, front of your face, back of head, down your neck, into your shoulders, back, chest, arms hands and through to your fingertips ... where the sand spills out down and away from you ... the warm sand continues to fill in from the top of your head, into the core of your body, down to your lower back, stomach, legs, thighs, knees, shins, calves, feet, through to the tips of your toes and fingertips where the sand spills out down and away from you.

### Light Imagery

With your eyes closed or your eyes softly looking down (if you prefer) use your mind to open up your imagination ... start by holding your hands open ... resting lightly on your lap. Imagine you are holding a large ball made out of light in the center of the palms of your hands. The ball is comfortably warm and heavy. Feel the weight and the warmth in the center of the palms of your hands. Sense the feelings of warmth and heaviness move into your hands, up your arms and into your shoulders. Feel this as a soothing sensation. Then imagine the light spills between your slightly parted fingers, down and away ... releasing.

Now imagine that you are an empty vessel ... again, let your imagination help you with this. Picture that light is slowly moving in from the top of your head, front of your face, back of head, down your neck, into your shoulders, the back, chest, arms hands and through to your fingertips ... where the light spills out down and away from you ... the light continues to fill in from the top of your head, into the core of your body, down to your lower back, stomach, legs, thighs, knees, shins, calves, feet, through to the tips of your toes and fingertips where the light spills out down and away from you.

- That's the starting point for the release exercise. I just want you to be able to work with this imagery as best as you can. You get better with it as we go along.
- I will also be asking you to use the release imagery to help you let go of emotions, thoughts, and body sensations associated with each focus point during this exercise as well.
- Remember, you will not need to recall any of the steps. I will guide you through the exercise each step of the way. Do you have any questions before we begin? Are you ok to begin this exercise? You can stop at anytime if you need a break, have any questions, or just need to stop for any reason.
- *[**If in an office setting with a client:** We will sit in a "ships passing in the night" arrangement – same as EMDR (2 chairs side by side – with forward chair legs at same parallel). **Or if on secure video session:** on screen direction will be provided.]*
- *[Clinician will use a pen or pointer to point out the focus point and hold it for the client.]*

**Script: Thematic Map & Release**

In TMR – we focus on very deliberate points to search for internal content:

- Thoughts
- Emotions
- Body sensations
- **Goal:** To access content that goes along with the themes/beliefs a person struggles with

**Steps summary**

1. Identify the theme or negative core belief – something that has been a negative driving force in life (i.e., I am unlovable)
2. Rate the theme or belief
3. Explain TMR and get permission to use
4. Watch the full/short TMR video
5. In order to assist you in developing this skill, we have included demonstration videos for you to review:
   - Long session demo video (Baranowsky, 2014a, November 3): see Video 27 in the supplementary material (or https://youtu.be/A9Lwly0hS2A)
   - Short session demo video (Baranowsky, 2014b, November 3): see Video 28 in the supplementary material (or https://youtu.be/GOafcmHQlZI)
- Remember, you will not need to recall any of the steps. I will guide you through the exercise each step of the way. Do you have any questions before we begin? Are you OK to begin this exercise? You can stop at anytime if you need a break, have any questions or just need to stop for any reason. Just let me know.
- *[If you receive approval begin, start with identifying the starting point … the Theme and SUDS level]*
- *[This is a Therapist Script and developed to help guide you in your client work with TMR.]* This is generally a thematic issue or negative conclusion or belief. This may be reinforced by many events from the past (i.e., life never works out for me, no one likes me, I will always be alone, etc.). Focusing on a theme vs. an event allows you to process through numerous events that might be related to a thematic belief system.
- *[Rate the theme on a Subjective Units of Distress Scale … SUDS (1 = neutral feeling – feels fine; 5 = sad/bad but can handle it; 10 = worst feelings of distress/upset).]*
- Now that you have identified the theme and rated it, let's begin with that and start with the focus point #1 (top right) … hold that focus point, hold that focus point and as you do allow whatever emotions, thoughts and body sensations associated with that focus point to surface … Try to be curious and interested rather than judgmental of what is arising. Just bear witness … being a compassionate observer of whatever surfaces and noticing without suppressing. Let emotions, thoughts and body sensations to surface – just noticing.
- Now close your eyes … and help me to understand what emotions, thoughts and body sensations are associated with that focus point … whatever you notice is fine … is helpful information for this exercise.
  - What emotions were you aware of … [clinician write out on template]
  - What thoughts were you aware of … [clinician write out on template]
  - What body sensations were you aware of … [clinician write out on template]
- *[Once you have gathered content from emotions/thoughts/body sensations … move on.]*
  - Keeping your eyes closed … we will begin the imagery part of this exercise. Bring your attention to your hands … rest your hands open on your lap and use your mind to harness your imagination.
  - Picture that you have a hand full of warm sand/large ball of light. The sand/light is warming the center of the palms of your hands. The sensation is soothing deeply into the hands … through to your fingertips and upward toward your arms and shoulders. Soothing and warming. Picture that the sand/light is dissolving and slowly spilling between your fingers down and away from you.
  - Now use that imagery to help you with the next part of this exercise to assist you in releasing.
  - Now imagine that you are an empty vessel, like an hourglass … again, let your imagination help you with this. Picture that warm soothing sand/light is filling in slowly from the top of your head … front of your face, back of head, down your neck, into your shoulders, the back, chest, arms hands and through to your fingertips …
  - Where the sand/light spills out down and away from you … the warm sand/light continues to fill into the core of your body, down to your lower back, stomach, legs, thighs, knees, shins, calves, feet, through to the tips of your toes and fingertips where the sand/light spills out down and away from you …

- Begin to picture that the emotions, thoughts and body sensations associated with that focus point begin to attach to the grains of sand/light … the sand/light continues to fill in slowly from the top of your head …. And as it does it moves through the body and the sand/light continues to attach to the emotions, thoughts and body sensations attaching and allowing them to flow down through to your fingertips and toes down and away from you, releasing, letting go of whatever no longer serves you … release whatever you no longer need.
  - Just release as best as you can in this moment, even one tiny drop.
  - Finally, bring your awareness back into the room and just notice how you feel right now [clinician write out on template].
- [Continue through each of the focus points. Always start by referencing the starting Theme, as described by the client. Go through each of the 6 focus points, using the same script above.]
- [At **Focus Point 7**, use the final script below:]
  - Look straight ahead with a soft and unfocused gaze. Reflect on the theme that we started with "XXXX". How would you rate the SUDS now? [Capture this on the TMR Template.]
  - Still with a soft gaze, ask yourself, what you learned from this exercise? And also, what can you take home with you from this exercise – what would you like to capture and use going forward?
  - Finally, just notice how you feel right now and compare it to how you felt when you started this exercise [clinician write out on template]
- [Capture the SUDS rating for the theme one final time.]

## Concluding the Session

Upon conclusion of an EMDR session, many feel a sense of relief and that the traumatic material has qualitatively changed to become less frightening, more manageable, and relegated to the past. However, not all sessions end with resolution and some end with the client still in mild-to-moderate distress. In these cases, EMDR training provides several protocols for containment and amelioration of this distress (e.g., "EMDR Safe Place Exercise," or "Light Stream Technique") or you may consult Phase I Exercises from this text to find a more suitable technique.

It is also worth noting, from our anecdotal experience practicing EMDR, that a significant amount of processing occurs in the days following an EMDR session, For this reason it is important for the clinician to invite contact from an EMDR client should troubling material arise.

## Research-Based Assumptions About Eye Movements

While there has been a great deal of research into the mechanisms of EMDR (i.e., bilateral stimulation), there is still much conjecture as to how and why EMDR works so efficiently. We can add to the research findings on EMDR below that the treatment also elegantly delivers all four of the previously discussed active ingredients shared by all effective treatments (therapeutic relationship; relaxation/self-regulation; exposure; and cognitive restructuring/psychoeducation).

- The ability to search for information stored in long-term memory may have developed from already-existing neural systems that enable the search for information in the visual environment (Ehrlichman & Micic, 2012).
- Your eyes move when you try to gather all the words, equations, and pictures that make up a coherent picture of an idea/thought.
- Psychologists have found that gaze shifts occur to free up cognitive resources – particularly when deeper thinking is required.
- Bergstrom and Hiscock (1988) found that your eyes move more frequently for things in long-term memory rather than working memory.
- Eye movements facilitate thinking, memory, and other cognitive functions (Ehrlichman & Micic, 2021; Bergstrom & Hiscock, 1988).

## USING THE TOOLS 24

**Thematic Map and Release**

**Theme** _____ **SUDS** (begin) = _____

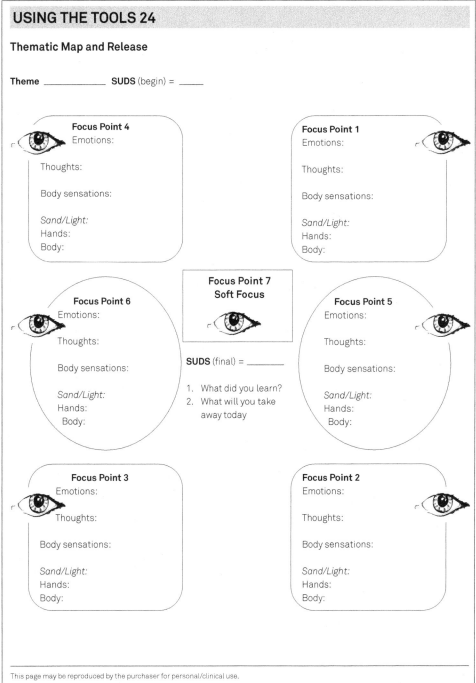

**Focus Point 4**
Emotions:

Thoughts:

Body sensations:

*Sand/Light:*
Hands:
Body:

**Focus Point 1**
Emotions:

Thoughts:

Body sensations:

*Sand/Light:*
Hands:
Body:

**Focus Point 6**
Emotions:

Thoughts:

Body sensations:

*Sand/Light:*
Hands:
 Body:

**Focus Point 7**
**Soft Focus**

**SUDS** (final) = _____

1. What did you learn?
2. What will you take
   away today

**Focus Point 5**
Emotions:

Thoughts:

Body sensations:

*Sand/Light:*
Hands:
 Body:

**Focus Point 3**
Emotions:

Thoughts:

Body sensations:

*Sand/Light:*
Hands:
Body:

**Focus Point 2**
Emotions:

Thoughts:

Body sensations:

*Sand/Light:*
Hands:
Body:

From: Anna B. Baranowsky & J. Eric Gentry, *Trauma Practice: A Cognitive Behavioral Somatic Therapy* (4th ed.). © 2023 Hogrefe Publishing

**USING THE TOOLS 24:**
Thematic Map and Release

# Grounding Lightstream (RE)

> **Time required:** 5–15 minutes.
>
> **Materials required:** None.
>
> **Indications for use:** Used when individual is experiencing a strong negative emotion and body felt sensation
>
> **Counterindications:** Physical exhaustion or when a greater focus on harnessing calm is required. This exercise can aid in stabilization but can also re-ignite some bodily felt distress.

The Grounding Lightstream exercise, adapted from eye movement desensitization and reprocessing (EMDR), is used to assist individuals who are experiencing a strong negative emotion and body felt sensation.

## Delivery of Approach

Instruct the participant to focus on an internal sensation of discomfort that exists in their body. If they don't feel anything right now, allow them to recall a time when they did, and allow the sensation to resurface just enough so that they're aware of it again. Continue to guide them through the exercise with the following questions:

- If the discomfort had a shape, what shape would it be?
- If the discomfort had a size, what size would it be?
- If the discomfort had a color, what color would it be?
- If the discomfort had a temperature, what temperature would it be? Hot or cold?
- If the discomfort had a texture, what texture would it be?
- If the discomfort had a sound, what sound would it make?

Instruct them to focus now on harnessing the power of their mind, and to open up their imagination. Picturing in their imagination, a soothing light coming down from above, and gently moving in, through the top of their head. This healing light is moving deeply in, and toward the discomfort in the body, wherever it lives.

Becoming aware of the color of the soothing light, and noticing that it is a different color than the source of their discomfort. This light feels healing and restorative to them, and it may even be their favorite color. Notice whether the light is warm or cool, and guide them to decide for themself what would feel best.

Using their imagination, picture the light coming in from above, through their head and into the body. Noticing that the light moves deeply into the shape that holds their discomfort, and just bearing witness with no judgement, as the light and the shape begin to move together. The light moves around the shape, shining through every inch of it. Noticing as it does this, what happens to the shape. Allow them to continue with this exercise watching the segment over and over again, until the shape begins to feel neutral. Or return to any of the earlier exercises to help them achieve this goal.

**WITH AUDIO:** A guided video demonstration of this exercise facilitated by Dr Baranowsky (2017, January 25) can be found on p. 227 in the supplementary material, Video 29 (also available at https://youtu.be/2Ymq4ov8Xyg).

# Phase III:
# Reconnection

*To be able to fill leisure intelligently is the last product of civilization.*

Bertrand Russell

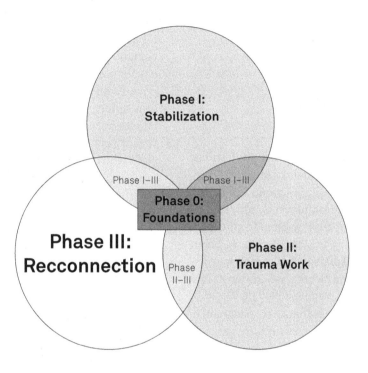

## Summary

As the trauma is addressed in recovery, the emotional constriction and withdrawal that was useful in the past for safety begins to lift. The final stage of recovery involves redefining oneself in the context of meaningful relationships and engagement in life activities. Trauma survivors gain closure on their experiences when they are able to see things that happened to them with the knowledge that these events do not determine who they are. Trauma survivors are liberated by the conviction that, regardless of what else happens to them, they always have themselves. Many survivors are also sustained by an abiding faith in a higher power that they believe delivered them from oppressive terror. In many instances, survivors find a "mission" through which they can continue to heal and to grow. They may even end up helping others with similar histories of abuse and neglect. Successful resolution of the effects of trauma is a powerful testament to the indomitability of the human spirit. After Phase II of trauma practice is completed, the personality that has been shaped through trauma must then be given the opportunity for new growth experiences that offer the hope of a widening circle of connections and the exploration of a broader range of interests. This is a time where posttraumatic growth (Tedeschi & Calhoun, 1996) opens doors and catalyzes the past adverse childhood and life experiences that undermine overall well-being. Dr. Jonice Webbs (2017) work on childhood emotional neglect and the concept of traumatic loneliness can further move the needle forward on the reconnection phase. Learn about the work of Dr. Jonice Webb on childhood emotional neglect and traumatic loneliness in four videos, see supplementary material Video 30 (see also Baranowsky, 2015, October 28, https://youtu.be/er2dUhNSghs); Video 31 (see also Baranowsky, 2015, October 14, https://youtu.be/6ZeR85s5oxl); Video 32 (see also Baranowsky, 2016, June 29, https://youtu.be/icWqqda2IYQ); Video 33 (see also Baranowsky, 2018, January 10, https://youtu.be/8HPAVongqpE).

# 1. Somatic

Many trauma survivors have spent a lifetime fighting the bodies they live in. They do not feel comfortable in their own skin. The behaviors they employed to keep themselves safe were often less than respectful to their bodies, or they just plain ignored their bodies. As they emerge from the emotional constriction of trauma, they begin the process of reconnection, including reconnection to their own bodies. Clients will find it useful to explore new ways to connect with themselves. Nutrition classes, exercise classes, Pilates, meditation, yoga, Tai Chi, Qigong, etc. are all useful and gentle ways to accomplish this. The following exercise is useful to help them "settle into their own skin" and begin the process of being aware of who they are.

## Centering (CR)

> **Time required:** As per Thich Nhat Hanh – forever.
>
> **Materials required:** None.
>
> **Indications for use:** Use when the primary need is to enhance physical, cognitive, behavioral, emotional, and relational coping skills in the Reconnection stage of trauma recovery.
>
> **Counterindications:** Inability to actively self-soothe.

This exercise springs from the increasingly familiar work on mindfulness or reflection and acceptance. Or, as Jon Kabat-Zinn (1990) explains in his ground-breaking book *Full Catastrophe Living*, "Mindfulness is cultivated by assuming the stance of an impartial witness to your own experience" (p. 33). He goes on to state that, as we begin to pay attention to the internal dialog, "It is common to discover and to be surprised by the fact that we are constantly generating judgments about our experience" (p. 33).

The next important piece of mindfulness is acceptance. Without this we will make no progress because we cannot live peacefully within our own bodies if we are unable to gracefully accept its natural fragility along with its strength. If we are plagued by chronic headaches following a traumatic event, we will certainly be worse off if we grow angry and frustrated every time we have a headache. Our anger and frustration will fuel our headache, feeding it into a much worse bodily-felt experience.

### Delivery of Approach

Thich Nhat Hanh (1990) explains a five-step process for centering that opens a dialog between the individual and their internal bodily-felt experiences. He recommends that we allow ourselves to get to know and reflect on our internal processes, whether it is fear, pain, sadness, confusion, irritation, etc.

1. Just notice what comes up, leaving judgment aside.
2. Greet the internal experience (e.g., "Hello sadness. What is happening with you today? Why are you here?"). This is in contrast to the common response which may be, "Hey, get out of here, sadness, you have no place inside of me! Who invited you?" In this way, we are no longer battling with ourselves. It becomes acceptable for us to feel whatever surfaces. The mindfulness is present and can moderate our internal experience of sadness – we are to just watch and let our attachment to judgment drop. Conscious breathing is an integral component to centering.
3. Coax an inner calmness just as you would soothe a young child who is feeling sadness or pain. You might say, "I am here, sadness, and I will not abandon you. I am breathing into my sadness with calm cooling breath." Being one with the feeling allows it the space and time to be nurtured, explored, expressed, and acknowledged, and provides the opportunity for respectful recovery.
4. Begin the process of releasing the feeling. You have faced the fearful emotion living in your body. It is now time to recognize that, as you add a calm mindfulness, the sadness begins to transform. You have taught your body to feel at ease, even in the presence of deep sadness. You have sent a new message to your body: you are ready to remain present and care for yourself even when faced with disturbing internal messages. Make a conscious decision to soften the feeling even more, noticing that it can become a gentler expression. Imagine yourself smiling calmly at your feeling and letting it go with willingness to release.
5. Take a deeper look. Bring your mindfulness to the source of the discomfort. Even if it has fully dissipated, the body will have a memory of its existence. Ask, "What is this feeling about? Where did it come from? What internal or external causes form this experience?" With questions like this, we can better understand ourselves. With understanding, we can find the source of our internal distress. We can offer our own wise counsel, offering words of kindness and support, self-acceptance, and transformation.

This is a self-mastery exercise, one that can add to the richness of anyone's life.

## Tame and Decode Bad Dreams (RE – CR)

**Time required:** 5–10 minutes.

**Materials required:** Pen or pencil, and paper

**Indications for use:** Use for an individual that has experienced a bad dream or nightmare that is causing continued stress, fear or anxiousness.

**Counterindications:** If the individual finds the dream too upsetting to revisit. Relaxation exercises such as deep breathing or listening to soothing music can be utilized to help.

There are many well-founded treatments for managing disturbed sleep and nightmares (i.e., medication such as Prazosin, CBT therapy using sleep hygiene, relaxation and breathing practices, and dream journaling). Research indicates that a trauma history is a known precursgrounor to clinical insomnia (Sinha, 2016). Sleep quality disruption is one of many ways that trauma can have a significant and prolonged impact on health and well-being, and this is largely because of the ways in which trauma can sensitize the central nervous system to become more hyperaroused. However, there are ways to mitigate this, improve sleep quality, and regulate the body's sleeping patterns again after trauma. An excellent article by Havens et al. (2019) outlines this research, and this has informed some of the exercise guidelines below.

For the purposes of this exercise we will focus on a unique protocol that is showing signs of being practical in relieving the strain of facing bad dreams.

The following guidelines are for an exercise that may help any individual with decoding their bad dream.

### Delivery of Approach

1. With eyes closed, instruct the individual to recall the dream.
2. Have the individual narrate a loud or write out the dream in as much detail as possible
3. Let the client know that next you will be reading the dream content back to them, and ask them as you do this, as best they can, to listen, practice self-compassion, and reflect on the content in a nonjudgmental way.
   a. If the individual is doing the exercise on their own, have them read the details out loud to themself, while maintaining commitment to practice listening with self-compassion and nonjudgmental reflection.
4. Ask the individual what they might learn from the dream content. Ask if there is any way in which this dream could teach them about something occurring in their life.
5. Start again at Step 1 and repeat the process 5–15 times, or until the meaning becomes clear, and the fear level associated with it is reduced. Advise that each repetition of this process is like peeling layers of an onion, before being able to arrive at the meaning.
6. The final steps of this exercise are drawn from image rehearsal therapy (IRT, or changing the ending) and dream journaling. The IRT (Tull, 2020) exercise is simple and requires the individual to write out a preferable new ending to the dream/nightmare. Once this is done either the therapist can read the new ending back to the client while they imagine the new ending in their

 **Script: Tame and Decode Bad Dreams**

My starting point with bad dreams, is that there is no universal meaning for what appears in your dreams and everything that appears is unique to you. Dream content is linked to your own life experience, and subconscious mind. Dreams are symbolic. It is up to the individual to decode dream meaning and how anything might tie into life.

You might dream about tigers chasing you, an impossible climb, or someone with a machine gun at your workplace that reminds you of something that occurred on the job …

When dream content repeats, it is often symbolic or representative of what needs addressing, rather than reflective of the actual problems in your life. For example, if in your life you are not getting along with a specific friend, your dream content might show you in a boat floating away from shore into murky water and away from a house that represents your connections and safety. You can see an array of animals growling on the shoreline as well as one cartoon character happily waving at you from one of the windows of the house. You don't need to live close to water or even in a house in order for the dream to have meaning for you or to relate to the struggle you might be having with a friend. Nothing needs to be an exact replica of events between you and your friend. Instead look at the content through the lens of "everything is an aspect of you".

In the example above, you are all elements. You are the murky water, the house you are leaving behind, you are the boat and the feelings you have being on the boat. You are all characters that you see. Given time and introspection, you can begin to notice how each element relates to you and your life themes and events.

mind's eye or they can read out the new ending while picturing this.

**WITH VIDEO:** Please watch a guided video demonstration of this exercise facilitated by Dr Baranowsky (2016, May 4), which can be found in the supplementary material, Video 34 (also available at https://youtu.be/Oi72TXnkEy4).

**WITH PODCAST:** Listen to the podcast below relating to managing difficult nightmares and dream content. https://annabaranowsky.com/taming-sleep-dreams-nightmares/

## Going Slow to Heal After Trauma (RE)

**Time required:** 5 minutes.

**Materials required:** Only the object of focus.

**Indications for use:** Having completed Phase I and II of trauma practice.

**Counterindications:** None.

Our bodies have an amazing capacity to heal, but often after experiencing trauma, can become stuck in a chronic state of reactivity responding to every perceived threat in a defensive self-protective manner. This hyperarousal, in combination with a modern lifestyle can produce a frantic pace and high level of stimulation. As a result, it can become challenging for the body to heal in a rested and relaxed state. The following exercise is one designed to allow the body to slow down, so that it can enter a relaxed state enabling greater access its own healing potential.

### Delivery of Approach

1. Have your client choose one go-slow activity that doesn't have a specific goal or outcome to measure, and have them practice this for 5 minutes. Examples can be activities like enjoying the smell/image of a lovely flower, gazing at a nice picture or piece of art, sitting in nature, etc. What is more important than the choice of activity is for the individual to remain fully present and immersed in the activity, without concern about outcome or result.

2. Ensure that distractions or disruptions such as phones are turned off or silent for these 5 minutes.

3. Have the individual observe how it feels to go slow in this way, and have them ask themselves what happens when they do this? Do they notice feeling more patience, clarity, or emotional calm? Or does the experience create agitation, discomfort, and intrusive thoughts. Both are acceptable, as we have an inner life that can surface in moments of slow. This exercise allows space for whatever is surfacing with self-appreciation and acceptance.

4. Encourage this 5-minute activity to become a daily practice for best positive impact.

**WITH VIDEO:** A guided video demonstration of this exercise facilitated by Dr Baranowsky (2015, January 2) can be found in the supplementary material, Video 35 (p. 227, or at https://youtu.be/v3IL9WZVLXI).

## Shake to Release (RE)

**Time required:** 5–10 minutes.

**Materials required:** A sturdy nonmoving chair or wall to lean on.

**Indications for use:** Use when stressed or feeling body-based hyperarousal/tension.

**Counterindications:** Any physical injuries that compromise mobility. Individuals should speak with their family doctors if they are uncertain if the exercise can be performed safely.

When we feel stress, we ignite the fight, flight, or freeze mechanism in our body, and this generally tends to create tension in the psoas muscle. The psoas muscle is a key hip flexor muscle that extends from the lumbar region, through the pelvis, and to the leg. This is important because not only is the psoas the only muscle that connects the spine to the legs, playing a large role in movement and posture, but it is also connected to the diaphragm, which as we know plays a large role in being able to activate calming responses in the body through deep breathing. Understanding that the large psoas muscle is implicated in any stress reaction is a useful realization, as the relaxation and release of this large and chronically tight muscle can create benefits in recovery after trauma. Improving psoas function can help reduce diaphragm dysfunction (Bordoni & Zanier, 2013), which will help the body in being able to better restore a sense of calm and relaxation.

One of the ways in which we can relax and release the psoas is with shaking exercises. If we shake, using a series of exercises that release tension in this part of the body, we can relieve feelings of tension, and engage a relaxation response to help resolve chronic stress.

## Delivery of Approach

Here is a list of several recommended shaking exercises that will help release tension in the body and in the psoas muscle particularly. It is recommended to go through the shake cycle of exercises 3–4 times in a row for best results. Please find a video link at the bottom, for a guided demonstration in the Shake to Release approach.

1. **Lift and shake the legs while seated exercise**
   - Have the individual begin the exercise seated at the edge of a steady chair that remain sturdy throughout movements.
   - Have them start with inhaling, and as they exhale, lift one knee and stretch the leg out in the air, holding it straight out in front of them, allowing the leg to start to shake. Then bring the foot back down to the ground.
   - While remaining seated, with heels on the ground, have them shake both legs for a few seconds, and then relax.
   - Repeat the last two steps with the other leg.
   - Repeat this series 2–3 more time for each leg, alternating which leg is lifted.

2. **Shaking the legs without lifting in seated position**
   - While remaining seated, have them point their toes in just slightly, while maintaining room for the legs to move. Have them shake their legs for about 5–10 seconds. Then have them stop and take a deep breath and let go of tension along with the exhalation.
   - Repeat this 2–3 more times

3. **Shaking until release - standing**
   - Have the individual now stand, while having a sturdy chair or a wall next to them to their side for support if needed, feet a little wider than hip distance apart, and with knees slightly bent.
   - Instruct them to allow their whole body to move while they shake from the feet up to the core, for about 5–10 seconds.

   - Take a deep breath, releasing tension in the body on the exhale.
   - Have them repeat this 2–3 more times.

4. **Chair/wall supported shake**
   - Instruct the individual to place their hands on something so they are solid and supported (like a sturdy and stable chair or wall), while leaning forward. Again, keeping the feet slightly more than hip width apart, with knees slightly bent.
   - Have them start shaking their legs from the base for 5–10 seconds.
   - Instruct them to take a deep breath, releasing tension in the body on the exhale.
   - Have them repeat this 2–3 more times.

▶ **WITH VIDEO:** Please watch a guided video demonstration of this exercise facilitated by Dr. Baranowsky and Frank Pasquill (Baranowsky, 2016, July 28) in the supplementary material, Video 36 (p. 227, or at https://youtu.be/iYAVAA10jjs). Frank Pasquill also provides a walkthrough of how laughter, or "emotional tuning," can be an additional help when integrated into the shaking exercise, which can also be found in a separate video (Baranowsky, 2016, July 21), see Video 37 (or at https://youtu.be/ebf6rJ_Y2wU).

# 2. Cognition

Even after resolving significant emotional reactions to trauma, clients are left with enduring patterns of how they think about themselves and the world. These are often very subtle patterns of thought that result in continued difficulties in reconnecting to others. Just like a fish never thinks about the water it swims in, people never think about why they think the way they think – they just do it. It takes effort to identify these thoughts and then more effort to change them. The first step is to become consciously aware of them. The following techniques are useful to help clients become aware of some of these enduring patterns of thought.

## Exploring Your Cognitive Map (CR)

**Time required:** A lifetime.

**Materials required:** Paper and pencil.

**Indications for use:** When one needs to identify the situations and triggers that result in less than useful thought patterns.

**Counterindications:** Inability to actively self-soothe.

The following exercise is adapted with permission from *A Language of the Heart: Therapy Stories that Heal* (Schultz, 2005, 2016). At first, clients are not accustomed to thinking about how they think. Life just happens. As they explore their cognitive map, they will begin to realize they are different under different circumstances. They are mostly unconscious that they are different. However, as they become more conscious of their thoughts, they will eventually become more aware of themselves in the moment and begin to recognize the triggers or prompts for being different. After they become more conscious, they can become more intentional.

### Delivery of Approach

There is printable handout material available for this exercise; see Using the Tools 25. What follows is a list of questions identified by others as significant in their development. The questions may help your clients begin to understand how they came to think about themselves and others and how they came to behave toward themselves and others. The questions cover different areas of early experience. The list is not exhaustive. For each question about an area of experience, your clients should ask themselves what impact these events had on their way of life. To what degree would they consider the impact to be positive or negative? How so? Specifically, have them consider the following questions when thinking about the impact:

1. What impact did these events have on your outlook, self-image, sense of safety, expectations, and relationships with others?
2. What are the beliefs about yourself that arose because of these events that you might question now?
3. What are the feelings the answers evoke and how do these relate to your current experience of the world?
4. What are the exact words you used to help you organize and understand the events to which they relate?
5. What are the exact triggers that remind you of these events?

As clients do this exercise, they should remember that the specific answer to each question is not as important as their own thoughts and emotional responses to the answer. Two people may have the same answer to the specific question, but very different thoughts and emotional responses to their own meaning attached to the answer. They may notice a specific emotional charge to some of the questions. Have them pay attention to these and ask themselves whether situations in the here-and-now are similar to past events. Are there cues such as tone of voice, word phrasing, etc., that remind them of these past events or feelings? Is there an emotional charge when they now experience these cues that perhaps triggers old thoughts and emotional responses?

## USING THE TOOLS 25

### Exploring Your Cognitive Map

Are there family myths surrounding your birth and early childhood (e.g., words describing you as a difficult birth, intentional/unintentional pregnancy, wrong gender, cranky temperament, beautiful baby, smart, slow, etc.)?

1. What are the exact words used to describe you as an infant, child, and teen?

   _____

2. What were the circumstances of your caregiving (e.g., breast/bottle fed, daycare, parents worked)?

   _____

3. How many siblings did you have and what was your birth order?

   _____

4. Were you adopted, raised by others than your parents, or did you live in foster care for any length of time?

   _____

5. Did either parent pass away while you were growing up?

   _____

6. What, if any, significant events occurred during the first 5 years, 5 to 10 years, 10 to 18 years of your life (e.g., family moved, went to hospital, went on vacation, death of someone close)?

   _____

7. What are your earliest memories? Are they pleasant or not so pleasant? Which stand out the most?

   _____

8. How would you describe your emotional interactions with each parent and sibling as an infant/toddler, when in primary/secondary school, as a teen, and as an adult?

   _____

9. Were there conflicts with any of the people in the above questions? How were they managed?

   _____

10. What are some of the exact words used in your communications with each in the above two questions?

   _____

11. With whom were you closest? Why?

   _____

12. With whom were you the most distant? Why?

   _____

13. Were you treated with respect and dignity? If not, who did not?

   _____

   _____

From: Anna B. Baranowsky & J. Eric Gentry, *Trauma Practice: A Cognitive Behavioral Somatic Therapy* (4th ed.). © 2023 Hogrefe Publishing

**USING THE TOOLS 25:**
Exploring Your Cognitive Map

14. Was anyone psychologically intrusive as you were growing up (e.g., head games, double messages, your feelings used against you, felt like you were not safe in your own mind)?

_____

15. What is your current relationship with the above persons?

_____

16. How did your parents discipline you? Under what circumstances?

_____

17. What were your responsibilities as a child (chores, taking care of siblings, etc.)?

_____

18. Were you ever left alone for periods of time?

_____

19. Were you ever frightened? What caused it? How did you and others respond to your fright?

_____

20. Were you ever in serious trouble at home, school, or elsewhere? What were the circumstances and outcomes?

_____

21. What were your friends like? Were they allowed to visit you in your home? Why or why not?

_____

22. How did your parents interact with your friends?

_____

23. Did your peers ever make fun of you or treat you in a disrespectful manner?

_____

24. How would you characterize the emotional atmosphere of your home (warm, tense, edgy, quiet, calm)?

_____

25. What were holidays like? Birthdays?

_____

26. How were gifts given in your childhood? Were there strings attached?

_____

27. How and from whom did you receive recognition?

_____

28. Were your parents ever divorced? More than once? With whom did you live?

_____

29. Did you have stepparents? What was your relationship with them like?

_____

From: Anna B. Baranowsky & J. Eric Gentry, *Trauma Practice: A Cognitive Behavioral Somatic Therapy* (4th ed.). © 2023 Hogrefe Publishing

30. Did either parent have a relationship with or live with a person to whom they were not married? What was your relationship with them like?

31. Did either parent have a previous family? What was your parent's relationship with that family like? What was your relationship with them like?

32. How did your parents communicate with each other?

33. Was there conflict? How did that look (e.g., passive, aggressive, violent, yelling, hitting, threatening)? Under what circumstances? What did you do when conflict occurred?

34. How did your parents demonstrate love to each other, your siblings, you, others? Under what circumstances? Were there favorites? How did that manifest?

35. Was either parent unfaithful? How did you know? What was the result?

36. Did your parents use alcohol or drugs? Was it a problem? How did it manifest?

37. Was either parent absent for long periods?

38. Were your parents outspokenly biased or prejudiced? How did that manifest?

39. Was either parent psychologically impaired? How so? Physically? How so?

40. Did you have physical or psychological problems? How were they addressed?

41. Would you consider either parent abusive (emotionally, physically, sexually)?

42. Have you experienced any form of abuse (emotional, physical, sexual) from family members or others?

43. Were you ever touched in a way that left you feeling uncomfortable?

44. Were you ever stared at or had comments made about your body, your development, or your looks in general?

From: Anna B. Baranowsky & J. Eric Gentry, *Trauma Practice: A Cognitive Behavioral Somatic Therapy* (4th ed.). © 2023 Hogrefe Publishing

45. When and how did you learn about sex?

46. When and how did you become sexually active?

47. Were you ever subjected to racist remarks or prejudice?

48. Were comments ever made about your intelligence or your abilities?

49. What were your experiences in school?

50. Did you have learning difficulties? If so, how did family and/or others respond to your difficulties?

51. What was your socioeconomic status?

52. Were you raised in a rural, small town, suburban, urban, or mixed community?

53. Did you work for money as a child? What were the circumstances?

54. What did you do for fun (activities: scouting, church groups, athletics, other)?

55. What was your weight and body build? Was it a problem?

56. Where you anorexic/bulimic, other?

57. Were you athletic?

58. Did your parents participate in outside activities with you? How was that experience?

59. What was your experience leaving home? Were you relieved, sad, anxious, excited?

60. Are there other areas not asked about in these questions that were a problem for you?

## Victim Mythology (CR)

**Time required:** Six structured sessions.

**Materials required:** Varies depending on the session progression. See Tinnin (1994).

**Indications for use:** Use when the primary need is to enhance cognitive coping skills in Phase III: Reconnection of trauma recovery.

**Counterindications:** Inability to actively self-soothe.

The concept of *victim mythology* was developed by Louis Tinnin, MD, a psychiatrist and professor at the West Virginia School of Medicine. Dr. Tinnin uses this concept to explain the cognitive and perceptual distortions that so often accompany traumatization, especially developmental trauma. In his TRI Model, now referred to as the instinctual trauma response model or ITT (https://helpfortrauma.com/trauma/), Dr. Tinnin utilizes six structured sessions to address and resolve this victim mythology in both outpatient and inpatient contexts.

Some of the symptoms associated with victim mythology include: diminished self-worth and esteem, desire to cause harm to oneself, seeking and perpetuating traumabonded relationships, distorted perception of true danger, foreshortened future, obsessive thinking, compulsive behaviors (addiction), fear of intimacy, and immature spiritual development. The ITT Model utilizes several different techniques to complete both a thorough trauma narrative and successful integration of the traumata to resolve intrusive and arousal symptoms. Dr. Tinnin believes that by resolving traumatic intrusions, the patient is increasingly able to focus upon and intentionally resolve cognitive and perceptual distortions. The six sessions use a combination of cognitive behavioral techniques to address and resolve these distorted thoughts and behaviors. Old patterns and beliefs of victim mythology are gently confronted and replaced with new, more fulfilling thoughts and behaviors.

The term *victim mythology* was coined by Louis Tinnin (1994) in the development of his treatment model for trauma (time-limited trauma therapy). Tinnin found that even after a trauma memory was resolved, many survivors clung to their posttraumatic beliefs that the world is a dangerous place and that the self is flawed. Tinnin believes that by helping the client understand the adaptive nature of the beliefs, by helping the client identify this mythology as part of the way that they coped with the overwhelming terror, pain, and grief associated with a traumatic experience, and by helping them to develop beliefs and meanings that are more adaptive to present-day life, the client is able to relinquish these traumagenic distortions.

Any therapy that helps the client identify distortions, script new, more adaptive self-talk, and rehearse these cognitions will work well toward helping the trauma survivor relinquish their victim mythology.

## Self-Compassion Reflection (RE – CR)

**Time required:** 10–20 minutes.

**Materials required:** Paper and pencil, timer, template; See video in Using the Tools 26 (Video 38 in supplementary material, or Baranowsky, 2014, March 12; see also Video 39, or Baranowsky, 2014d, August 25).

**Indications for use:** Use when the primary need is to enhance cognitive and emotional coping skills in the Reconnection stage of trauma recovery.

**Counterindications:** Client clearly confused, unmanaged stress, actively dissociating or dissociates during exercise.

This is an excellent exercise for building internal resources that can leave the individual have a greater sense of peace, acceptance, and relaxation.

### Delivery of Approach

There is printable handout material available for this exercise; see Using the Tools 26. In this exercise, the individual is asked to identify a person whom they can easily feel a positive sense of compassion toward. They then use this as the basis of understanding compassion which they eventually direct toward themselves, building the resource of self-compassion. Increased feelings of self-compassion are known to be related to lessened feelings of stress, depression, and anxiety.

The goal of the Self-Compassion Reflection Exercise is to help plant the seed of self-kindness. It is important to develop a sense of appreciation for yourself and what you have gone through. Many people with a history of trauma also tend to be quite personally unforgiving, often carrying the burden of harsh negative self-talk. This exercise is a gentle solution to this challenging habit.

---

### USING THE TOOLS 26

**Self-Compassion Reflections**

1. Start by reflecting on someone you know (alive or no longer – person or animal) for whom you can easily feel a sense of appreciation and open-hearted warmth and acceptance. Write down the names of those to whom this sensation applies.

   _____

   _____

   _____

2. Next, reflect on the center of your heart, allowing for the beginning of a full-bodied, warm, positive emotion to be present while you recall the person or animal. Close your eyes and hold this feeling for a few minutes as best as you can. This begins the practice of learning about compassion, and, as a result, increasing your ability to understand the way in which it expresses itself through your body, mind, and spirit.

3. Now repeat the following three phrases, silently in your mind three times:
   - _May you have kindness in your life_
   - _May you have peace in your life_
   - _May you have health in your life_

4. Write out your reflections on what it feels like for you to hold this feeling of compassion toward another in your own heart.

   _____

   _____

   _____

5. Now close your eyes and return to the heart-felt, open, and warm sensation and this time allow yourself to shine this full feeling on yourself. Hold it as best you can, allowing yourself to release any negative thoughts that surface. Again, place yourself fully within the heart-felt, open, and warm self-regard of which you are learning. Simply notice any feelings of resistance and release this as well allow it to be replaced by the new sensation of self-compassion.

6. Now repeat the following three phrases, silently in your mind three times:
   - _I embrace kindness in my life_
   - _I embrace peace in my life_
   - _I embrace health in my life_

7. Reflect on and then write about the feelings you experience when you attempt to embrace a sense of self-compassion. If you notice that this ignites strong negative feelings at first, rest assured that it is not unusual to initially resist self-compassion and that it gets easier with practice. Write about these feelings and practice items 2–7 above again until you are better able to sit comfortably with feelings of self-compassion. The goal is to eventually work through any negative feelings, allowing them to be gradually replaced with a warm feeling of self-compassion, acknowledgement, and acceptance. Use extra paper as needed to capture your reflections.

   _____

   _____

 **WITH VIDEO:** A guided video demonstration of this exercise facilitated by Dr Baranowsky (2014, March 12) can be found in the supplementary material, Video 38 (also available at https://www.youtube.com/watch?v=VjierSla_tw)

**USING THE TOOLS 26:**
Self-Compassion Reflections

---

Kristine Neff (2011), a writer and researcher in the newly emerging field of self-compassion, found that those who achieve a higher degree of self-compassion tend to have a reduced risk for symptoms of depression, anxiety, and stress. Since posttraumatic stress disorder is a trauma and stress-related disorder, the practice of learning self-compassion may prove to be preventative, as well as an aid in trauma recovery. This is especially true when we struggle with self-defeating internal monologues that disable our learning and coping strategies. A recent systematic review of studies shows that higher levels of self-compassion is consistently associated with reduced levels of PTSD symptomology (Winders et al., 2020)

## Letter to Self (CR)

**Time required:** One or more sessions.

**Materials required:** Paper and pencil.

**Indications for use:** Use when the primary need is to enhance cognitive and emotional coping skills in Phase III: Reconnection of trauma recovery.

**Counterindications:** Unresolved trauma.

### Delivery of Approach

This technique is a way to both center oneself and address victim mythology.

1. Have the client write a letter to the self that experienced the event. In the letter they should first make sense in detail of the earlier self's actions and emotions with the understanding they have achieved through therapy.
2. Move the client toward forgiveness of the self for their actions and emotions both during and subsequent to the event.
3. Help the client welcome that self home into an integrated sense of self. This means they begin to incorporate the experiences of that self as valid information.
4. Finally, have the client make a detailed commitment to self-care, outlining their plans to keep themselves healthy and safe.

## Wellness Mind Map (RE – CR)

**Time required:** 15–30 minutes.

**Materials required:** Paper, drawing utensils (pen, pencil, colouring pencils, or whatever your client prefers to use). Alternatively, some may opt to create the mind-map digitally on a computer.

**Indications for use:** Progressing into Phase III exercises and prepared to integrate approaches for reconnecting with meaningful life activities and self-care.

**Counterindications:** Visual impairment or not yet prepared to work on Phase III: Reconnection exerices.

A wellness mind map is a visual map of tools, resources, practices, and healthy habits that can help move your client towards recovery. Often in times of stress or triggers, the rational mind can be over-run with a fear response that blocks logical thinking areas in the brain, which can make it very difficult to think clearly, leading to the practice of unhelpful or destructive coping habits and thought patterns. The mind map can help re-enforce helpful tools, resources, practices and habits in these times or at anytime, and is a helpful asset in recovery.

### Delivery of Approach

To create a wellness mind map, have your client use a piece of paper (or computer if they prefer to create digitally), and draw a visual representation of themselves, with lines connecting them to different tools, resources, practices, and healthy habits that are helpful to them in recovery or keep them going on the path that they desire for themselves.

As a therapist, you can brainstorm ideas with them going over tools or practices that have been helpful and demonstrated positive results in their recovery. The visual representations can be drawn images or words that for them symbolize the helpful tools, resources, habits, or practices. For an example, see Figure 13.

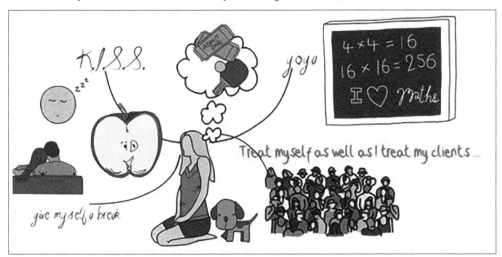

**Figure 13.**

Example of a wellness mind map.

**WITH VIDEO**: A guided video demonstration of this exercise facilitated by Dr Baranowsky (2015, July 22) can be found in the supplementary material on p. 227, Video 40 (also available at https://youtu.be/qqEXDp3IX6k).

## Your Heart's Desire (CR)

> **Time required:** 10–60 minutes.
>
> **Materials required:** Template.
>
> **Indications for use:** Use when trauma history is no longer a troubling or overwhelming element and instead the focus is on moving into a more invigorated approach to life beyond trauma.
>
> **Counterindications:** Unresolved trauma or re-evoked trauma triggers.

Working through our trauma history, frees up energy and allows us to sit with greater comfort with ourselves. It also has the unsettling effect of opening up time and space and leaving us to wonder "what now ... what next ... what do I really want?"

Well, the "what now ... what next ... and ... what do you really want ..." is all about reconnecting with the deepest part of the true self and one's heart's desire.

Children who grew up in distressing/traumatic/neglectful homes or adults living and/or working within systems that are challenging or traumatic mean that there is no time or space for one's truest heart's desire. We are in survival mode and this demands all of our resources. We cut off from that which is our deepest longing, our hopes and dreams. When we begin to heal and recover, there is finally time and space for this but truly it can be confusing to figure out what you really want. This is especially true when a person has spent a lifetime pushing those thoughts, hopes, and dreams away just to survive.

This exercise is designed to help your client get in touch with their heart's desire.

### Delivery of Approach

There is printable handout material available for this exercise; see Using the Tools 27.

## USING THE TOOLS 27

### Your Heart's Desire

Children are born to play and dream. In fact, this is how children learn and we are all born with this capacity.

Imagine a time and place where you recall being a child playing. Any memory that evokes a pleasant, peaceful time is good. This might only be a tiny moment that you can recall and that is perfect for this exercise. Try to picture everything you see, hear, feel.

If the memory evolves to something challenging or unresolved, then this is not the memory to work with.

Instead, just resettle and find the earliest memory you have that evokes a playful and happy memory. Stay with this for a few moments, reflecting with your eyes closed imagining everything and noticing the inner feeling you have when being with this past moment in time. Write out the details:

_____

_____

_____

_____

_____

Just notice if there was a feeling of being very content with some element of that memory? Did you recognize a love of music, a desire to dance, or a pleasure of the tactile experience of finger painting? Did you love nature, climbing a tree, singing with friends? Just find one precise element that stands out for you and describe everything you can about what brought you the deepest sense of pleasure in that childhood play.

_____

_____

_____

_____

Reflect on whether there is any way in which you can bring this feeling into your adult life? No judgment, just encouraging a willing playfulness in bringing this element into your life. Do you want to take a writing class, learn how to sew, use a high-powered telescope to star gaze, garden, or take up rock climbing? Whatever it is, you can start with simple investigation with the willingness to say "yes," when in the past the answer would have been a definitely "no."

Remember, you now have more space and time as your energies are not fully immersed in getting through or dealing with trauma. It is time for you to celebrate a bit and free yourself up to do things that are about your heart's desire.

List a few activities that you feel evoke the feelings above. Stay open even if this feels a bit strange or even scary. Notice that excitement and fear can feel similar but that being excited has a hopeful feeling attached to it. This is an experiment in moving toward your heart's desire. The more you practice this the more you will connect with the feeling and begin to move toward the pleasure of this state of flow.

From: Anna B. Baranowsky & J. Eric Gentry, *Trauma Practice: A Cognitive Behavioral Somatic Therapy* (4th ed.). © 2023 Hogrefe Publishing

**USING THE TOOLS 27:**
Your Heart's Desire

Make your list here:

_____

_____

_____

_____

Give yourself the freedom to investigate, explore, test, and try out anything or all the things on your list. There is no right or wrong, only the willingness to give yourself freedom to explore. You are just testing things out and there is no need or expectation for an activity to be a perfect fit but rather for you to have the space to figure it out as you go along. Enjoy and reach toward your heart's desire. It's time to reclaim your love of play.

From: Anna B. Baranowsky & J. Eric Gentry, *Trauma Practice: A Cognitive Behavioral Somatic Therapy* (4th ed.). © 2023 Hogrefe Publishing

# 3. Behavior

A therapist can guide clients through the recovery process and help them think about and talk about their lives differently. Clients can think and talk about changing, but until their behaviors actually change they will not move into a healthierand balanced lifestyle. For recovery to be fully integrated into their lives, they must *do* things differently. This is accomplished by them taking the initiative to change their own behaviors. Therapists and clients can prepare for life after therapy by discussing a plan to participate in healthier and adaptive behaviors. The following technique is just a small example of the various resources useful to that end.

## Self-Help and Self-Development (CR)

**Time required:** One or more sessions.

**Materials required:** Varies.

**Indications for use:** Use when the primary need is to enhance cognitive and emotional coping skills in Phase III: Reconnection of trauma recovery.

**Counterindications:** None.

There are literally thousands of books, audio/video tapes, organizations, and websites that are designed to facilitate empowerment through knowledge and connectedness for trauma survivors. One of the most important goals of CBT, or any psychotherapy, is helping the client to find their own resources and answers – to become self-sufficient and symptom free.

We note some website addresses for your use below, which include excellent resource for all things related to trauma and recovery from traumatic events. Feel free to pass these along to your clients! However, be aware that this is simply a starting point and not at all meant to be the final word on great tools to find.

### Web Pages

- BouceBack: https://bouncebackontario.ca/
- The LifeLine Canada Foundation: https://thelifeline-canada.ca/
- The Trauma Foundation: https://thetraumafoundation.org
- Gift From Within (nonprofit organization for survivors of trauma and victimization): http://www.giftfromwithin.org & https://www.giftfromwithin.org/html/trauma_support_pages_directory.html

- Traumatology Institute: *http://www.psychink.com and*https://psychink.com/resources/free-tools/FUS Department of Verterans Affairs National center for PTSD: https://www.ptsd.va.gov
- David Treleaven: https://davidtreleaven.com/the-truth-about-mindfulness-and-trauma/
- Sidran Institute for Traumatic Stress Education and Advocacy: http://www.sidran.org
- Trauma Practice for Healthy Communities (TPHC) – a charitable organization offering online group programs and resources for trauma survivors in the community: https://traumapractice.org/
- The Trauma Practice Research Project (TPRP) – developed in collaboration with York University to track the efficacy of the Trauma Practice approach: https://traumapractice.net/
- David Baldwin's Trauma Information Pages: http://www.trauma-pages.com/
- https://whatisptsd.com/

### YouTube

- The Trauma Foundation video "Trauma and the Nervous System – A Polyvagal Perspective:" https://youtu.be/ZdIQRxwT1I0
- Traumatology Institute YouTube channel "What Is PTSD:" https://www.youtube.com/c/Whatisptsd

## Picture Positive (RE – C – CR)

**Time required:** 20–30 minutes.

**Materials required:** Internet access, template.

**Indications for use:** Use when the primary need is to enhance a sense of having new resources to cope with everyday life demands in the Reconnection stage of trauma recovery.

**Counter-indications:** Client clearly confused, unmanaged stress, actively dissociating or dissociates during exercise.

This resources-building tool enhances the individual's sense feeling good about the skills they are developing, along with a sense of calm that with practice they get stronger daily.

### Delivery of Approach

There is printable handout material available for this exercise; see Using the Tools 28. This work is built upon the new brain science field of neuroplasticity. In Hanson's book *Hardwiring Happiness* (2013), he reflects on the very powerful notion that we are wired to think about the bad because, from an evolutionary perspective, it kept us alive. Every one of us had an ancestor who remained watchful and careful, and, as a result, was able to successfully share their genes with us as a result of this survival instinct. However, we now live in a world that allows for a greater degree of resources and safety for a large number of people. This means fear-based living is failing us by leaving us anxious, worried, and depleted. Instead, we can use the power of our minds to harness positive feelings and practice the sensation of good feelings to create a foundation of resources that grow over time with practice (Seligman, 2002; Allen et al., 2012; Shaffer, 2016;

Tabibnia & Radecki, 2018). The burgeoning field of neuroplasticity continues to amaze clinicians, who see endless possibilities in using the brain in an intentional manner to re-shape our fearful responses into a state of calm resourcefulness.

This exercise is like a launching pad for clients who are ready to move toward a happier and more fulfilling life.

We start by identifying an area where the individual would like to feel a greater sense of satisfaction (i.e., greater comfort in relationships, being able to drive in a more relaxed state, say no in a positive manner, sense of calm or gratitude at home or work, etc.).

A commonly used phrase in neuroplasticity states that "neurons that fire together wire together" and this means that if we practice a state of resourcefulness – even in our imagination – the resource state becomes more of a possibility. In contrast, tending to think negatively (i.e., people don't like me) leads to a wiring of this belief state. The more we practice the negative, the more vulnerable we feel towards this old belief. It is important to recognize that very lovely individuals who are well-liked can hold beliefs about being unloveable. This does not mean that no one loves them but rather that the belief is driving their feelings about themselves regardless of how much affection other may actually have for them. That is truly problematic as they then fail to feel the warmth and affection from others as a result of the negatively held beliefs they carry within. This means that the only approach that would really work is a whole-hearted inside challenge.

Using self-directed neuroplasticity (intentional practice of the positive) we can begin to break old habits and begin to build a new resource kit. In Picture Positive, we untilize the immense picture bank of search engines to help us with the task.

## USING THE TOOLS 28

### Picture Positive

1. Start by selecting a desired state or outcome (i.e., calm with family, appreciated at work, relaxed driving my car, or any other state of being).

2. Type in the catch phrase or key words into the image section of a search engine. You will see a series of images. Select images that positively capture the desired state.

3. Have the individual describe the scene and the people or person in the image.

4. Ask them to describe feelings, actions, expressions, and whatever else is in the pictures without judging or adding negative interpretations (i.e., they are smiling but probably faking it). That is the old negative thinking habit resurfacing.

5. Once they capture a positive individual experiencing their desired resource state (i.e., I am comfortable with my co-workers and enjoying my work) ask the individual to close their eyes and "Be that person ... Allow yourself to be in that positive moment and feel what you would feel ... Tell me when you have that feeling."

6. When they have the feeling, encourage them to enjoy it for a moment, then open their eyes.

7. You now move onto another image, or, if there was a particularly difficult image to embed, redo that one if it would be beneficial.

8. Continue to follow the picture positive steps – reinforcing the learning that goes along with wiring the new picture positive images.

9. End by inquiring about the feelings they have in the moment following the exercise. Do these feelings more closely reflect the desired state or the positive images that they had been reflecting upon? If yes, then Picture Positive has helped the individual to harness that state. If no, then it is time to reflect on what is getting in the way and to return to a stabilization exercise to end the meeting.

From: Anna B. Baranowsky & J. Eric Gentry, *Trauma Practice: A Cognitive Behavioral Somatic Therapy* (4th ed.). © 2023 Hogrefe Publishing

**USING THE TOOLS 28:**
Picture Positive

# 4. Emotion/Relation

Humans are social animals not only by culture and environment, but also biologically. We are genetically programmed to connect to others. As previously discussed, trauma has the effect of preventing us from successfully connecting to others. The process of trauma recovery is not about forgetting what happened and simply forcing ourselves to behave differently. It is about integrating what happened into a personal story of victory and overcoming the obstacles created by trauma. Reconnecting emotionally is the final victory, accomplished by remembering what happened, learning the lessons of sadness, and relearning to fearlessly love. It is a courageous act of intentionally reentering the world of social connection with an open heart and a clear head. The following techniques help clients remember with intention, mourn their experiences with intention, and reconnect with intention.

## Memorials (CR)

Time required: 15 minutes to multiple hours, if developed as a comprehensive experience.

Materials required: Art supplies, community, etc.

Indications for use: Use when the primary need is to enhance emotional and relational coping skills in Phase III: Reconnection of trauma recovery.

Counterindications: Inability to actively self-soothe.

The goal of memorials is often to make a bridge from the horrific past to the hopeful future. Memorials provide a ceremonial reconnection between those who have experienced great loss or trauma and their communities through acceptance and acknowledgement – a time to offer mutual support, an honoring for those left behind, and a testimony to those no longer present. This is a chance for closure. Memorials offer a moment for sharing positive restorative memories and a time to reinterpret tragic events. All these things can be integrated into a memorial. It can have a powerful and reconstructive quality.

### Delivery of Approach

There is printable handout material available for this exercise; see Using the Tools 29. Memorials can take the form of clients participating in prayer circles, erecting monuments, taking down walls, singing together, burying or burning symbols of a traumatic event, or ritualistically divorcing abusers. There are many forms and few absolute rules. Can you recall meaningful memorials you have attended, developed, processed, or heard about?

There are many approaches to reconnection memorials. Please use the time during this section to recall or imagine a memorial that you have used, witnessed, or are aware of that seems meaningful to you. Use the space available in this book to describe memorials that you would like to collect for future use.

## USING THE TOOLS 29

### Memorials

Take a moment to reflect upon your journey. What parts of your life need to be memorialized? What losses do you need to commemorate so that you can move on? Take a moment to allow yourself to identify these parts of your life, people, things, and beliefs that need to be identified and write a brief memorial to them all.

_____

_____

_____

_____

_____

_____

_____

_____

_____

_____

_____

_____

_____

_____

_____

_____

_____

_____

_____

_____

_____

_____

_____

_____

_____

_____

From: Anna B. Baranowsky & J. Eric Gentry, *Trauma Practice: A Cognitive Behavioral Somatic Therapy* (4th ed.). © 2023 Hogrefe Publishing

**USING THE TOOLS 29:**
Memorials

## Connections with Others (RE – CR)

> **Time required:** 20 minutes or more for research and a lifetime for implementation.
>
> **Materials required:** Varies.
>
> **Indications for use:** Use when the primary need is to establish meaningful connections with others and enhance cognitive and emotional coping skills in Phase III: Reconnection of trauma recovery.
>
> **Counterindications:** None.

There is printable handout material available for this exercise; see Using the Tools 30. It is easy to become overly focused on life's demands and forget to include joyful pursuits, but it is often these joyful pursuits that act as buffers against the pressures of our work and life. Engaging in meaningful activities while connecting with others creates a road back to a healthy life filled with new opportunities and choices. It is common to hear from people that they no longer enjoy the activities they pursued at earlier times in their lives. They no longer sing in a choir, play baseball, read poetry, attend a book club, take acting classes, or run marathons. But why not? What is the meaning of all our hard work and dedication if we are not also ensuring meaningful engagement in life? At this stage of trauma practice, recovery is part of the picture, and ensuring that we stay on track means investing in today and connecting to our communities and with people around us in shared and meaningful activities. A supplementary video (Baranowsky, 2016, September 21) that further explores and discusses this topic can be viewed in the supplementary material, Video 41, titled "The Importance of Community & Connection" (or at https://youtu.be/Iv9-TQBZQkI). The video can be used as a lead into the following exercise that can be used to nurture community and connection with others..

## USING THE TOOLS 30

### Connections with Others

The rules are as follows:

1. Identify two to three activities of interest within the following four domains: physical, intellectual, creative, and spiritual.

2. Ensure that all selected activities occur within a social context with other people.

3. This is an experiment, so keep it fun.
   Stage I: Simply investigate options or activity areas within each domain.
   Stage II: Select one activity from at least three of the four domains to try.
   Stage III: Try the activity.
   Stage IV: If you like it, continue; if not, choose another to try.
   Stage V: Continue moving through your options until you find three or four that you truly enjoy and wish to continue.

**For Phase III: Reconnection in the tri-phasic model of trauma treatment, there are four connections:**

### Connections with others

Identify activities that may interest you within each of the four cluster areas that include a social component. Investigate what activities are available in your vicinity or create your own group. Select two or three items to get involved in at least once each month. Develop your social life and become involved in your community. Decide if a given activity is a good fit for you only after attending at least three or four times. If not, move on to the next.

1. Physical (e.g., walking club, yoga class, bowling)

   _____

   _____

2. Intellectual (e.g., book club, university/college course, astronomy club)

   _____

   _____

3. Artistic/Creative (e.g., painting class, pottery class, scrapbooking)

   _____

   _____

4. Spiritual/Religious (e.g., join a religious church/temple, learn to meditate, volunteer in a homeless shelter)

   _____

   _____

*The key to happiness is realizing that it's not what happens to you that matters,*
*it's how you choose to respond.*

K. D. Harrell

**USING THE TOOLS 30:**
Connections with Others

## Codependency Revolution (CE – CR)

> **Time required:** 10–60 minutes.
>
> **Materials required:** Template and internet access (https://codacanada.ca and https://coda.org).
>
> **Indications for use:** When the focus of growth is on building relationships and stretching into healthy connections.
>
> **Counterindications:** Unresolved trauma or re-evoked trauma triggers.

Essentially, codependency is all about unhealthy relationship boundaries. We become codependent when our primary caregivers raised us in an environment with trauma, emotional neglect, addiction, narcissistic abuse, or when our caregivers struggled with unresolved mental health issues or were wounded by trauma themselves (Webb, 2017).

This means that we may have had to survive a childhood that failed to provide us with the nourishment to feel it was safe to be ourselves, or the self-esteem to select people who would treat us kindly. It may take years to arrive at a point where our clients are able to truly look closely at themselves and recognize that the patterns that they bring into relationships and that their relationship choices are not the best fit for healthy connection.

Sometimes, we don't have any idea that we have codependent tendencies until we have progressed in our own trauma healing. Often, born out of a need to survive; there may not be enough energy to look beyond the trauma stories or to confront our own behavioral patterns. Early on in our recovery journey, it may simply be too hard to reflect on ourselves and what we are bringing to our relationships, and we have to wait until our ship is steady enough to contemplate our own inner make-up and how we have been shaped.

In other cases, it might take a major life event (i.e., accident, illness, trauma) to wake-up to the unhealthy choices we have made. In these situations, we are dealing with a devastating and significant life event, combined with a deep dive into the dissatisfaction that goes with recognizing unhealthy, narcissistic, abusive relationships with those around us, sometimes for the first time. I recall working with a woman who was diagnosed with cancer and for the first time in her life, she was unable to do everything for everyone else in her life. Right now, she needed help, support, kindness. Instead, she had to face the reality that the people in her life were unwilling or unable to show up for her in the way that she had always supported them.

The harm of old behavior and relationship patterns, can go on far too long, leaving one feeling alone even in our "closest" connections. This is especially true if we are afraid of being seen for fear of being rejected, or if you never learned to value yourself. Codependency author Lisa Romano (Romano, 2020) suggests the following four elements as reflective of active codependency:

1. Codependents focus on others rather than themselves
2. Codependents lean toward self-sacrificing behaviors
3. Codependents address conflict/struggles by employing controlling behaviors to manage the situation and people
4. Codependents constrain their emotions or rein themselves in hiding their true feelings

Please remember that codependency is established as a mechanism of survival, not because someone is trying to be difficult. Challenging codependency within ourselves is an act of courage and one that will likely result in greater freedom and flexibility to live life more authentically.

When working on codependent tendencies we embrace ourselves and our inner experience rather than rejecting our feelings, thoughts, and reflections. Coming to that new place means truly grappling with your deepest inner wounds. These wounds were structured to see oncoming danger and to scramble to the known strategy (i.e., fawning over abusers, pretending you want to do something when you do not so you will not be alone, putting another's happiness and comfort ahead of your own, etc).

An article in the Huffington Post (Borresen, 2018) illustrates ten warning signs given by experts on codependency that you are in a codependent relationship (also note that "partner" is interchangeable with any connection, friend, sibling, co-worker, etc):

1. You say yes without reflecting on your own feelings.
2. You compensate for your partner's behavior even when you know it does not feel right to you.
3. Your main priority is your partner's happiness at the expense of your own.
4. You enable your partner by fixing, saving and repairing on their behalf, keeping them from taking responsibility for their own actions.
5. You have lost any sense of your own needs, desires or preferences.
6. You are frequently manipulated to serve the preferences of your partner.
7. You give so much of yourself without having much coming back from your partner.

8.  Your tendency for generosity, kindness, concession is taken for granted and given too freely.
9.  You do everything to reduce any pain or strain that your partner might experience by carrying the burden yourself.
10. You are not in a balanced relationship but rather one where you are coerced, controlled, or only loved when your partner is getting something from you.

Reinforcing these concepts, clinical psychologist Dr. Nicole LePera (2021) outlines codependency signs as follows:

- Feeling responsible for the well-being, emotions, or actions of others
- Saying "yes" when you want to actually say "no"
- Consistently feeling like you're being taken for granted and resentful for giving more than you receive
- Obsessively (unconsciously) attempting to control the behavior of others

## Delivery of Approach

At this point in recovery, I hope it is clear that the deep work that needs to be done to really address codependency should not be done alone or in a vacuum. This is work best done in community, where one can see and hear the kind words of support and comfort of another victor on the journey of recovery or clear perspective and wisdom from someone further along on this codependency recovery journey.

Co-Dependents Anonymous Canada (codacanada.ca) and Co-Dependents Anonymous (coda.org) offer a wealth of resources and programming both online and in person.

The impressive effort of these two organizations has provided tools, resources, and well-structured road maps for those ready to do the work. As a starting point, it seems best to begin with some initial meetings to familiarize yourself with the language, the steps, and the recovery process. Study meetings are particularly interesting as they form an ongoing structure from which to engage in deeper reflections of personal responsibility taking within a supportive, structured, and established framework.

In Phase III of trauma practice, the task is to continue with your growth on this journey of evolving into the person you are meant to be, beyond the trauma story. This is one approach that many have found particularly fruitful.

# Integrative and Clinician Self-Care Models

*Opportunities are usually disguised as hard work,
so most people don't recognize them.*

Ann Landers

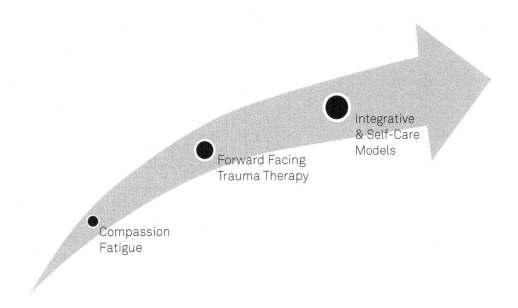

Compassion
Fatigue

Forward Facing
Trauma Therapy

Integrative
& Self-Care
Models

**Summary**

This chapter on Forward-Facing® Trauma Therapy (FFTT) introduces a safe, effective, and accelerated method of treating trauma that does not require the survivor to revisit painful memories in order to heal the distress they experience from their past. Instead, drawing upon recent research from brain science, physiology, stress studies, and trauma treatment, FFTT teaches users to monitor and regulate their own over-enervated and dysregulated nervous systems. By helping trauma survivors to confront the perceived threats of their daily lives in the present using the pairing of exposure and relaxation to desensitize the negative effects of past traumas, clients can enjoy immediate relief from their symptoms. FFTT fully exploits this integral component of all effective trauma treatment to help survivors to heal their traumatic stress – and all stress – by a simple set of skills practiced in the present. In addition, survivors who develop this disciplined process of confronting perceived threats begin to find themselves able to lessen their reactivity and begin to live intentional and fulfilling lives.

# Forward-Facing® Trauma Therapy

*Between stimulus and response there is a space. In that space is our power to choose our response.*
*In our response lies our growth and our freedom.*

Viktor Frankl (1963)

## Introduction

Until the early 1990s, the treatment of traumatic stress for many survivors was as bad or worse than the symptoms they experienced. The popular treatment during the early years was informed primarily by psychodynamic psychiatry and utilized a process of abreaction and catharsis during which the therapist guided the survivor through the painful re-experiencing of their traumatic memories. This treatment was called "flooding" or "implosion therapy," and involved the telling and re-telling of the most painful parts of the traumatic experience until a catharsis was achieved. It was theorized that the patient would complete desensitization and integration of their traumatic memories following these abreactions. It was an arduous and painful process for survivors who were already challenged and compromised in their functioning. It is no wonder many trauma survivors during this period chose to keep their symptoms instead of enduring the rigors of this difficult treatment.

This model of treatment, which has evolved into what is now called prolonged exposure (PE; Foa et al., 2007), remains frequently utilized and is identified by the Department of Veterans Affairs/ Department of Defense (VA/DoD) as one of the evidence-based treatments for PTSD (Foa et al., 2009; Management of Posttraumatic Stress Disorder Work Group, 2017; American Psychological Association, 2017). While evidence for the effectiveness of this method has been demonstrated, dropout rates as high as 30% have been reported in some studies using this method (Ironson et al., 2002; Belleau et al. 2017). A recent meta-analysis of 22 studies showed a mean dropout percentage for PE of 22% (Lewis et al., 2020). While it may be effective, this archaic and draconian treatment is not elegant, efficient, or easily tolerated by many survivors of trauma.

The 1990s saw explosive growth, development, and maturation in the understanding and treatment of traumatic stress. The groundbreaking article "Abreaction Reevaluated" by Van der Hart and Brown (1992) was one of the catalysts that began this evolution of trauma treatment. In this article, they urged a gentler path of helping trauma survivors resolve their painful pasts and articulated that the integration of the dissociated memory fragments was more important than strenuous emotional upheaval. They advocated for helping survivors construct and share narratives of their traumatic experiences while remaining relaxed through hypnosis as a primary emphasis for healing posttraumatic conditions.

Van der Hart and Brown (1992) gave language to the idea that if we can help trauma survivors imaginally confront their traumatic memories and integrate the dissociated and repressed memory components through the use of relaxation and narrative, survivors could resolve their symptoms of PTSD with minimal distress. These authors pronounced that survivors could complete these important tasks and heal their PTSD with minimal pain and suffering throughout treatment. Since the publication of that article, many treatments have emerged that maximize efficiency and effectiveness while, simultaneously, minimizing distress for our clients. It was during this time that eye movement desensitization and reprocessing (EMDR; Shapiro, 1989, 1995; Shapiro & Solomon, 1995) matured from an experimental treatment into one of the most utilized and researched treatments (Berliner et al., 2019; Valiente-Gómez et al., 2017) in the history of our field. In that same year, Judith Herman (1992) published *Trauma and Recovery*, which prescribed a tri-phasic model of treatment that minimized retraumatization while developing with the survivor a battery of skills for better managing their lives and successfully navigating treatment. Several other approaches that utilize narrative combined with relaxation to maximize efficiency and minimize distress, such as cognitive processing therapy (CPT; Resick & Schnicke, 1992; Watkins et al., 2018), visual-kinestheric dissociation (VKD; Dietrich, 2000; Gray 2011), and traumatic incident reduction (TIR; French & Harris, 1998), also emerged during that time.

In the 42 years since PTSD first appeared in DSM-III (American Psychiatric Association, 1980), many in our field have been steadily evolving our treatment processes, making them increasingly effective while also lessening the distress and duration that had previously been associated with trauma treatment. These newer treatments are becoming progressively efficient with the utilization of exposure, relaxation, and memory integration. They help survivors rapidly resolve their distress and integrate the fragmented memories of their traumatic experiences so that they can more quickly return to productive and satisfying lives following trauma.

This section introduces and proposes another evolutionary leap in the understanding and treatment of posttraumatic stress. It is a method of treatment that can resolve the negative effects of historical trauma without the need for survivors to revisit their painful pasts. It is an accelerated method designed to ameliorate the symptoms of PTSD without the backwards-facing regression and arduous processing of trauma memories that is central and essential to every evidence-based method currently utilized for treating traumatic stress. Instead of the therapist directing the survivor through the labyrinth of their painful memories, this method outlines a stepwise process for the therapist and client to collaborate and together resolve the effects of trauma in the here and now, through present-day principle-based living. This method helps survivors begin to immediately optimize their lives and, in doing so, minimize their posttraumatic symptoms. This treatment is called Forward-Facing® trauma therapy (FFTT).

FFTT is a unique combination of accelerated psychotherapy/counseling, performance coaching, and maturational processes designed to help individuals heal the effects of past trauma while at the same time developing skills for optimizing their lives. The exciting thing about this method of trauma resolution is that it does not require the strenuous and often painful process of accessing and processing trauma memories. Instead, it focuses upon desensitizing the present-day effects of trauma by confronting intrusions from past trauma with a regulated autonomic nervous system and relaxed body. This novel utilization of reciprocal inhibition (i.e., exposure + relaxation; Wolpe, 1968), a common factor for *all* effective treatments of anxiety and trauma disorders, resolves the current painful effects of trauma while simultaneously helping the survivor to evolve into resilience and optimal functioning in a very short time. Traditional methods of trauma resolution, such as CBT and EMDR, require a significant period of safety and stabilization to teach clients the skills required to navigate their trauma memories. These traditional methods then require the therapist and survivor to engage in a form of "archeology" – digging up, sifting through, and processing trauma memories – to resolve the symptoms associated with traumatic stress. Many survivors find this revisiting of their memories too painful and demanding for them to continue treatment.

Studies exploring prolonged exposure treatment methods have reported very high dropout rates (Belleau et al., 2017; Lewis et al., 2020), in part due to this demand upon the survivor to wade through the memories of the past (Ironson et al., 2002). FFTT allows the therapist and survivor to begin gainful treatment from the very first session. The skills utilized in this model, in addition to ameliorating the negative effects of past trauma, also help survivors to rapidly stabilize and improve their current functioning.

This simple treatment method combines the features of evidence-based CBT – developing a good therapeutic relationship, psychoeducation, cognitive restructuring, self-regulation/relaxation, and *in vivo* exposure (Carbonell & Figley, 1999; Foa et al., 2000; Follette et al., 1998; Gallo, 1996; US Department of Veteran Affairs & Department of Defense, 2017) – with intentionality, personal integrity, and internalized locus of control. This combination forms an integrated strategy to address the symptoms of traumatic stress, anxiety, and depression. This accelerated approach also allows participants to avoid some of the pain, costs, demands, and stigmatization that are frequently associated with traditional psychiatric treatment. Instead, it provides a simple path for anyone – but especially survivors of trauma – to engage in a powerful process to help individuals turn away from a life dominated by painful symptoms and reactivity, and toward a healthy and disciplined lifestyle based upon their own individual purpose and principles. FFTT helps participants to create, articulate, and rapidly begin living in fidelity to their own "moral compass." By developing this principle-based intentionality through the practices of self-regulation central to this treatment, participants enjoy the added benefit of reducing stress-related symptoms. While it may never replace traditional psychotherapy, it does provide a complimentary approach that has effectively accelerated treatment and life satisfaction for scores of clients and hundreds of workshop participants.

FFTT was born from a broad, eclectic mix of ideologies, disciplines, and protocols to form a simple, clear, commonsensical approach to counseling, maturation, and living that helps people migrate from the reactivity of anxiety, depression, and traumatic stress to the comfort and maximal functionality of living with intention. It is rooted in and focused on helping individuals to live intentionally in the present as a way of rapidly healing their past. FFTT may be less a treatment, and more a blueprint for living with integrity that has the by-product of symptom reduction. One of the primary benefits of this model is helping people to understand how their past painful, fearful, and traumatic experiences led them to perceive a threatening and dangerous world in the present (Holbrook et al.,

2001). It also helps them to see how present-day intrusions from these difficult past experiences contaminate their current perceptions, causing them to perceive threat where there is no danger. Helping participants to understand the negative and symptomatic consequences of autonomic nervous system dysregulation caused by the chronic perception of threat motivates participants to develop an internalized capacity for self-regulation. By maintaining relaxed bodies in the context of these perceived threats, normally functioning adults can quickly find physiological and psychological comfort, maximize neocortical (thinking) functions, and regain intentional, principle-based behavior, even while we are confronting these threats (Bremner, 2000; Bremner et al., 2000; Breslau & Kessler, 2001; Critchley et al., 2001; Lanius, 2014; Porges, 2007). Additionally, it is well-documented that relaxation is a crucial ingredient for the resolution of traumatic stress symptoms and an effective agent in lessening anxiety symptoms (Scotland-Coogan & Davis, 2016; Friis & Sollers, 2013; Meichenbaum, 1994, 2012; Shalev, Bonne, & Eth, 1996; Wolpe, 1954).

For all its CBT underpinnings, however, FFTT is probably best defined as developmental in its approach to healing trauma, because it helps people to restart, continue, and accelerate their natural maturational processes. Painful and traumatic past learning, along with the subsequent adaptations resulting from these traumatic experiences, may cause normal, healthy maturation to become thwarted in deference to the constant attention and action that perceived threats demand (Bonner & Rich, 1988; Falconer et al., 2008; Scaer, 2005; Schnurr et al., 2004; Sherin & Nemeroff, 2011; Dennis et al., 2017; Dunkley et al., 2018). The learning and adaptation that survivors develop from their painful and traumatic history often afflicts them with a heightened perception of threat, even when there is no real danger. Depending on the frequency and intensity of past experiences, these perceptions of threat can frequently be ubiquitous, chronic, and symptom generating (Spilsbury et al., 2007; Stoppelbein et al., 2006; Maeng & Milad, 2017).

Once survivors discover how to reduce the tension in their muscles, calm their nervous systems, and put this knowledge into practice, they can restart their thwarted natural maturational trajectory (Doublet, 2000; Shusterman & Barnea, 2005; Sherin & Nemeroff, 2011; Dennis et al., 2017). This regulation allows them to "get out of the way" of their natural healing processes, leave behind symptoms (Holland et al., 1991), and find satisfying lives based on their own intention and principles, no matter what the external circumstances or conditions (Hamarat et al., 2001). By helping participants to articulate their

intention (defined by Merriam-Webster Online as: *a determination to act a certain way*) while simultaneously helping them to relax their bodies when they encounter perceived threats, FFTT enables survivors to begin to live their lives with fidelity to their principles *and* lower their level of stress-related symptoms (Benson, 1997).

FFTT utilizes three phases, or sections, over multiple sessions:

Phase I:    Education
Phase II:   Intentionality
Phase III:  Practice (coaching and desensitization)

These three phases of FFTT are developed and thoroughly discussed later in this section.

The first phase of FFTT is dedicated to helping clients understand how traumatic and painful learning can result in an increase in perceived threats in the present, and how perceiving these threats can cause subsequent dysregulation of the autonomic nervous system. This phase also includes learning the self-regulation skill of relaxing one's muscles while confronting these perceived threats. This important skill helps participants internally attenuate their own levels of arousal instead of becoming stressed out by the external and often capricious happenings of their lives. By practicing this skill, hundreds of clients and thousands of workshop participants have found that they are able to enjoy comfort in their bodies and successfully manage their stress levels no matter the external stimuli. As this skill is matured, individuals find themselves able to attenuate their energy level to allow the exact amount required for the task at hand and no more. The more survivors develop and practice this capacity, the more optimally they function in all situations in their lives.

The second phase of the FFTT focuses upon helping participants to develop intentionality. This is achieved by first helping them construct their own personal Covenant (see Using the Tools 32) and a Code of Honor (Using the Tools 33) in clear, succinct language. The Covenant is the articulation of our purpose for living – a personal mission statement. The Code of Honor is a statement of the principles that we choose to govern our lives – each person's individual moral compass. In addition to the construction and sharing of these declarations, the second phase also coaches participants through exercises designed to assist them in identifying the situations and circumstances where they habitually fail to maintain these principles – instances where they "act out" and breach their integrity. As participants gain the insight to see that this reactivity is simply the result of allowing the autonomic nervous system to become and remain dysregulated after an encounter with a perceived threat, they become increasingly motivated to practice the relaxation strategies of self-regulation when encountering these perceived threats. Relaxing the body, which resets the autonomic nervous system back to optimal functioning, allows the individual to regain comfort, maximal brain functioning, and intentionality in these circumstances and situations, usually within a few seconds (Critchley et al., 2001; Lanius, 2014; Porges, 1999, 2007; Scotland-Coogan & Davis, 2016). Said differently, intentional behavior is achieved simply by holding intention in mind and relaxing the body while navigating through the "haunted house" of perceived threats that emerge hundreds of times each day. The simple elegance of this formula has become the primary engine of change and transformation in FFTT.

The final activity of this second phase is facilitating a shift from an external to an internal locus of control. This shift is accomplished first by the therapist helping the survivor to discover the myriad of situations where they become reactive, "act out," and breach their integrity. The therapist then helps the survivor to understand that it is not the environmental stimuli that is causing distress and reactive behavior. Instead, the survivor begins to see that it is the dysregulation of their ANS – what is happening inside the body – when confronting these environmental stimuli that are both the problem and the solution. Finally, the therapist helps the survivor to develop and practice self-regulation strategies for lessening arousal while confronting the perceived threats in their life. As the survivor grows in their capacity to confront these perceived threats with a relaxed body, they are no longer a victim of past trauma or present adaptations. Instead, the survivor has become free to pursue the life they choose.

The subsequent work in this treatment, which comprises the third and final phase, is essentially the practice of continually confronting triggers while maintaining a relaxed body so that participants can become progressively intentional in a greater number of contexts in their lives. The more practiced at self-regulation participants become, the more they find themselves able to retain fidelity to their Covenant and Code of Honor. Moreover, the more relaxed and intentional (i.e., parasympathetically dominant) a person remains, the fewer symptoms they experience. In other words, while focusing on intentional living by confronting perceived threats with a relaxed body, the individual will likely lessen many of the symptoms of anxiety, depression, and traumatic stress.

However, most clients participating in this treatment have found at least one situation (more for those who have severe PTSD symptoms) in which, no matter how strenuous the commitment to remain self-regulated and relaxed, they still find situations that produce nearly immediate reactivity. It is likely that this acute reactivity is caused by one or more past experiences of traumatic learning intruding into the individual's perceptual system with such intensity and ferocity that the SNS spikes to immediate dominance and brain functioning is rapidly compromised (Herman, 1992; Breslau & Kessler, 2001, Sherin & Nemeroff, 2011). The space between stimulus and response has collapsed. These intrusions thwart the ability to self-regulate as the SNS is already strongly compelling the survivor into a fight-or-flight response. Those who experience this bewildering inability to self-regulate in particular situations will need to revert to traditional methods of desensitization and reprocessing (exposure, narrative, and relaxation) with a trained professional. They will need to find a therapist who can help them to access and desensitize these past painful/traumatic experiences. It should be noted that the primary function and purpose of these traditional methods – eye movement reprocessing and desensitization (EMDR, Shapiro, 1989, 1995; Shapiro & Solomon, 1995; Valiente-Gomez et al., 2017) is utilized and recommended the most – is to desensitize and reprocess past experiences sufficiently so that the intrusion of perceived threat is diminished to a level such that the participant can now self-regulate in the context of the reminders or triggers associated with these memories. Complete desensitization and reprocessing of the memory is not required – just enough to allow for survivors to intentionally relax and regulate themselves the next time they confront those particular triggers. Most clients find that after a few successful sessions of desensitization and reprocessing with past memories, they are better able to keep their bodies relaxed in future situations in which they confront perceived threats associated with these and different memories.

Many have found themselves developing a level of proficiency with self-regulation and a modicum of success in confronting and navigating through stressful situations with comfort and intentionality within the first couple of weeks of practicing these skills. As they continue to employ self-regulation in the contexts of perceived threats, they often find themselves amazed at the simplicity of maintaining intentionality, comfort, and principle-based living. However, each and every person who has ever practiced this model will quickly point out that the simplicity of the concepts and skills does not mean easy implementation. While it is simple to understand that relaxing one's body in the context of perceived threats yields comfort, maximal intelligence, and the ability to remain intentional, this capacity requires constant monitoring and regulation while engaged in the moment-to-moment activities of daily life. Maintaining this state of bodyfulness demands ongoing focused attention to areas of the body

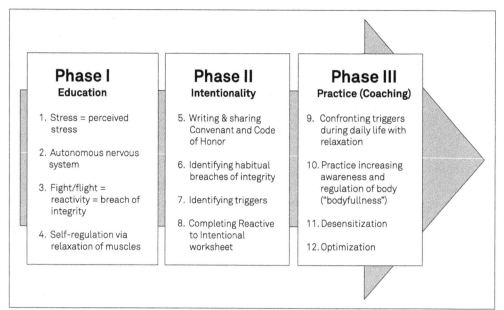

**Phase I**
**Education**

1. Stress = perceived stress
2. Autonomous nervous system
3. Fight/flight = reactivity = breach of integrity
4. Self-regulation via relaxation of muscles

**Phase II**
**Intentionality**

5. Writing & sharing Convenant and Code of Honor
6. Identifying habitual breaches of integrity
7. Identifying triggers
8. Completing Reactive to Intentional worksheet

**Phase III**
**Practice (Coaching)**

9. Confronting triggers during daily life with relaxation
10. Practice increasing awareness and regulation of body ("bodyfullness")
11. Desensitization
12. Optimization

**Figure 14.**
Forward-Facing® Trauma Therapy

to which many people have rarely paid attention in the past. Many soon discover that, as they lose conscious awareness of their bodies, it is not long before their muscles are again clenched and they are once again ratcheting upwards toward sympathetic dominance, reactivity, and symptoms.

As was previously stated, FFTT is implemented in three phases or stages (see Figure 14). It is important for individuals engaging in this treatment to be stabilized to the degree that they are not experiencing frequent abreactions or suicidal ideation before beginning any treatment. It is also important to understand that successful outcomes for participating in this program, like all healing, will be primarily contingent upon the quality of the relationship the individual builds with their therapist and the degree to which the individual is able to maintain a positive expectancy – hope – that this treatment will work for them. To maximize the quality of the relationship and positive expectancy, it is recommended that individuals choose a therapist who has demonstrated the capacity for overcoming difficulty and hardship in their own life. Additionally, a FFTT therapist should be someone with whom the participant is able to connect and who is able to maintain this supportive connection with warmth, assertiveness, compassion, empathy, and challenge. Ideally, a participant will choose someone who is working this model, or something like it, in their own life. It is recommended that therapists utilize feedback-informed therapy (FIT; Miller et al., 2013; Winkeljohn Black et al., 2017) with FFTT to assure the development and maintenance of a good therapeutic relationship.

## Phase I: Education

The first phase of the FFTT can usually be completed during a single session. However, the information shared with clients during this first phase will be reviewed and re-taught throughout the course of treatment. This is also true for readers who may wish to practice this process in a self-help model outside of traditional therapy formats.

One strategy that has been effective in transitioning from the well-trodden landscape of traditional psychotherapy into the realm of the FFTT has been to offer participants the following challenge:

*Would you be interested in learning, over the next 30 minutes, how to be stress free for the rest of your life?*

Or, if the clinician wishes to engage a more conservative approach, they may ask:

*Would you be interested in learning, over the next 30 minutes, how to significantly lessen stress in your life?*

(Note – this intentionally provocative statement is designed to heighten interest and participation from clients. The clinician is about to embark upon a psychoeducational dialog with their client to help them to understand that, in FFTT, intentional relaxation of the muscles in the body *is* the operational definition of "stress-free.")

Most clients cannot resist the temptation to hear how the clinician is going to manage this seemingly impossible task. Even the most recalcitrant clients can usually muster enough willingness and open-mindedness to at least listen, albeit skeptically, for the next half hour. At this juncture, clients are asked to identify the sources of stress or stressors they perceive in their lives. Most clients

## Causes and Effects of Stress

| Causes | | Effects |
| --- | --- | --- |
| Work | | Anxiety |
| Finances | | Depression |
| Health Concerns | | Irritability |
| Relationships | → | Fatigue |
| Aging | | Sleep Problems |
| Children | | Over/Under Eating |
| Politics | | Isolation |
| Demands | | Somatization |

**Figure 15.**
Example listing of stress causes and effects.

recite a litany of objects, people, and activities they believe to be the causes of their stress. These might include things like: finances, relationships, work, traffic, the economy, etc. Following the creation of this list of causes, the therapist can now elicit the effects of stress from their client: *What effects are all these stressors having in your life?* The answer to this question is usually a summary list of the symptoms for which the client has sought treatment. Effects such as somatic problems (e.g., headaches, GI disturbances, chronic pain, etc.), anger/irritability, sleep problems, over/under eating, substance abuse, relational problems, and anxiety are the more commonly reported effects of these stressors.

*Exercise:* Take a moment to list in a table the causes of stress in your life and then the effects that these stressors have upon you (see Figure 15).

This next step in the therapy is precarious and needs to be offered with equal parts of compassion and humor. The clinician holds up these two lists and, pointing to the lists of causes, says:

*These are NOT the causes of your stress. As long as you believe that these are the causes of your stress, there is a good chance you will keep having these (pointing now at the list of effects).*

Occasionally, clients may become a little irritated with this confrontation and the clinician will need to assure them that they have offered this with compassion and ask them for permission to continue to pursue the REAL cause of their stress. Most clients, by this point, are very much engaged and interested in what is coming next.

Continuing, the next important step is to reveal the true cause of stress, that is: *STRESS = PERCEIVED THREAT.* Perceived threat is the single cause of all stress in human beings. The reason that we experience stress when we encounter financial or relational difficulties or when we are at work or in traffic is because we have learned, through painful or fearful past experiences, to perceive threat in

these circumstances. Stress is simply the body and mind's reaction to a danger (Cox, 1992; Hamarat et al., 2001; Becker & Rohleder, 2019). It makes no difference in our response whether this danger is real or only perceived. Perceived threat (real or imagined) activates the sympathetic nervous system, and a discussion about the changes that take place in the body and brain when the SNS becomes activated is the next step of this first phase of the FFTT (see Figure 16).

When we perceive threat, our SNS activates. Only during these periods of perceived danger is the SNS active and, if we stay in the context of the perceived threat, then the SNS will remain activated to become dominant (Yartz & Hawk, 2001; Yaribeygi et al., 2017). When we do not perceive threat, or when we intentionally relax our bodies, our parasympathetic nervous system (PNS) becomes and remains dominant (De Champlain et al., 1999; Tindle & Tadi, 2020). Parasympathetic dominance may best be described as being "comfortable in our own skin."

The physiological hallmarks of sympathetic dominance include increased heart and respiration rate, decreased peripheral circulation, muscle tension, and increased energy (Sapolsky, 1996). In addition to the physiological changes that occur when we perceive threat, our brain also changes (Critchley et al., 2001; Lanius, 2014; Porges, 2007; Scaer, 2006; Sherin & Nemeroff, 2011, Becker & Rohleder, 2019). The middle part of our brains (thalamus), our brain stems and basal ganglia – often referred to as the "reptilian brain" – become more active when we perceive threat. While in the context of a perceived threat, these parts of our brain increase activity, and while these reptilian parts of our brain are increasing activity, the neocortex, or thinking part of our brain, is becoming recessive. The neocortex includes the frontal lobe, the temporal lobe, and other associated structures. These structures have been demonstrated to be the housing for our higher and executive functions (Goldberg, 2001). These

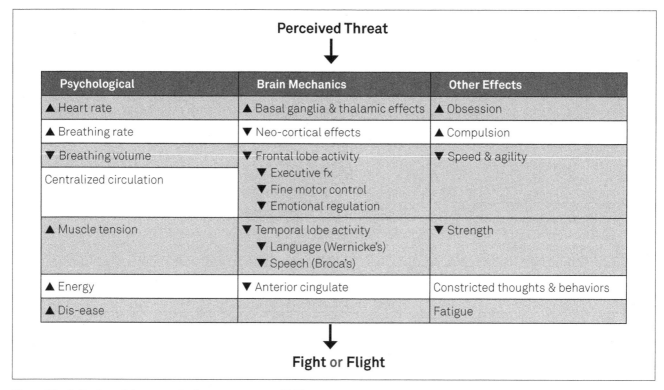

**Figure 16.**  Activation of the sympathetic nervous system (SNS)

functions include: judgment, reason, discernment, fine motor control, identity, time management/ conceptualization, language, speech, and the ability to discriminate between real vs. perceived threat. When we look into these processes, we begin to see that the longer we spend in the context of a perceived threat without intentionally relaxing our bodies, the more we compromise the cognitive and performance areas of our brains. We become progressively less able to think clearly and rationally, compromised in our language and memory skills, less agile and graceful, unable to creatively solve problems, and incapable of being ourselves when we remain in the context of a perceived threat without relaxing our bodies.

Before we impugn the SNS, however, let's look at some of the benefits of sympathetic *activation* (activation vs. dominance). The SNS gives us energy and strength, helps us to focus, supplies excitement, and affords us with joy, anticipation, and ecstasy. It's only when the SNS gets stuck in the "on" position that it causes us problems (Sapolsky, 1996; Scaer, 2006; Mariotti, 2015). Let us imagine we are automobiles and recognize that we are meant to idle at less than 1000 RPMs (PNS) and cruise at 2500 RPM (balanced PNS + SNS) and occasionally move up into the higher registers of RPMs when we need to pass another car or get somewhere in a hurry (SNS). However, many of us who chronically perceive threat and do not

intentionally and regularly relax our bodies are like cars that have the accelerator pedal mashed to floor, in gear, with another foot on the brake. We are spending our days with our RPMs red-lined, going fast but getting nowhere while we burn out the components of our engines. There is an increasing amount of research that points to this phenomenon as a cause for many diseases and immune dysfunctions (Yaribeygi et al., 2017; Mariotti, 2015; Rothschild, 2000; Scaer, 2006; van der Kolk, 1996a, 1996b).

In 1908, psychologists Robert M. Yerkes and John Dillingham Dodson demonstrated the relationship between arousal and performance. This original research has evolved into the Yerkes-Dodson Law (Yerkes & Dodson, 1908; Diamond et al., 2007; Chaby et al., 2015) to help professionals improve performance in business, athletics, and entertainment. This law describes how optimal performance is in a curvilinear relationship with arousal (see Figure 17). Low levels of arousal are required for good performance – no one runs quickly, plays blistering guitar solos, or successfully negotiates multi-million dollar deals while they are napping. This measured and regulated low-level arousal is associated with optimal performance or "flow" (Csikszentmihalyi, 1997; Norsworthy et al., 2018). However, once the energy in our bodies becomes dysregulated and climbs beyond optimal levels, there is a precipitous drop in performance capacities – cognitive and

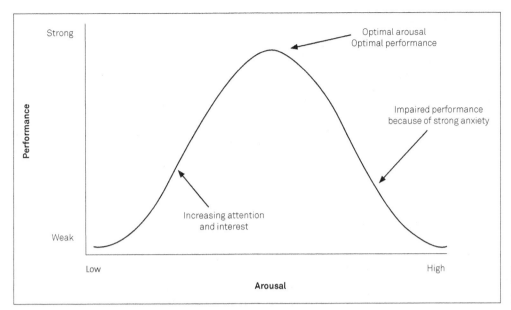

Figure 17.
Yerkes-Dodson Curve (Yerkes-Dodson Law, 1908).

motor. Not only do we experience lessened capacities when we allow the energy in our bodies to escalate without conscious regulation beyond optimal levels, we also begin to find ourselves fatigued, wrung out, and overwhelmed during and after these tasks. Research has illustrated this relationship a little more finely by showing that performance capacities begin diminishing at lower levels of arousal when completing complex and challenging tasks when compared with more mundane tasks (Dovan, 2013; Taylor, 2012). From this research we can theorize that the more complex and challenging the task, the more we need to lessen our levels of arousal. This principle is central to FFTT – teaching our clients how to confront the tasks of their lives with regulated energy in their bodies so that they can discover, in vivo, elevated capacities and performance during these tasks.

*How did we get so anxious?* Good question. In 2007, the World Health Organization published an article on personal safety in the twenty-first century. In this article they indicated that in high-income countries (North America, Europe, some of Asia, some of South America), we are the "safest" generation to ever live on Earth. We are less likely to become a victim of warfare, pestilence, famine, disease, disaster, crime, and several other indices of safety than any previous generation. However, with the never-ending parade of trauma across the evening news, it doesn't feel very safe, does it? While we may indeed be the safest generation to walk the planet, we also seem to be the most afraid. *What is different about our generation than any preceding it? That's right...the media. We bear witness to exponentially more trauma and traumatic occurrences than did any of our ancestors through the constant bombardment from*

*the media. In 1990, Linda McCann and Laurie Pearlman in their landmark work with vicarious traumatization, demonstrated to us that one need not be the survivor of a traumatic event to become traumatized by it – we need only witness it.*

To illustrate this phenomenon, often in workshops we ask participants: *How many of you in this room have ever been attacked in a parking garage?* Usually no one raises their hand. If someone does, we ask them to sit out on answering the next question: *How many of you find yourself on-guard and anxious when you are in a parking garage?* In almost all cases, all the hands in the room go up. When asked why they experience this anxiety, we can almost see the light bulb switch on as we hear answers like: *the evening news, CSI, the newspaper, my friend was attacked.* These folks witnessed trauma in a parking garage, and the next and future times they found themselves in that context they perceived threat in a parking garage – where there was no real danger. Add to this the phenomenon of state-dependent learning, which teaches us each and every time that we experience something painful, fearful, or uncomfortable that there is a good possibility that we will perceive future situations that remind us of this original event as threatening. So, said differently, if a person is the **survivor** of a significantly traumatic experience (abuse, rape, natural disaster, motor vehicle accident, etc), they are more likely to perceive generalized threat in the future. If they are the **witness** to a traumatic event, through the media, hearing stories, reading, or however that person learns about something traumatic happening to someone else, that person is likely to perceive threat and be afraid in situations that are similar to those witnessed. And, finally, if we **experience** painful, fearful, or uncomfortable incidents in our lives, through the process of association, we are likely to perceive threat in situations that remind us of these occurrences (e.g., putting our hands on a hot stove, receiving criticism, encountering periods of financial hardship). All these past learning experiences have the potential to cause us to perceive threat in the present when there is no danger. Again, the SNS does not care whether the threat is real or imagined, it will activate in either instance. If we stay in the context of this threat (i.e., parking garage) without intentionally relaxing our bodies, our SNS will become dominant and we will begin to experience the array of symptoms generated by the SNS (e.g., anxiety, panic, difficulty concentrating, irritability, somatic discomfort, etc.). It does not take much insight into this process before we begin to see that, for many of us, threat perception is ubiquitous and chronically occurring hundreds, or even thousands, of times each day.

The original goal of the SNS was survival – to help our ancestors recognize and rapidly respond to threat. However, over tens of thousands of years, we humans have developed a frontal lobe that has given us the capacity for reasoning and discernment. Without the capacities of a neocortex, it is imperative that animals recognize and respond to every threat to its survival since it cannot tell the difference between a real and a perceived threat. However, once we are able to discern this difference, it is no longer imperative, or even useful, to respond to *perceived* threat with an SNS response. There is data to support the compromise of important capacities and skills when the SNS is dominant for extended periods of time. In addition to diminished cognitive and language skills, we can also lose strength, agility, and speed. Any athlete or performance artist will confirm that their best performances occur when they are relaxed and PNS dominant. And any martial artist will confirm that they are better prepared to protect themselves and disable an attacker when they are also relaxed.

*What is RIGHT ACTION, the right use of one's will, when one perceives a threat but is in no real danger?*

Answer: RELAX one's body. This is the most important question asked because from the right answer flows intentionality, comfort, and maximal performance. Often in workshops, we hear participants tell me that the right action is to change our perception, and we whole-heartedly agree. However, it is nearly impossible to change perception when the SNS is dominant due to diminished neocortical functioning. So, best to relax our bodies for 20–30 seconds and allow our SNS to dissipate and the frontal lobe to engage so that we can: (a) be comfortable in our bodies; (b) maximize our intelligence and bring to bear all our past learning (i.e., change perception); and (c) shift from reactive fight-or-flight behaviors to intentional and principle-based actions.

## Intentionality vs. Reactivity

If we continue to perceive threat without relaxing our bodies, then our SNS will become and remain dominant, flooding our bodies with energy and chemicals (Yaribeygi et al., 2017; Mariotti, 2015; Katz & Yehuda, 2006; Yehuda, 2001). All that muscle-clenching, heart-racing, and shallow breathing is compelling us toward one of the two inexorable goals of the SNS – fighting or fleeing (Cox, 1992; Sapolsky, 1996; Goldstein, 2010). With the SNS dominant, we are increasingly compelled to fight or flee, and we are continuing to gradually lose neocortical function (Critchley et al., 2001; McNaughton, 1997; Shusterman & Barnea, 2005; Arnsten, 2009; Yaribeygi et al., 2017). As this energy continues to ratchet upwards and our neocortical functioning continues to lessen, we will soon find ourselves acting in ways we do not want to act – compulsively and against our wills (Takahashi et al., 2005: Yartz & Hawk, 2001; Yaribeygi et al., 2017).

For example, let's say that someone criticizes you at a meeting and you perceive this criticism as a threat (later, we will explore and make good sense of why we perceive these threats during seemingly innocuous occurrences and while we are perfectly safe). Your face flushes, fists clench, and jaws tighten as you think of several ways to defend yourself. You decide to say nothing, thinking that it is best to just allow the remark to pass, and choose instead to remain focused on the content of the meeting and compassionate towards your co-workers. However, you notice that you are still uncomfortable (e.g., flushed face, clenched fists, tight jaw) as you become progressively more irritated by the remark that occurred a few moments ago. Continuing to perseverate on the comment (therefore remaining in the context of the perceived threat) your SNS continues to ratchet upward while, at the same time, you are losing frontal and temporal lobe functioning. Presently, while still in the meeting, you find yourself targeting angry looks and making sniping comments towards the offender (fight). After the meeting is over, you find yourself actively avoiding contact with this person for days, weeks, months, or even years (flight).

*What happened?* Your intention was to simply ignore the critical comment and stay true to your intention of being compassionate, tolerant, and attendant to your work. You did not want to get drawn into these interpersonal politics and you certainly don't want to develop and hold on to resentment, knowing that it is causing you more harm than it is anyone else. However, it feels as though you were powerless to stop yourself even with your best effort.

This concept is the central pillar of FFTT – helping people to understand and make good sense of why they act like they do, and then to help them transform from entrenched, reactive, fight-or-flight behaviors to principle-based intentionality with comfort in their bodies. Those of us who chose to live lives of intention quickly learn that strife and willpower are rarely effective tools towards facilitating this transformation. In the example above, with which most of us can resonate, a **threshold** was crossed and we became compelled, against our will, to fight or fly (see Figure 18). When we have lost too much of our neocortical functioning and the energy in our bodies compels us to act, we can no longer hold on to our intention and instead we find ourselves involuntarily protecting ourselves from a danger that is rarely real. We act out, involuntarily, with the SNS now in control. We say things we don't mean, we hurt those we care about, we isolate, we over-eat, we over-spend, we drink and/or use drugs, and we engage in other forms of self-destructive behaviors to either run, fight, and/or soothe the discomfort of SNS dominance. All behavior directed by the SNS will have the goal of either getting away from or neutralizing the threat. Again, it does not matter if the threat is real or perceived. As long as we continue to perceive a threat without relaxing our bodies, we are destined for reactive behaviors. What's even worse is, prior to acting out against our principles and breaching our integrity, we will have endured several moments to several hours of uncomfortable SNS

dominance. This is the very definition of stressed out! (Hoffman et al., 1982).

Anytime a person acts against their will, breaches their integrity, or does anything of which they are ashamed, chances are that the person was engaged in these actions while their sympathetic nervous system was dominant (Takahashi et al., 2005). It is likely that these behaviors were, in some form, an attempt to achieve safety from a perceived threat by fleeing or fighting. Clients who participate in this process find early in their work that they are frequently acting in ways that they do not want to act. They are fighting with spouses they love, yelling at children they cherish, and dreading work they chose as their mission. In this treatment, they learn that many, if not all, of the myriad of symptoms they are experiencing result from chronic SNS dominance. In our experience, we have seen this factor at the center of symptom generation and the distress that an overwhelming majority of our clients bring into therapy.

For those whose symptoms are caused by some organic cause – a structural anomaly or biochemical issue – some form of organic treatment is usually required (e.g., surgery, medication, diet, lifestyle change, etc.). They may still benefit from psychotherapy, but it may be insufficient when the cause of the symptoms is organic in nature. For those clients whose symptoms are a result chronic SNS dominance, there is much hope. In our nearly 40 years of working with troubled and traumatized clients, we have discovered an interesting truism among the 10,000+ clients we have seen: We humans cannot live in habitual,

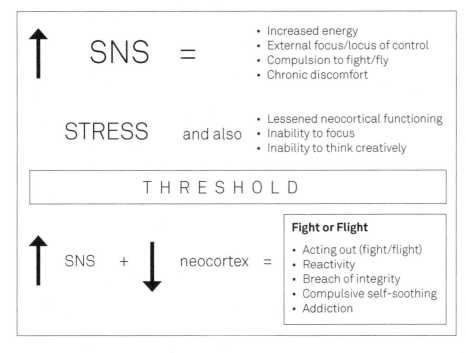

**Figure 18.**
Threshold crossing leads to fight or flight reaction.

willful, and chronic breach of our integrity without suffering symptoms. People who are the most symptomatic also seem to live in frequent betrayal of their own integrity. We breach our principles and fail to maintain intentional behavior because we have failed to relax our bodies and regulate our ANSs in the context of perceived threats. As we teach our clients to develop and maintain relaxed bodies in the context of perceived threats, not only do they begin to find themselves able to maintain their principle-based behavior – being the people they intend to be and acting the way they choose – but they also find themselves becoming progressively less symptomatic. They are prohibiting SNS dominance and instead are enjoying the relaxed comfort of PNS dominance, no matter the external situation or circumstance. Intentional, principle-based living achieved through relaxation in the context of perceived threats lessens our symptoms.

---

### Clinical Note

Clinical professionals who wish to facilitate clients' successful navigation through FFTT will want to develop this previous material into language that is comfortable for themselves and their clients. Having mentored several clinicians through the process of becoming skilled in this model, we have discovered that it takes some time to develop mastery over the complex information. It is recommended that readers take some time to familiarize themselves with the literature in the bibliography, speak with experts in the area of the human nervous system's functioning and disorders, and practice for themselves these principles. Six to twelve months is not an uncommon period of time required to gain mastery with the psychoeducational concepts and ideas contained in this model.

---

## Self-Regulation

The final component of the Educational Phase of FFTT is teaching self-regulation (Gentry, 2002, 2016, 2021; Perry, 2007; Perry & Szalavitz, 2007; McClelland et al., 2018). The use of the term "self-regulation" is different from "relaxation," even though relaxation is a crucial part of self-regulation. Self-regulation, for use in FFTT, is defined as: *the intentional and conscious process of monitoring and relaxing one's body while in the context of a perceived threat, preventing the SNS from achieving dominance.* This means an individual must develop sufficient mastery of a set of relaxation skills that they can implement at anytime to shift their arousal downward from SNS toward PNS dominance – no matter what the external circumstance or situation. It also requires individuals to develop the capacity

to monitor themselves for SNS activation and then implement these relaxation strategies to prevent the SNS from achieving dominance. Said differently, self-regulation is the development and ultimate mastery of the ability to internally attenuate our own level of arousal, anxiety, and stress (i.e., SNS dominance) to a level of comfort that facilitates maximal neocortical and motor functioning allowing for intentional principle-based behavior. Said even more simply: Stop clenching the muscles in your body!

Traditional relaxation approaches employed in the service of mental health treatment have proven to be useful but require attention, dedication, and are not always immediately effective with every individual. Most of these techniques are designed to achieve a relaxed body but fall short in helping our clients to maintain this relaxation. Maintaining a relaxed and comfortable body while engaged in the activities of daily life – especially when those activities involve frequently confronting perceived threats – is extremely challenging. Progressive relaxation, paradoxical relaxation, meditation, autogenesis, even diaphragmatic breathing all require clients to disengage from their current activities to some degree while they attempt to bring about relaxation by one of these methods, making concurrent, sustained attention on work or other activities of daily living extremely difficult. These methods work wonderfully when a person has ample time and space to engage in these deeper relaxation protocols (Sadigh & Montero 2013; Mandle et al., 1998; Jacobson, 1938). It is recommended that individuals who practice these and other methods continue their practice. However, FFTT asks them to add the skill of self-regulation to their toolkits.

Self-regulation, as defined and employed in this treatment, is simple, but it is not easy. It involves a commitment to life-long practice of discovering and then relaxing constricted muscles in one's body in a disciplined and consistent way. Many people who have developed these skills find that they need to attend to their body in a regular and ongoing process at a frequency of once every five minutes or so to maintain stress free living and maximal performance. This is especially true during engagement with demanding activities. The more demanding the activity, the more we need to attend to regulating the energy in our bodies.

We have called this ongoing identification and regulation of muscle tension "bodyfulness." While mindfulness challenges the client to disengage from trying to control thoughts and just notice them while attempting to relax, the bodyfulness of self-regulation asks them to not attend to thoughts at all, but instead maintain an awareness and relaxation of their muscles (Jamison, 1999; Kabat-Zinn &

Hanh, 2009). Good mindfulness begins with a relaxed body *before* attempting to address cognitive functioning.

There are a myriad of ways a person can achieve a relaxed body in the context of perceived threats. Different people will find different ways that work best for them. One way we have found effective to demonstrate the simplicity of self-regulation is to ask audiences in our workshops to take five seconds to become a "wet noodle" or "wet dishrag." We ask them to simply relax all the muscles in their body. At the conclusion of the five seconds, we say, "You have now demonstrated to yourself that you have the capacity for self-regulation." We further explain to them that what they have not attempted, up until now, is to develop and maintain this physiological state of relaxation while confronting the high-demand and perceived threatening contexts of their lives. This intentional use of reciprocal inhibition – pairing exposure (to perceived threats) with relaxation – is the engine of *all* effective treatments of trauma, including FFTT.

Whenever a person is intentionally monitoring their body to discover constricted muscles and then intentionally releasing and relaxing these muscles, they are practicing self-regulation. FFTT challenges clients to become increasingly aware and intentional in this process. If a person becomes aware of tight muscles in their neck while sitting in a meeting and then relaxes these muscles, they are practicing self-regulation. If a person is driving and notices that the muscles in their lower back have been tense for a period of time and then releases this tension, that person is practicing self-regulation. Developing this skill is a life-long process that produces immediate results in lessening stress. However, if the client embraces this discipline, they begin to find that not only are their symptoms lessened, but that person has also begun to optimize their life.

The muscles of the pelvic floor and, more specifically, the psoas muscles, have been clearly indentified as an important area for the regulation of anxiety and stress (Berceli, 2005; 2007; 2009; Heim et al., 1998). Relaxation of the pelvic muscles can bring about an immediate and profound relaxation of the entire body – often within a few seconds. Slower and deeper breathing, reduced heart rate, relaxed core and peripheral muscles, and reactivation of neocortical function are all benefits of a relaxed pelvic floor (Staugaard-Jones, 2012). It is difficult, if not impossible, to generate the visceral effects of fear and SNS (e.g., elevated heart rate, clinched muscles, shallow breath, diminished cognitive functioning) when the pelvic muscles remain relaxed. In other words, if you can keep the muscles between your waist and thighs relaxed and unclenched, the rest of you will likely be comfortable and PNS dominant, no matter what is happening around you. We have had reports from many clients, before they learned pelvic floor relaxation, who were so phobic or scared that they could not engage in certain activities (flying, driving over bridges, getting shots, and even skydiving). As they learned and began practicing self-regulation by relaxing the pelvic muscles, they were able to engage in these activities and reported that they had no sense of discomfort or fear. Probably the most important point about pelvic floor relaxation as a strategy for self-regulation is that people can do it while they are engaged in other activities. It takes practice and determination, but after a few months most clients who have practiced this method find that they can effectively attend to the dual activity of relaxing their pelvis while engaging in work, performance, school, relational encounters and the other activities of life. However, pelvic floor relaxation never seems to become automatic and requires constant intention and attention, or bodyfulness. Individuals wanting to remain comfortable, maximally functioning, and intentional will need to willfully practice this simple skill of pelvic relaxation moment-to-moment for the rest of their lives. Simple, but not easy.

*Why does the relaxation of the pelvic floor muscles result in profound systemic relaxation that affects both body and brain?* Well, we're not certain. We discovered this technique from emergency medical technicians (EMTs) when we learned their protocol for assisting a person who is suffering an attack of tachycardia, or dangerously fast heart rate. Paramedics are taught to use a process that is called a *val salva* maneuver, which triggers a *vaso-vagal* response (Lim et al., 1998; Waxman et al., 1980). This response is accomplished by having the patient bear down, with a gentle downward and outward pressure, as though they are having a bowel movement. This action, in most patients, produces a significantly precipitous bradycardic (slowed heart rate) response within a few seconds (Kinsella & Tuckey, 2001). This response is known to occasionally cause heart attacks with geriatric patients when they go to the bathroom (Sikirov, 1990). We became increasing curious as to how manipulation of the configuration of the muscles in one's pelvis could have such a profound effect upon heart rate. While we have been able to find precious little information or data regarding these muscles and the effects they have, except in the area of incontinence, what we have found has led to the vagus nerve (Lanius, 2014; Porges, 1992, 1999, 2007, 2011a, 2011b). The vagus nerve is the 10th cranial nerve. It is the longest nerve in the human body, hence its name – *vagus* is Latin for "wanderer." It is connected to the roof of our mouth, follows the carotid artery into the chest and terminates at the perineum (where the legs join together). The vagus nerve is intricately connected to the regulation of the PNS and the SNS, as it controls and/or regulates many of these functions in both our bodies and our central nervous systems. We know vagal nerve stimulation can and does have a profound effect on mood and is a growing treatment for some of the most recalcitrant mood disorders. We also know that mild manipulation of the vagus nerve can cause a person to pass out, have extreme heart rate variability and, during periods of extreme stress, has been linked to paralysis (i.e., conversion disorder) and dissociation (George et al., 2000).

We have much to learn about the vagus nerve and, after multiple attempts at scouring the literature, we have been unable to find any articles that give a satisfactory explanation for the mechanics and relationship between pelvic floor relaxation, the vagus nerve, and PNS vs. SNS dominance. We are unable to provide a good citation that supports the notion that when you relax your pelvic muscles, the rest of your body relaxes, and you are able to think clearly and act intentionally. While there are multiple websites that advocate and provide instruction for pelvic floor relaxation as a treatment for anxiety, we were unable to find a single empirical article after an exhaustive search. We do, however, invite you to try it. If it works for you, then you may wish to continue to utilize it as a method for self-regulation. It will certainly cause no harm. Scores of clients and thousands of workshop participants have reported to us that the quality of their lives transformed from practicing the simple skill of relaxing their pelvic muscles when they experience perceived threat. Comfort, maximal functioning, and intentionality follow in its wake.

A detailed explanation of self-regulation, SNS vs. PNS dominance, and the procedure for pelvic floor relaxation is contained in Appendix 1: Self-Regulation at the end of this book. We make copies of this handout available to all our clients and workshop participants. Please feel free to print out and disseminate this handout. It is recommended that you practice the exercise contained in the handout and complete 30 seconds of totally relaxing your pelvic floor muscles. When you have completed the 30 seconds, notice how you feel. You will likely notice that you are comfortable, sleepy, relaxed, your breathing will have slowed, and the muscles elsewhere in your body will have released. For those people having some difficulty establishing a felt sense of their pelvic floor muscles (anecdotally, this is about 10% of the clients and workshop participants), we do a Kegel exercise with them (Kegel, 1951). This is done simply by asking a person to tighten for five (5) seconds the muscles they would use if they wanted to stop urination mid-flow. Tighten these muscles as tight as you can for the five seconds and then release with a deep breath. Take a second even deeper breath and then release these muscles even more profoundly. We ask participants to then memorize this sensation of pelvic relaxation and to replicate it anytime they feel tense, perceive a threat, or are aware of any stress in their bodies. For those that continue to have difficulty establishing a felt sense of their pelvic muscles, we will refer them to a physiotherapist, neuromuscular therapist, or doctor of osteopathic medicine and tell them to ask for help in locating their psoas and Kegel muscles. A good practitioner of kinesiology will be able to help you to locate and release these muscles.

## Clinical Note

When working with clients at the conclusion of this session of treatment, and after a client has been able to successfully get and keep their pelvic muscles relaxed for a short period of time, we congratulate them on learning one of the most important skills they will ever learn. Before they leave the session, we playfully ask them the following question:

*So, are you leaving this session knowing how to never experience stress again... for the rest of your life?*

From most of our clients we get a grumble, a smile, and something like, "Yeah, but I didn't know it was going to take this much work." As they leave the session, we take heart knowing that we have given maximal attention to both the therapeutic relationship and positive expectancy – the two most powerful predictors of positive change. They (and now you also) have been equipped with powerful and necessary information to help them live lives of comfort and intention.

Whether it takes one or two sessions to complete this Educational Phase of FFTT, with its completion you will likely witness a growing sense of hope and anticipation from your client. As you reinforce for them the understanding that as they practice relaxing their bodies, in the form of pelvic floor relaxation, they will be able to enjoy immediate comfort, maximal functioning, and be able to live with fidelity to their own principles and morality, it is likely that they will be excited about continuing the work towards developing and maintaining this capacity. With the completion of this phase, we ask our clients to complete, as homework, the FFTT exercises that will help them to articulate their Vision, their Covenant, and their Code of Honor. We ask them to find 60–90 minutes of contemplative time where they can work on these exercises without interruption or encroaching demands. Templates for these exercises can be found at the end of this chapter (see Using the Tools 32, 33, 34, and 35. Use the templates to construct and complete a statement of your Vision (see Using the Tools 32), Covenant (see Using the Tools 33), and Code of Honor (see Using the Tools 34). You should be as succinct and clear as possible in the completion of this exercise.

## Phase II: Intentionality

Emphasizing intentionality (see Box 3) aims at helping the individual to heal trauma with intentional living rather than remaining caught in reactivity.

**Box 3.** Intentionality.

**Case Example:
Intentionality & The Appalachian
Trail (J. Eric Gentry)**
2168 miles, 2,000 bug bites, 21 blisters, hypothermia, and a stress fracture.

In 1996, I thru-hiked the Appalachian Trail from Mount Katahdin, Maine to Springer Mountain, Georgia. I spent the first night of the six-month hike at Daisy Pond Shelter, 2.3 miles south on the AT from Mt. Katahdin. It was the first of hundreds of three-sided sleeping shelters that dot the trail about every six miles all the way from Maine to Georgia. I was cold, scared, and alone. I discovered in that shelter, like the hundreds that were to follow, a notebook that was maintained for each hiker to write whatever thoughts or information that they would like to leave for future hikers that would pass through the shelter in the days and weeks to come. These notebooks became an important source of news, entertainment, information, connection, and comfort for me on the AT. Sometimes funny, sometimes sad, and sometimes poetic, these notebooks were savored at the end of the day at each shelter, and most days I added my thoughts and feelings to this patchwork narrative. On that first night in that first shelter I opened and read the first page of that first notebook. Here is what it said: *The first step of a journey is great not for the distance it covers but for the direction it heralds.* I spent that night meditating on this truism – on what a first step declares and the potency of that declaration. After all was said and done, that first step provided me with enough momentum and commitment to take the next five million and complete what only 5% of those who take that first step complete – a thru-hike of the Appalachian Trail.

This second phase of the FFTT begins with helping the individual to articulate and share their Vision, Covenant, and Code of Honor. This first meeting is an important moment in the trajectory of the participants' healing and self-actualization. With the completion of these exercises, your clients are emerging, stepping forward as best they can with declarations of who they are and how they *choose to be. We will want to lend to this moment all the gravitas that it deserves. Additionally, a few moments spent discussing with your client the process of writing their Vision (see Using the Tools 32), Covenant (see Using the Tools 33), and Code of Honor (see Using the Tools 34) is time well spent. A conversation that includes difficulties, challenges, and triumphs are all worthy of discussion in this early part of the first meeting with your partner.*

Next, you can discuss with your client some of their experiences with self-regulation. *Did they attempt to self-regulate during times of anxiety, stress, and perceived threats? What were the outcomes of these attempts? Do they need some remediation for self-regulation skills?*

At the conclusion of this section, there is a worksheet that will assist you in navigating through the concepts, activities and exercises of this second phase of FFTT (see Using the Tools 35). Contained in the Reactive to

**Clinical Note**

The comment we most often hear in these early sessions is that our clients were able to find comfort, relaxation, and had some minor success *when they remembered to relax their bodies.* However, most will have only practiced self-regulation a few times between sessions. It is important for the clinician to begin with encouragement and good motivational interviewing techniques. One example of this might look something like the following: *So, you were able to self-regulate during a few experiences over the past week and you were able to be comfortable in your skin and act like you wanted to?* [Client acknowledges] *Hmm. And when you forgot to self-regulate, you were uncomfortable and acted out, right?* [Client acknowledges] *Where am I going with this?* This playful confrontation reinforces for the client that they are able to choose to act differently, but must do so by remembering to first relax their body instead of trying to think their way through.

For clients who fail to complete the FFTT exercises, some time should be spent discussing the meaning of this shortcoming. Are they committed? Do they wish to negotiate to complete these exercises for the next or future session? Is there something else more emergent that needs attention? Is there something that is thwarting their belief that they can change? These are all appropriate discussions for those who fail to complete the exercises. For those who articulate a desire to continue but, for whatever reason, were unable to complete the exercises, we help them to complete an abbreviated version of their Covenant and Code of Honor. We ask them to identify three words that best describe their purpose for being alive, and then we ask them to identify three words which represent the principles they choose as their own personal code – their moral compass. We then use these six words to help them move through the following exercises of the session.

Intentional Worksheet are the five main components of this phase of the program. These are:
1. Covenant/Code of Honor
2. Reactive Behavior/Breach of Integrity
3. Intentional Actions
4. Triggers
5. Narratives

This portion of the work in FFTT addresses each of these five components in relation to one or more reactive behavior, helping you to prepare to transform this habitual reactivity into intentional, principle-based behaviors. Please print and have ready to utilize the Using the Tools 35: Reactive to Intentional Exercise for this portion of the work. Figure 19 shows an example of the intentionality rehearsal with the worksheet.

**1. Covenant/Code of Honor.** The worksheet Using the Tools 32 will help your client to identify a few principles from their Covenant or Code of Honor that they habitually breach during the course of a day or week. *What are the primary points of this moral compass? How do you want to act at home, at work, at school?* You may want to ask your client to write a few words that define the principle behind their intentions (e.g., kind, friendly, helpful). In the example in Figure 19, you can see the example is "compassion." For this example, we are using the scenario that was discussed earlier in this section during which the subject was criticized in a meeting and then engaged in reactive behavior.

**2. Intentional Actions.** To complete this second box, you can help your client find behaviors alternative or opposite to their breaches of integrity – behaviors that they would like to practice instead in the similar situations. These behaviors should be actions that represent fealty to their Covenant and Code of Honor. In the example above, in which you were criticized in a meeting, "speaking assertively" to the criticizer represents intentional behavior. This is contrasted with the harboring of contempt that is identified as the reactive behavior which, when you engage in it, breaches your integrity.

**3. Reactive (Acting Out) Behaviors.** In this third box, you can ask your clients to identify their reactive behaviors – the instances where they habitually breach either their Covenant or Code of Honor. This is simply facilitated by helping them to select one of the tenets of their Covenant or one of the principles of their Code and asking them: Where do you find yourself failing to be _____ (compassionate, frugal, honest,

trustworthy, kind, etc). The therapist usually offers an example of such a breach from their own life (one of the authors Covenant sits framed on a table in their office). Eric Gentry frequently shares with clients is: *Every morning I wake up and make a petition to be an instrument of love and peace on this planet... then I get behind the wheel of my car* [smile]. *It is hard to reconcile the intention of being an instrument of peace while yelling at someone to get out of my way.* In addition to getting a smile from his client, this disclosure usually helps them understand the look and feel of these instances of reactivity. Another metaphor that is helpful is that of a train on its tracks. The Covenant and Code of Honor are the "tracks" that you have laid that say, "This is my path... this is who and how I choose to be." You are the train, chugging along the rails of your intention. Describing the ways in which you end up "in the ditch" is a helpful aid in understanding reactivity. Whatever way you use is fine as long as you are able to describe the specific behaviors in which you engage that are repetitive and reactive and represent a breach of your integrity. Contempt is identified as the reactive behavior in Figure 19.

**4. Five Common Triggers.** Explaining and helping clients understand and identify their triggers may be the most challenging part of this approach. Triggers are the real-world objects or occurrences that we experience as perceived threats. Triggers can be anything perceived by the five senses – something felt, heard, seen, smelled, or tasted – that activates the SNS. We usually encounter triggers a few seconds to a few minutes before engaging in reactive behavior, although this latency period can be longer. Triggers most often addressed with clients tend to be relational encounters, but they can be anything from an old song to a particular date (i.e., anniversary) or time of day (i.e., bedtime). Triggers are present remembrances or little flashbacks associated with previous experiences of pain, fear, and/or trauma, causing us to perceive threat when we encounter these objects or occurrences. They are intrusions of past painful learning into our present perceptual system, causing us to perceive threat where there is no danger. Failure to relax our bodies in the context of one or more of these triggers leads to SNS dominance that, in turn, can lead to reactive behavior and breaches of integrity. We want to begin to recognize our triggers and confront them with intentionally relaxed bodies. If we can keep our bodies relaxed during and immediately after an encounter with a trigger, then we can confront these situations with: (1) a comfortable body without stress, (2) maximal neocortical functioning with creative intelligence for problem-solving, and (3) the ability to maintain

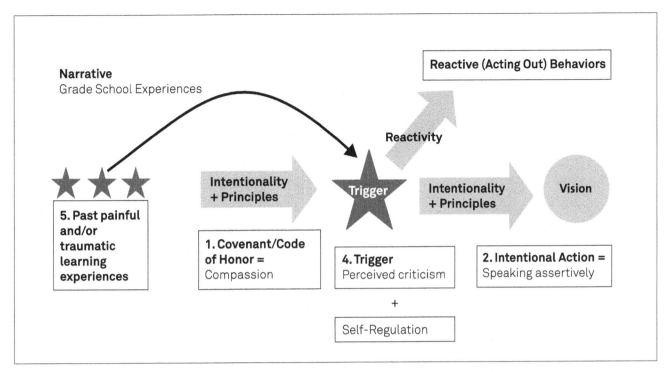

**Figure 19.**  Healing trauma with intentional living.

intentional behavior where previously we have been reactive.

The best way to discover and confront triggers is by developing an ongoing awareness of tension in our muscles – or, as we have called it, bodyfulness. If our muscles are clenched, then we have encountered a perceived threat. Tracing backwards in time from the moment of awareness of our tightened muscles to find whatever we have encountered that might have been perceived as a threat will help us to grow this capacity for finding triggers. Being reminded that stress is caused by perceived threat and that every time we experience stress during our day we are perceiving some kind of threat (real or imagined) will help us orient toward looking for the triggers that precede and precipitate this uncomfortable condition (see Figure 15. Example listing stress causes and effects). As we develop this capacity for bodyfulness, we begin the transformative process of migrating from an external locus of control in which we are victims of the capricious whims of our environment and circumstances to intentional and principle-based living with internal control of our anxiety and fear. We are healing the trauma of our pasts here, in real time.

After encountering a trigger, we find that we have a window of opportunity in which we must relax our bodies if we want to maintain intentionality. Depending upon the individual, a few seconds to a few minutes of experiencing the heightened arousal resulting from sustained threat perception will lead to progressive SNS dominance and diminished frontal lobe functioning. In this state of constriction, we become increasingly compelled to fight or fly while, concurrently, we will experience loss of intention, memory, language skills, and creativity. We revert to procedural memory instead of being able to think logically, creatively and solution-oriented (Crowder et al., 2012). It does not take long in this condition for us to lose the ability to intervene for ourselves in a productive manner and, once again, we may find ourselves acting out, "in the ditch," and repeating the same mistakes of our pasts. For most people, and the authors include themselves here, it takes a significant number of times of ending up "in the ditch" and harvesting the pain, frustration, and shame that comes from these reactive behaviors before we become willing to apply the simple solution of relaxation to the problem. Said differently, many of us have to fight and struggle with these situations long and hard until we have suffered enough pain that we can finally surrender to this simple solution (see Figure 20).

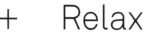

## Perceived Threat

## + Relax

= Comfort in body
= Increased thinking capacity
= Ability to live with integrity

**Figure 20.** Formula for Hope #1.

### Clinical Note

This insight can become a useful motivation tool for later sessions with our clients when we can ask them: *Have you had enough pain yet or do you need some more?* This question should always be attenuated with compassion and loving-kindness, not with sarcasm or aggression. However, the judicious use of this question will help underscore for your client that they now have a choice – where before they were condemned to repeat these same mistakes, they can now choose to relax their body for 20–30 seconds to regain comfort and intentionality.

**5. Past Learning (Narratives).** This may be the most exciting part of this method – helping individuals attach narratives and meaning to their triggers and helping them make good sense of their perceived threats. We have made a well-supported argument previously in this text that narratives are one of the most elegant and powerful ways to help our trauma-survivor clients to complete the exposure component of effective trauma treatment. When we help our clients revisit their traumatic memories and turn them into narratives (verbal, pictorial, or graphic) while relaxing their bodies, we are helping them successfully complete reciprocal inhibition and therefore desensitizing the distress associated with these memories. This exposure + relaxation is at the core of every effective treatment for trauma, many of which use a narrative process (e.g., cognitive processing therapy, traumatic incident reduction, visual-kinesthetic dissociation, and other hypnotic methods). However, each of these treatments, for which there exists evidence of their effectiveness, are regressive and therapist-facilitated. This means that, in using these models, the therapist and client have to agree upon which trauma will be the focus of today's therapy session and then begin the arduous process of constructing then sharing these narratives before the client can gain relief from these memories.

In the FFTT, our clients get immediate relief – as soon as they relax the muscles in their bodies. They do not need to revisit and retrieve their painful memories to achieve reciprocal inhibition and the resulting desensitization. All they have to do is relax their bodies in the context of the perceived threat while they are being intruded upon by these past memories. It is not the restaurant that is causing the combat veteran's heart rate to spike to 100 bpm. Instead, it is the intrusion of their combat memories into their current perception of all the possible dangers while they are out having a meal with family. Helping these veterans to learn to relax their bodies while they are in these situations will afford them immediate relief while they are with their families and, simultaneously, help them to heal their traumatic pasts.

As with the example above, there are always good reasons why we perceive threat where there is no current danger. The reason that we perceive threat in the present while encountering objects or situations that hold no real danger for us is not because we are crazy, but because of the intrusion of past painful or traumatic experiences into our present perceptual systems. Any painful past experience, no matter how brief or seemingly innocuous, can erupt into present consciousness causing us to perceive threat where there is none. There are literally thousands of these past painful experiences by the time we reach adulthood. Any object or activity that simulates one of these past painful learning experiences can precipitate the intrusion of perceived threat into our present-day consciousness. For some of us, these experiences include trauma proper while, for others among us, our current-day threat matrix is comprised entirely of these painful (but not traumatic) learning experiences. Add to this fertile and fomenting compost the experiences of secondary traumatic stress we experience through the media – or, for those of us who are caregivers, our work – and it is obvious that there are an infinite number of potential past experiences that shape the perceptions of objects and activities of our daily adult lives towards that of perceived threat.

Before beginning this process of maturation, most of us, when we encountered a trigger, did one of two things: – we tried to either alter or avoid the thing or situation we perceived as threatening. For many of us this was an instinctual and unconscious action. We rarely, if ever, confronted the trigger with relaxed bodies. The cost of this avoidance strategy was that we remained anxious, reactive, and diminished in our functioning every time we encountered these triggers. We became victims of our environment, having to fight or flee to manage stressful circumstances. The hidden costs of this strategy were even greater. Every time we encountered a perceived threat, we experienced a certain level of SNS activation and, if we remained in the context of this threat for a period of time, SNS dominance. Then we employed some form of attack or avoidance. This meant that the level of arousal we experienced when and if we ever confronted a trigger remained high, not ever diminishing because we had not yet successfully relaxed our body in the context of these triggers. One single experience of confronting a trigger with a relaxed body begins the process of desensitization. After the first time of keeping our bodies relaxed throughout an encounter with a trigger (20–30 seconds), the trigger will never again produce as much arousal as it did in previous encounters. The more occasions on which we relax in the context of the trigger, by the process of reciprocal inhibition or desensitization, the less intense the arousal will be in subsequent encounters. We become less reactive in our behaviors and more comfortable in our bodies as past experiences have less and less effect upon our present functioning. Said differently, **we heal our past by relaxing our bodies in the present**. This is the primary transformational engine of FFTT – knowing that we can unchain ourselves from the trauma and painful learning of the past with simple self-regulation.

In the past, when we encountered triggers with SNS dominance and diminished neocortical functioning, we were unable to use language very successfully. We forgot the things we learned, we stumbled over our words, and we experienced a never-ending loop of obsessive, less-than-helpful thoughts. This diminished neocortical functioning, accompanied by the compulsion of the SNS to get us out of danger, pre-empted any attempts we might have made to understand why we were so afraid when there was no real danger. As we begin to bring relaxation to the equation and remain PNS dominant through an encounter with a trigger, we can begin to ask ourselves: *Why am I so frightened? What experience(s) from my past has/have caused me to perceive a threat in this situation?* We begin to mine the experiences that have led us to perceive threat in the present. We begin to make good sense of why we are so afraid. As we are able to make sense and understand why our SNS has become activated and why we perceive threat in the present – honoring the experiences of the past where we learned through pain, fear, and trauma – we begin to experience some compassion and respect for ourselves. We discover that we were not sick or defective; we were simply adapted to a world where pain, fear, and trauma were normative. We are no longer in need of this adaptation, and we can begin to let it go; finding comfort, maximal functioning, and intentionality instead.

Helping survivors of trauma to construct and share their narratives has a powerful ameliorative effect upon the symptoms of traumatic stress, especially the re-experiencing symptoms (e.g., flashbacks, nightmares, psychological or physiological arousal with cues). FFTT creates a simple and naturalistic method for individuals to begin to construct and understand these narratives for themselves. As we practice relaxing our bodies and confronting triggers instead of avoiding them while engaged in the activities of our lives, we can begin to pay attention to the narratives that will spontaneously emerge.

An excellent example of this process is illustrated by an experience with a recent client. A 30-year-old married female who is employed full-time and is also a full-time student had been in therapy with one of the authors for six sessions. Her complaints upon intake were uncontrollable crying, compulsive behaviors, and dysthymia, or chronic low-grade depression. We had been navigating through this forward-facing process and she reported having some success with developing and maintaining relaxation. She reported finding some degree of comfort and ability to be intentional in situations in which she had previously engaged in compulsive behavior. She also reported that she was having difficulty remembering to relax her body but when she did remember, she said that her quality of life was getting much better. At the seventh session she presented for therapy and reported that her husband was experiencing depression and had spent several days of the past week on the couch, refusing to look for work or engage in any activities. The client reported that, in the past, this behavior would make her angry and she would attempt to coerce her husband into gainful action. However, she said that this time she sat down with her husband on the couch and said the following: "*When I was a child and my mother was depressed and despondent, it meant that I was soon going to be cold, hungry, or dirty. I am an adult now. I know that I will not be cold, hungry, or dirty, when you are not present with me. I love and desire you no matter what.*" There were tears in both the eyes of the client and the therapist as she related this story. This experience is a perfect example of the elegance with which clients can find resolution of their painful pasts without having to engage in regressive therapy to desensitize the memory. Instead, she was able to bring a modicum of healing to her past, present, and future by relaxing her body in the present and practicing intentionality – it was part of her covenant to love and desire her partner no matter what he did or did not do.

The Intentionality Phase of FFTT is concluded by completing the Using the Tools 35: *Reactive to Intentional* Worksheet in which your client will identify some of their triggers that you will likely be helping them to confront over the next period of time (i.e., week). Extra copies of the worksheet can be copied so that your client can work towards self-regulation, intentionality, and narrative construction on several reactive behaviors simultaneously. It is also suggested that you coach your client to maintain a journal in which they can record their thoughts, feelings, insights, and narratives as you navigate through this process.

## Phase III: Practice (Coaching and Desensitization)

### Practice

The third phase of FFTT is the least structured. For many clients this phase and subsequent sessions will look more like support or performance coaching than psychotherapy. It will simply involve more of what has already been done – helping them identify triggers, encouraging them to practice self-regulation, and helping them to make good sense of how their past experiences have resulted in perceived threats in the present. Additionally, we will want to make ample opportunity for them to share their narratives of trauma, pain, and fear and support whatever affect comes with these narratives. For clients who have minimal to moderate levels of posttraumatic stress, this version of FFTT is often sufficient. They are frequently ready to terminate therapy with satisfaction in 6–12 sessions.

This third phase also works well in a small group format (5–8 participants) of 60–90 minutes, during which each participant can take a turn to discuss successes and challenges they encountered during the intersession between group meetings. The support and identification participants experience in a group format is even more potent than individual meetings with a therapist or partner.

This phase of participation in FFTT, however, often takes on a different timbre for individuals who have significant levels of posttraumatic stress. They often find themselves - after successfully completing the first two phases - frustrated, angry, and sometimes hopeless that their progress in this third phase has not been more bountiful. It is important for the participants who encounters early difficulties with FFTT not to give up. Often these early difficulties are simply pointing to a more intensive traumatic and traumatized past that will need some focused clinical work - usually of a short duration - before they find themselves becoming successful in their ability

to confront perceived threats while maintaining a relaxed body.

For participants of FFTT who experience these setbacks in the third phase and are unable to negotiate the confrontation of triggers while keeping their bodies relaxed, and who are finding themselves continuing to act in ways that are breaches of their integrity, there is still much hope! If your client is one of these people who are simply unable to get and keep their bodies relaxed when they confront the perceived threats they encounter during their day, then you will likely need to shift your focus of treatment to more traditional methods for a short time. Likely, what is occurring for your clients is that the traumatic memories of their past are intruding with such intensity and ferocity that they are unable to find enough space between stimulus and response to get their bodies relaxed. The memories are still so raw that their nervous systems are immediately kicking into survival mode and they are unable to focus on anything else except finding safety. For these clients, you will want to help them desensitize these memories in more traditional ways using evidence-based treatment methods (i.e., trauma-focused cognitive behavioral therapy). Eye movement desensitization and reprocessing (EMDR; Shapiro, 1989, 1995; Shapiro & Solomon, 1995, Valiente-Gómez et al., 2017; Berliner et al. 2019) dovetails very nicely with FFTT to accomplish this task. The purpose of employing these traditional methods is not to completely resolve trauma memories. Instead, the value of these methods is in their ability to help your clients to desensitize their trauma memories just enough that they can begin to successfully relax and keep relaxed their bodies in the context of the perceived threats they encounter throughout their day.

As participants continue to practice the skills of FFTT, they begin to find themselves able to remain intentional, inside of comfortable bodies, with increased simplicity – even though self-regulation continues to require ongoing bodyfull awareness. It is at this juncture that participants begin to discover the ultimate simplicity of FFTT that is summarized in the Formula for Hope #2" in Figure 21:

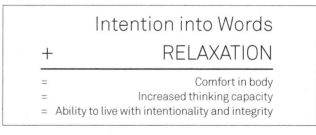

**Figure 21.** Formula for Hope #2.

## Clinical Note

For clients who need to revisit trauma memories to lessen the intensity of their present day triggering, clinicians will want to take great care to normalize this process. Utilizing good relational skills, the therapist can reassure their clients that this is simply part of the process of healing, and some brief additional therapeutic activities need to be completed before they will be able to enjoy the full benefits of their hard work. Helping them to make sense of why they are not able to remain self-regulated and intentional during the activities of their lives is valuable for both the client and for maintaining the therapeutic relationship. It is crucial to help clients gain the insight that they are being intruded upon by their trauma memories with such ferocity that they are becoming immediately overwhelmed, SNS dominant, and reactive. It is also the therapist's task to help them understand that this continued reactivity is not a moral failing on their part. It is, instead, a testament to the intensity of the injury they suffered, and continue to suffer, from the traumatic experiences of their past.

Using the worksheet Using the Tools 35, we can point to Square #5 and explain to our clients that the intrusions from their past traumatic experiences are coming forward into present consciousness with such intensity (lightning bolt on the worksheet) that they are preventing them from being able to practice self-regulation when they encounter certain triggers. We ask them to identify the triggers they have experienced over the recent past that produced reactive behaviors. We then explain to them that it is likely that these triggers represent a memory or group of memories that were traumatic or painful experiences. We further explain that their adaptation to these traumatic and painful experiences was to orient themselves to avoid anything in the future that reminded them of these experiences. Anytime they encountered a reminder this was perceived as a threat, activating their SNS, resulting in them frequently attempting to avoid contact with this reminder.

Work over the next few sessions will focus upon helping our clients to desensitize and reprocess the trauma memory(ies) associated with the trigger(s). The goal of this desensitization and reprocessing work is to diminish the intensity of the intrusions – the perceived threats – sufficiently so that our clients can begin to self-regulate and remain relaxed when confronting these triggers. In FFTT, this is always the single goal of regressive desensitization and reprocessing work with our clients. We do not employ our therapeutic skills to develop insight or to trigger abreactions or to change beliefs. While all these may occur as byproducts of this work, the goal remains only to desensitize and reprocess the memory sufficiently so that our clients can practice self-regulation without being overwhelmed in the present. It is important that the clinician work with whatever method of desensitization with which they enjoy a sense of mastery. CBT (e.g., direct therapeutic exposure, dialectical behavioral therapy, prolonged exposure, cognitive processing therapy, etc); neuro-linguistic programming (NLP)/hypnotic methods; traumatic incident reduction (TIR); narrative therapy; and the TRI Method all have been the subjects of published studies that report effectiveness with PTSD symptoms. EMDR, however, is the recommended method of treatment for this phase of treatment. The procedure and philosophy of EMDR fits perfectly with FFTT. For those who are aware of the EMDR protocol, the triggers from FFTT easily become the target for the EMDR set-up. EMDR, better than the other methods mentioned above, facilitates the client to desensitize and reprocess multiple trauma memories that may be associated with a particular trigger inside a single session. The other methods, while all being of value, require that each trauma memory be addressed individually, and the use of one of these other models may require a longer treatment trajectory to achieve sufficient desensitization.

Clients who are able to successfully desensitize and reprocess a set of trauma memories and find that they are now able to effectively relax their bodies in the context of triggers that had previously been overwhelming often gain a renewed sense of hope and commitment to therapy. As they experience themselves successfully maintaining intentionality, where they previously capitulated to their fear, clients begin to believe that they just might be able to find a life that is no longer based in fear, pain, avoidance, and despair. They begin to see the possibility of living a life of principle-based intention and a pathway to a future where, truly, anything is possible for them. Lost dreams awaken.

## Conclusion

By confronting perceived threats that we encounter over the course of a day with relaxed bodies and regulated nervous systems, we can heal the trauma of the past – here and now, in present time. Not only can we heal the negative effects of our past but we can also learn to be free from strife in the present while optimizing our physical and cognitive functioning by employing simple relaxation skills.

This is the essence of the FFTT approach. Teaching clients about how our autonomic nervous systems conspire with our learning processes so that when we encounter painful situations in our lives any future event that is similar to this previous experience is likely to be perceived as threatening helps clients to make sense of why they are so dysregulated in their current situations. As they learn that they do not have stressful lives but, instead, they have lives that are peppered with a myriad of perceived threats, then their locus of control shifts from external to internal. Finally, as we teach and coach our clients to confront these perceived threats with relaxed bodies, instead of brute force, they begin to find relief from their symptoms. But that is only the beginning. As clients are continually coached in the principles and skills of FFTT, not only do they find their symptoms dissipating, they begin to find themselves living more and more satisfying and productive lives. They find that they are able to remain intentional in situations where they were previously reactive. They find that they are able to make sense of their pasts and see it as a training ground for helping to live a good life in the present. They make peace with their pasts and find themselves able to make it through their days with fidelity to their principles and intention. They find themselves hopeful and excited about the future, many for the first times in their lives.

FFTT has provided relief from chronic fear, anxiety, obsessive thoughts, compulsive behavior, traumatic stress, and depression for scores of clients and hundreds of workshop participants. While there is yet no published research on the effectiveness of this method, it is built upon and around protocols and principles of CBT that have demonstrated effectiveness for treating anxiety, depression, and traumatic stress. This program is not offered here as a substitute for traditional therapeutic approaches. It is, however, offered as a framework within which an individual can augment and accelerate traditional approaches to psychotherapy. For some, FFTT will allow them to make significant gains in symptom reduction and intentional living with minimal need for traditional psychotherapy.

The main difference between this method and traditional trauma-focused psychotherapy is that the goal of FFTT is to help clients live an intentional, principle-based life in alliance with their own personal intention. The goal of traditional psychotherapy is symptom reduction. As we have attempted to demonstrate in this section, FFTT accomplishes symptom reduction as a byproduct of its utilization instead of as the goal of treatment. This shift in focus and process produces a significantly different feel to psychotherapy. Instead of the allopathic model in which the therapist is the doctor who brings healing to patient; in FFTT the therapist is more of a midwife or coach who supports the process of natural healing while assisting the client in removing the impediments to their own maturational trajectory. As this method begins to prove itself as an effective method for treating traumatic stress, it will open the door for paraprofessional and self-help applications in the successful resolution of traumatic stress.

FFTT will help individuals to establish a safe and effective pathway towards intentional living and to begin to become the people they have always wanted to be, living the way they want to live, regardless of their history or present day situations. It may provide a pathway of healing for some individuals that will allow them to completely circumvent traditional psychotherapy. Others may need a little help from a caring and competent professional throughout their process.

Said a little differently, as survivors navigate successfully to and through the Practice Phase they have essentially moved their work on optimal living and healing from their past into a self-help process. They may still wish to seek the occasional guidance and assistance of their therapist but may survivors will be able to use FFTT as a template for disciplined and intentional living that they can utilize for the rest of their lives.

As a self-help model FFTT is poised to become the first of its kind to show effectiveness in treating the symptoms of traumatic stress, anxiety, and depression. No self-help models have been discovered in the literature reviewed for this section that demonstrate effectiveness while significantly lowering the symptoms traumatic stress. It will be interesting to see whether FFTT will be able to provide this lessening.

While FFTT, as a treatment for traumatic stress, has only annectdotal evidence for its effectiveness, The Forward-Facing® Professional Resilience (FFPR) protocol has multiple peer-reviewed empirical studies detailing effectiveness with work-related stress and compassion fatigue symptoms (Flarity et al., 2021; Flarity, Moorer, & Jones, 2018; Flarity et al., 2016; Flarity, Rhodes, & Rechard, 2016; Cocker & Joss, 2016; Craigie et al., 2016; Potter, Pion, & Gentry, 2015; Flarity, Holcomb, & Gentry, 2014; Potter et al., 2013). It is reasonable to assume that FFTT – which utilizes the same primary mechanisms of self-regulation and intentionality – will enjoy these ameliorative benefits as well.

We have watched countless clients lower their symptoms and, much more importantly, begin to live principle-based lives with which they are satisfied through practicing the simple principles of this program. We have received literally hundreds of emails from workshop participants who, after one day of training, have told us that their lives have transformed as a result of implementing these principles and practices. Currently the use of FFTT as both an adjunct to psychotherapy and as a self-help protocol is experimental. We are unable to make any scientific claims as to its effectiveness or to its safety – although it is difficult to see how it could be harmful. We are in the process of beginning research on this model and only time and careful data collection will be able to demonstrate conclusively whether FFTT is effective for symptom reduction or in facilitating intentional living, leading individuals to greater satisfaction with their lives. We do, however, expect that positive results will follow. You are invited to conduct your own research (see USING THE TOOLS 31 on p. 196). If you find the practice of the principles and exercises of FFTT helpful, then continue to utilize this program, free of charge, for as long as you find it helpful. If you do not find it useful, you have lost precious little in your attempts. If you do choose to apply FFTT to your life, we would appreciate hearing from you, whether the program has been helpful or not. Our contact information appears at the end of this section.

The single most exciting thing about FFTT, for us, is its immediacy for hope. Clients and clinicans find it frequently staggering how they can move away from years of suffering after a single session, with the symptoms of traumatic stress and anxiety brought on by the chronic dominance of the SNS changing to the comfort and intentionality of parasympathetic dominance. To witness the dawn of hope upon the faces and in the hearts of those suffering survivors who sit across from us and for whom there has been no hope, sometimes for decades, count among the greatest experiences of our lifetimes. Since beginning to employ the principles of the FFTT, witnessing transformation among our clients has become an ever more frequent occurrence.

If there is any way that we can assist a reader of this section in helping to implement this process in their lives or the lives of others, we welcome your contact.

Send inquiries and comments about FFTT to:
J. Eric Gentry, PhD
Forward-Facing® Institute, LLC
PO Box 937
Phoenix, AZ 85001
USA
www.forward-facing.com

## USING THE TOOLS 31

### Algorithm for Forward-Facing® Trauma Therapy

**Develop, Maintain & Enhance Therapeutic Relationship**
- Utilize feedback-informed treatment (FIT)
- Maximize positive expectancy

**Teach Tools for Hope**
- Perceived threat
  - Painful past learning = perceived threat in present
  - Perceived threat = SNS activation
  - Chronic perceived threat = SNS dominance = stress
- The autonomic nervous system
  - Parasympathetic nervous system
  - Sympathetic nervous system
    + Physiological effects of SNS dominance
    + Brain/cognitive effects of SNS dominance
    – Regulation = Optimal
- Self-regulation
  - Constricted muscles = SNS / Relaxed muscles = PNS
  - Monitoring body for constriction then softening muscles
  - Demonstrate and teach "wet noodle"
  - Teach peripheral vision
  - Teach pelvic (core) muscle relaxation
  - Lessening energy in body via relaxing muscles (more demanding task = more need for lessened energy)
  - Confronting perceived threats with relaxed muscle
- Intentionality
  - Discuss principle-based living as method of treatment
  - Help survivor to identify intentions in daily life
  - Teach breach of integrity = autonomic dysregulation (increased energy in body + lessened neocortical functioning)
  - Vision Statement, Covenant, and Code of Honor exercises
  - Complete Reactive to Intentional Worksheet
  - Identify triggers
  - Pair relaxed body with confrontation of triggers

**Practice**
- Individual and/or group
- Discussion of recent breaches of integrity
- Discover specific trigger(s) for these breaches
- Plan for maintaining relaxed body while confronting triggers
- Assist survivor with narrative (i.e., making sense of the trigger)
- Continued practice
- Transition to traditional evidence-based trauma memory processing for survivors who are unable to achieve relaxed body when confronting trigger(s)

From: Anna B. Baranowsky & J. Eric Gentry, *Trauma Practice: A Cognitive Behavioral Somatic Therapy* (4th ed.). © 2023 Hogrefe Publishing

**USING THE TOOLS 31:**
Algorithm for Forward-Facing®
Trauma Therapy

## USING THE TOOLS 32

### Vision Statement Exercise

Your vision statement is an extremely important tool in developing and maintaining a principle-based life. Your vision describes the outcome and payoff of all your hard work. It is where you will end up if you follow your mission and stay true to your principles. Your vision articulates who you are and what you are doing when you are where you want to be. This exercise is designed to help you articulate your vision.

#### Preparation

Use the Retirement Party Visualization exercise from the CD *The Accelerated Recovery Program for Compassion Fatigue: A Self-Guided Resiliency & Recovery Series* (Baranowsky & Gentry, 2010). Psych Ink Resources. https://youtu.be/K9hRsjhwKwg?t=4561). This exercise will help you visualize yourself at your own retirement party and allows you to see yourself having already arrived at you vision. This exercise is an excellent way to stimulate your thinking and emotions toward writing a perfect vision statement.

If you are unable to acquire the CD, then take a few moments (2–3 minutes) to clear your mind and begin to imagine yourself getting where you want to be, doing what you want to do, and, most importantly, being the person that you want to be. Jot down a few notes.

#### Suggestions

1. A vision statement should be contained within a 2–5 sentence paragraph, written in the present tense (i.e., "I am financially secure," instead of, "I will achieve financial security.").
2. A vision statement should be global instead of specific (i.e., "I am a national leader in the field of financial planning," instead of, "I have 450 active clients.").
3. A vision statement should be written in the first person (i.e., "I am a successful and respected corporate attorney.").
4. A vision statement is your achievable dream – your carrot dangling from a stick that keeps you moving and on track. Make certain that the vision statement you write provides you with sufficient motivation and inspiration to keep you committed to your mission during the lean and difficult times.
5. Your vision statement articulates you achieving and fulfilling the purpose of your life – the reason for your being.
6. Make certain that your vision statement is for you – not for your spouse, your parents, your children, your boss.
7. Write your vision statement without regard to fear or risk – who would you be if you never experienced fear?
8. Remember your vision will become more refined the better you know yourself and your mission. Write your vision today with all the information you have available to you knowing that it is possible that it may change tomorrow. There is no wrong way to write a vision statement. Get writing.

**USING THE TOOLS 32:**
Vision Statement Exercise

## USING THE TOOLS 33

### Covenant/Mission Exercise

A Covenant (or "Mission" if that is more comfortable for you) is designed to provide its author with direction, purpose, and motivation towards actualizing all of their potentials – professional and personal. It is written in an active and declarative voice and should empower its writer with a clear vision of their perceived "best self" (the preferred persons we are becoming). This exercise is designed to help you bring into focus this best self and to identify pathways to facilitate the continued evolution toward this goal.

### An Empowering Covenant/Mission:

1. Represents the deepest and best within you. It comes out of a solid connection with your deep inner life.
2. Is the fulfillment of your own unique gifts. It's the expression of your unique capacity to contribute.
3. Is transcendent. It's based on principles of contribution and purpose higher than the self.
4. Addresses and integrates all four fundamental human needs and capacities. It includes fulfillment in physical, social, mental, and spiritual dimensions.
5. Is based on principles that produce quality-of-life results. Both the ends and the means are based on "true north" principles (i.e., what is true and right for you).
6. Deals with both vision and principle-based values. It's not good enough to have values without vision – you want to be good, but you want to be good for something. On the other hand, vision without values can produce a Hitler. An empowering mission statement deals with both character and competence – what you want to be and what you want to do in your life.
7. Deals with all significant roles in your life. It represents a lifetime balance of personal, family, work, community – whatever roles are yours to fill.
8. Is written to inspire you – not impress anyone else. It communicates to you and inspires you at the most elemental level. (Covey, Merrill, & Merrill, 1997, p. 107)

From: Anna B. Baranowsky & J. Eric Gentry, *Trauma Practice: A Cognitive Behavioral Somatic Therapy* (4th ed.). © 2023 Hogrefe Publishing

**USING THE TOOLS 33:**
Covenant/Mission Exercise

**Preparation**

Time-limited exercise. Take five minutes and complete the following questions:

1. Why are you alive? What is your purpose for being on this planet?

 

 

2. What do you want to be when you grow up?

 

 

3. What dreams do you have for yourself that are yet unfulfilled?

 

 

4. What is REALLY important to you?

 

 

5. What are your greatest strengths?

 

 

**Stop.** Review the above answers and circle the top five in each category. What does this tell you about yourself? Where are you in alignment with your values and principles? Where are you out of alignment? Take a moment to simply write down your thoughts after reviewing the above answers:

 

 

From: Anna B. Baranowsky & J. Eric Gentry, *Trauma Practice: A Cognitive Behavioral Somatic Therapy* (4th ed.). © 2023 Hogrefe Publishing

**Practice**

(adapted from: Covey, S. R., Merrill, A. R., & Merrill, R. R. (1997). *First things first*. Simon & Schuster, p. 107)

Practice with the following sentence forms to start creating your vision and mission for yourself. Take one minute to complete each unfinished sentence.

It is my covenant:

To live: _____

_____

_____

To work: _____

_____

_____

To continue: _____

_____

_____

To love: _____

_____

_____

To be: _____

_____

_____

To become: _____

_____

_____

_____

From: Anna B. Baranowsky & J. Eric Gentry, *Trauma Practice: A Cognitive Behavioral Somatic Therapy* (4th ed.). © 2023 Hogrefe Publishing

To believe: _____

_____

_____

To promote: _____

_____

_____

To strive: _____

_____

_____

To seek: _____

_____

_____

**Now write your Covenant/Mission**

From: Anna B. Baranowsky & J. Eric Gentry, *Trauma Practice: A Cognitive Behavioral Somatic Therapy* (4th ed.). © 2023 Hogrefe Publishing

**My Covenant/Mission**

## USING THE TOOLS 34

### My Code of Honor

This exercise is the last of three in helping you to establish the foundations of a principle-based life. If your Vision Statement (Using the Tools 32) represents the destination of your life and your Covenant/Mission statement (Using the Tools 33) represents your purpose, then the priniciples listed in My Code of Honor are the methods that you utilize to perform your mission and to achieve your vision. Your principles articulate your integrity – by what laws and rules you will choose to live. Use a train metaphor: your Vision statement is the destination, your Covenant/Mission statement is the train and its fuel, and your principles in the Code of Honor are the tracks upon which the train glides. The better you are at remaining on the tracks of your principles, avoiding derailment, the more quickly and effortlessly you will achieve your vision.

### My principles

Below is a list of words that can be constructed into Code of Honor principle-based statements (e.g., Honest = "I am honest in all dealings with others and myself.").

| | | |
|---|---|---|
| Honest | Conservative | Effective |
| Challenging | Liberal | Scientific |
| Approach vs. avoidance | Moderate | Creative |
| Ethical | Tolerant | Detailed |
| Frugal | Conservative | Compassionate |
| Faithful | Outspoken | Resilient |
| Sense of humor | Assertive | Powerful |
| Commitment | Service | Responsible |
| Hopeful | Thrifty | Productive |
| Joyous | Efficient | Just |
| Courage | Leader | Passionate |
| Truth/truthful | Facilitative | Secure |
| Parenting | Optimistic | Loving |
| Nonviolent/peaceable | Farsighted | Strong |
| Fearless | Self-confident | Active |

Pick 10–12 words from the above list and write sentences that describe you living these principles perfectly all the time (i.e., "I remain hopeful in all situations"). It is understood that you will not be able to maintain these principles 100% of the time and that they are the focus of our work. You will, however, become progressively more efficient in living within your principles as you practice some of the tools you learn in FFTT. Remember, with this exercise you are laying the tracks toward your vision upon which you will practice with your covenant/mission day in and day out, so make certain that the principles you choose are really true for you. *To thine own self be true*

From: Anna B. Baranowsky & J. Eric Gentry, *Trauma Practice: A Cognitive Behavioral Somatic Therapy* (4th ed.). © 2023 Hogrefe Publishing

**USING THE TOOLS 34:**
My Code of Honor

## USING THE TOOLS 35

**Reactive to Intentional Worksheet**

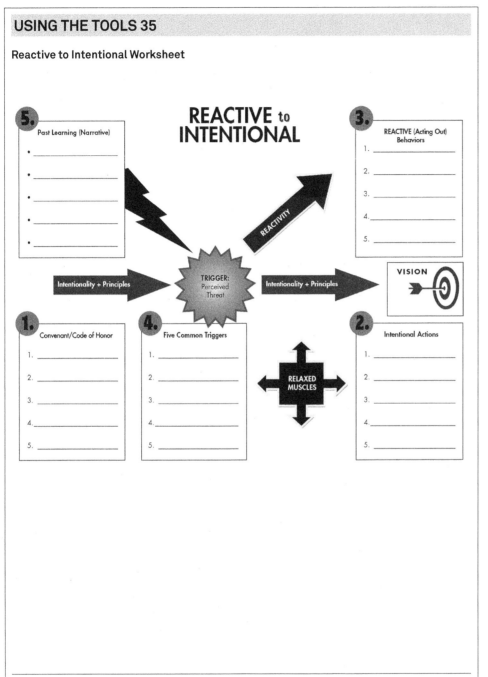

**5.** Past Learning (Narrative)
- _____
- _____
- _____
- _____
- _____

**REACTIVE to INTENTIONAL**

**3.** REACTIVE (Acting Out) Behaviors
1. _____
2. _____
3. _____
4. _____
5. _____

REACTIVITY

Intentionality + Principles

TRIGGER: Perceived Threat

Intentionality + Principles

VISION

**1.** Convenant/Code of Honor
1. _____
2. _____
3. _____
4. _____
5. _____

**4.** Five Common Triggers
1. _____
2. _____
3. _____
4. _____
5. _____

RELAXED MUSCLES

**2.** Intentional Actions
1. _____
2. _____
3. _____
4. _____
5. _____

From: Anna B. Baranowsky & J. Eric Gentry, *Trauma Practice: A Cognitive Behavioral Somatic Therapy* (4th ed.). © 2023 Hogrefe Publishing

**USING THE TOOLS 35:**
Reactive to Intentional Worksheet

## USING THE TOOLS 36

### Individualized Compassion Fatigue Resiliency Plan

1. **Self Regulation.** Ability to switch from the SNS to the PNS after you have determined that you are safe from threat. Requires relaxation of pelvic (psoas) muscles. Identify two methods that you can employ to relax and keep relaxed this area of your body.

   a. _____

   b. _____

2. **Intentionality.** The ability to follow your mission or Code of Honor to within your integrity. The ability to follow the path in which you aim yourself. Identify two areas where you perceive threat, habitually respond reactively, are derailed from your mission, and breech your integrity (can be professional or personal). Make commitment to self-regulate during these periods.

   a. _____

   b. _____

3. **Self-Validated Caregiving.** The ability to give yourself acknowledgement and validation for the work that you do. Resolving the threat perceived and remaining relaxed when client and/or peer is angry or judgmental with you. Ability to monitor and provide self with physical, emotional, and spiritual needs. Identify two situations in your personal or professional life in which you find yourself "caving in" to the perceived demands of a client or peer. Identify situations where you become anxious about the way that you might be perceived by another. Practice relaxation and positive self-supervision in these situations.

   a. _____

   b. _____

4. **Connection/Support.** The employment of three or more peers to serve as a support for you. These persons should be educated in how to best help you and should be able to listen without judgment or interruption. You will want these peers to be safe for you and trusted enough that you can share uncomfortable information. These support persons should be used with intention for you to both narrate traumatic experiences (primary and secondary) and expose secrets. Identify three people who you will request to become members of your support family.

   a. _____

   b. _____

   c. _____

From: Anna B. Baranowsky & J. Eric Gentry, *Trauma Practice: A Cognitive Behavioral Somatic Therapy* (4th ed.). © 2023 Hogrefe Publishing

**USING THE TOOLS 36:**
Individualized Compassion
Fatigue Resiliency Plan

**5. Self-Care.** What activities refuel you? You should identify at least one aerobic activity in which you will engage three times weekly. You should also identify an integrative activity (e.g., learning a musical instrument, learning an art or craft, learning a sport) that contains both the learning and discipline of mastering the rudiments (e.g., scales, tools, drills) as well as ample time to participate in playing in this activity. The remaining three should be activities that replenish you and give you a sense of joy, reconnecting you with life, hope, and wonder. Identify five activities that will help you face each new day with fullness and potency.

a. (aerobic) _____

b. (integrative) _____

c. _____

d. _____

e. _____

From: Anna B. Baranowsky & J. Eric Gentry, *Trauma Practice: A Cognitive Behavioral Somatic Therapy* (4th ed.). © 2023 Hogrefe Publishing

# References

Abramowitz, J. S., Tolin, D. F., & Street, G. P. (2001). Paradoxical effects of thought suppression: A meta-analysis of controlled studies. *Clinical Psychology Review, 21,* 683–703. https://doi.org/10.1016/S0272-7358(00)00057-X

Adenauer, H., Catani, C., Gola, H., Keil, J., Ruf, M., Schauer, M., & Neuner, F. (2011). Narrative exposure therapy for PTSD increases top-down processing of aversive stimuli-evidence from a randomized controlled treatment trial. *BMC Neuroscience, 12*(1), 1–13. https://doi.org/10.1186/1471-2202-12-127

Allen, M., Dietz, M., Blair, K. S., van Beek, M., Rees, G., Vestergaard-Poulsen, P., Lutz, A., & Roepstorff, A. (2012). Cognitive-affective neural plasticity following active-controlled mindfulness intervention. *The Journal of Neuroscience, 32*(44), 15601–15610. https://doi.org/10.1523/JNEUROSCI.2957-12.2012

American Psychiatric Association. (1980). *Diagnostic and statistical manual of mental disorders* (3rd ed.). (DSM-III). American Psychiatric Association.

American Psychiatric Association. (2000). *Diagnostic and statistical manual of mental disorders* (4th ed., text rev.). American Psychiatric Association.

American Psychiatric Association. (2013). *Diagnostic and statistical manual of mental disorders* (5th ed.). American Psychiatric Association.

American Psychological Association. (2017). *Clinical practice guideline for the treatment of PTSD.* Guideline development panel for the treatment of PTSD in adults. https://www.apa.org/ptsd-guideline/ptsd.pdf

Andersson, M. A., & Conley, C. S. (2013). Optimizing the perceived benefits and health outcomes of writing about traumatic life events. *Stress Health, 29*(1), 40–49. https://doi.org/10.1002/smi.2423

Anker, M. G., Duncan, B. L., & Sparks, J. A. (2009). Using client feedback to improve couple therapy outcomes: A randomized clinical trial in a naturalistic setting. *Journal of Consulting and Clinical Psychology, 77*(4), 693–704. https://doi.org/10.1037/a0016062

Antonovsky, A. (1979). *Health, stress, and coping.* Jossey-Bass.

Antonovsky, A. (1987). *Unraveling the mystery of health: How people manage stress and stay well.* Jossey-Bass.

Arnow, B. A., Steidtmann, D., Blasey, C., Manber, R., Constantino, M. J., Klein, D. N., Markowitz, J. C., Rothbaum, B. O., Thase, M. E., Fisher, A. J., & Kocsis, J. H. (2013). The relationship between the therapeutic alliance and treatment outcome in two distinct psychotherapies for chronic depression. *Journal of Consulting and Clinical Psychology, 81*(4), 627–638. https://doi.org/10.1037/a0031530

Arnsten A. F. (2009). Stress signalling pathways that impair prefrontal cortex structure and function. *Nature Reviews: Neuroscience, 10*(6), 410–422. https://doi.org/10.1038/nrn2648

Asmundson, G. J. G., & Taylor, S. (2009). PTSD diagnostic criteria: Understanding etiology and treatment. *The American Journal of Psychiatry, 166,* 726–726. https://doi.org/10.1176/appi.ajp.2009.08121799

Asmundson, G. J. G., Thorisdottir, A. S., Roden-Foreman, J. W., Baird, S. O., Witcraft, S. M., Stein, A. T., Smits, J., & Powers, M. B. (2019). A meta-analytic review of cognitive processing therapy for adults with posttraumatic stress disorder. *Cognitive Behaviour Therapy, 48*(1), 1–14. https://doi.org/10.1080/16506073.2018.1522371

Australian Government, National Health and Medical Research Council (n.d.). *Australian PTSD guidelines.* https://www.phoenixaustralia.org/australian-guidelines-for-ptsd/

Baer, L. (2001). *The imp of the mind.* Dutton.

Baldwin, D. V. (2013). Primitive mechanisms of trauma response: An evolutionary perspective on trauma-related disorders. *Neuroscience & Biobehavioral Reviews, 37,* 1549–1566. Retrieved from http://www.trauma-pages.com/a/dvb-2013.php https://doi.org/10.1016/j.neubiorev.2013.06.004

Baldwin, S. A., & Imel, Z. E. (2013). Therapist effects: Findings and methods. In M. J. Lambert (Ed.), *Bergin and Garfield's handbook of psychotherapy and behavior change* (6th ed., pp. 258–297). John Wiley.

Bandler, R., & Grinder, J. (1979). *Frogs into princes.* Real People Press.

Baranowsky, A. B. (1997). *Layering: A mastery approach to disturbing physical and emotional sensations.* [unpublished manuscript]. Psych Ink Resources.

Baranowsky, A. B. (Ed.). (2000). Special issue on neoteric treatment approaches in traumatology. *Traumatology E Journal, 5*(4).

Baranowsky, A. B. (2010). *Recovery now: Trauma* [Audio Recording]. Psych Ink Resources.

Baranowsky, A. B. (2010, May 11). *Breath training: 3-6 breathing: The window into the nervous system* [Video]. YouTube. https://youtu.be/lR0cV9vOIRM

Baranowsky, A. B. (2012). Silencing response. In C. Figley (Ed.), *Encyclopedia of trauma: An interdisciplinary guide* (pp. 628–631). Sage.

Baranowsky, A. B. (2013, November 27). *Manage stress and anxiety with your breath* [Video]. YouTube. https://youtu.be/PyifRngs4jY

Baranowsky, A. B. [What Is PTSD]. (2014, March 12). *Day 31 self-compassion reflection* [Video]. YouTube. https://www.youtube.com/watch?v=VjierSla_tw

Baranowsky, A. B. [What Is PTSD]. (2014a, August 25). *Comfort on palms of your hands (M4-GE)* [Video]. YouTube. https://youtu.be/_g1gUcjY28I

Baranowsky, A. B. [What Is PTSD]. (2014b, August 25). *Layering (M4-GE)* [Video]. YouTube. https://youtu.be/qWCLQbF6A50

Baranowsky, A. B. [What Is PTSD]. (2014c, August 25). *Paced breathing (M3-GE)* [Video]. YouTube. https://youtu.be/VDasBQQxqNE

Baranowsky, A. B. [What Is PTSD]. (2014d, August 25). *Reflection on self compassion (M6-GE)* [Video]. YouTube. https://youtu.be/SWQ59_juTcg

Baranowsky, A. B. (2014a, November 3). *Thematic Map and Release: Full Session* [Video]. YouTube. https://youtu.be/A9LwIy0hS2A

Baranowsky, A. B. (2014b, November 3). *Thematic Map and Release: Short version* [Video]. YouTube. https://youtu.be/GOafcmHQlZI

Baranowsky, A. B. [What Is PTSD]. (2015, January 2). *Go slow to heal after trauma. Ask Dr Anna S.2.E.1* [Video]. YouTube. https://youtu.be/v3IL9WZVLXI

Baranowsky, A. B. [What Is PTSD]. (2015, April 12). *Improve sleep, relax deeply & embed positive messages. Ask Dr Anna S.2E.16* [Video]. YouTube. https://youtu.be/ZQmfCEtzvEE

Baranowsky, A. B. [What Is PTSD]. (2015, April 16). *Learn about ddrenaline & cortisol to help manage stress. Ask Dr Anna S.2.E.17* [Video]. YouTube. https://www.youtube.com/watch?v=rHpLoK4ZhQQ

Baranowsky, A. B. [What Is PTSD]. (2015, July 8). *Embrace positivity with a hope box. Ask Dr Anna S.2.E.25* [Video]. YouTube. https://youtu.be/1zbudRJ5muU

Baranowsky, A. B. [What Is PTSD]. (2015, July 15). *How to create a containment vessel to deal with difficult situations. Ask Dr Anna S.2E.26* [Video]. YouTube. https://youtu.be/du5MaQk-w3M

Baranowsky, A. B. [What Is PTSD]. (2015, July 22). *How to create a wellness mind map. Ask Dr Anna S.2.E.27* [Video]. YouTube. https://youtu.be/qqEXDp3IX6k

Baranowsky, A. B. (2015a, August 23). *3-6 Breathing* [Video]. YouTube. https://youtu.be/fmjoLMHPCHQ

Baranowsky, A. B. (2015b, August 23). *Diaphragmic breathing* [Video]. YouTube. https://youtu.be/ys3AuHFTKQg

Baranowsky, A. B. (2015c, August 23). *Grounding & containment 5-4-3-2-1* [Video]. YouTube. https://www.youtube.com/watch?v=mwnzg4aJih4

Baranowsky, A. B. (2015d, August 23). *NLP anchoring* [Video]. YouTube. https://youtu.be/fiQJ2KXRvmQ

Baranowsky, A. B. [What Is PTSD]. (2015e, August 23). *Relaxation autogenics* [Video]. YouTube. https://youtu.be/OUlJAsO3XQE

Baranowsky, A. B. [What Is PTSD]. (2015a, September 9). *Day 17: Making peace with your sleep in the trauma recovery program online* [Video]. YouTube. https://youtu.be/5HjzyLMsygM

Baranowsky, A. B. [What Is PTSD]. (2015b, September 9). *Make peace with your sleep (M2-GE)* [Audio]. YouTube. https://youtu.be/n9BRRCdj0s4

Baranowsky, A. B. [What Is PTSD]. (2015, September 24). *Day 7: Relaxed breathing guided practice in Trauma Recovery Program online* [Video]. YouTube. https://youtu.be/XxoLhLvdscw

Baranowsky, A. B. [What Is PTSD]. (2015, October 14). *Emotional Neglect & Traumatic Loneliness. Ask Dr. Anna S.2.E.36* [Video]. YouTube. https://youtu.be/6ZeR85s5oxI

Baranowsky, A. B. [What Is PTSD]. (2015, October 28). *How to Overcome Emotional Neglect with Dr Webb. Ask Dr. Anna S.2.E.38* [Video]. YouTube. https://youtu.be/er2dUhNSghs

Baranowsky, A. B. [What Is PTSD]. (2015, November 11). *The emotional brain lays a landmine of frightening memories. Ask Dr Anna S.2.E.40* [Video]. YouTube. https://youtu.be/sL-kJSleE_c

Baranowsky, A. B. [What Is PTSD]. (2016, February 3). *Use the Body Scan to help you recover. Guided body scan exercise* [Video]. YouTube. https://youtu.be/zYf_4tJva2M

Baranowsky, A. B. [What Is PTSD]. (2016, April 13). *Simple grounding and containment exercise* [Video]. YouTube. https://youtu.be/zpKOW0ylsfY

Baranowsky, A. B. [What Is PTSD]. (2016, May 4). *Tame and decode bad dreams* [Video]. YouTube. https://youtu.be/Oi72TXnkEy4

Baranowsky, A. B. [What Is PTSD]. (2016, June 29). *You CAN recover from Childhood Emotional Neglect* [Video]. YouTube. https://youtu.be/icWqqda2IYQ

Baranowsky, A. B. [What Is PTSD]. (2016, July 21). From fear to shake and laughter: Emotional tuning with Frank Pasquill [Video]. YouTube. https://youtu.be/ebf6rJ_Y2wU

Baranowsky, A. B. [What Is PTSD]. (2016, July 28). *Try this shake to release stress exercise with Dr. Anna Baranowsky and Frank Pasquill* [Video]. YouTube. https://youtu.be/iYAVAA10jjs

Baranowsky, A. B. [What Is PTSD]. (2016, September 21). *The importance of community and connection* [Video]. YouTube. https://youtu.be/Iv9-TQBZQkI

Baranowsky, A. B. [What Is PTSD]. (2017, January 25). *Find calm using the grounding light stream exercise!.#.* [Video]. YouTube. https://youtu.be/2Ymq4ov8Xyg

Baranowsky, A. B. [What Is PTSD]. (2017, July 19). *Inherited family trauma with Mark Wolynn* [Video]. YouTube. https://www.youtube.com/watch?v=WzQ5FM3hCgo&t=1061s

Baranowsky, A. B. [What Is PTSD]. (2017, July 26). *Traumagram and epigenetics: Healing power of traumagram* [Video]. YouTube. https://youtu.be/TQUOjoAODAo

Baranowsky, A. B. [What Is PTSD]. (2018, January 10). *Healing Relationships after Childhood Emotional Neglect* [Video]. YouTube. https://youtu.be/8HPAVongqpE

Baranowsky, A. B. [What Is PTSD]. (2018, July 17). *Deep stress release with hands over heart space exercise* [Video]. YouTube. https://youtu.be/Ah46XMY1YpA

Baranowsky, A. B. (2019). *Thematic map and release (CR-RE-R)*. Psych Ink Resources. https://psychink.com/wp-content/uploads/2019/07/Thematic-Map-and-Release-2019.pdf

Baranowsky, A. B. [What Is PTSD]. (2019, April 8). *Deep relaxation with safe place visualization* [Video]. YouTube. https://www.youtube.com/watch?v=rMIAgTY_-Fc

Baranowsky, A. B. [What Is PTSD]. (2020, December 5). *Recovery now TRAUMA* [Audio]. YouTube. https://www.youtube.com/watch?v=DvzwJ614frM

Baranowsky, A. B., & Gentry, J. E. (2010). *Compassion fatigue: A self-guided resiliency & recovery series* [Audio]. https://podcasts.apple.com/us/podcast/compassion-fatigue-resiliency-recovery/id1463793962?i=1000510544225

Baranowsky, A. B., & Gentry, J. E. (2011a). *Compassion satisfaction manual*. Psych Ink Resources.

Baranowsky, A. B., & Gentry, J. E. (2011b). *Workbook/journal for a compassion fatigue specialist*. Psych Ink Resources.

Baranowsky, A. B., & Gentry, J. E. (2015, August 23). *Circle of support* [Video]. YouTube. https://youtu.be/CcbJz4CZTbM

Baranowsky, A. B., Gentry, J. E., & Schultz, D. F. (2005). *Trauma practice: Tools for stabilization and recovery*. Hogrefe.

Baranowsky, A. B., & Lauer, T. (2013). *What is PTSD? 3 Steps for healing trauma*. Traumatology Institute.

Barlow, D. H., Boswell, J. F., & Thompson-Hollands, J. (2013). Eysenck, Strupp, and 50 years of psychotherapy research: A personal perspective. *Psychotherapy, 50*(1), 77-87. https://doi.org/10.1037/a0031096

Bean, R. C., Ong, C. W., Lee, J., & Twohig, M. P. (2017). Acceptance and commitment therapy and trauma: An empirical review. *The Behavior Therapist, 40*, 145-150.

Beck, A. T. (1967). *Depression: Causes and treatment*. University of Pennsylvania Press.

Beck, A. T. (1976). *Cognitive therapy and the emotional disorders*. International Universities Press.

Beck, J. G., McNiff, J., Clapp, J. D., Olsen, S. A., Avery, M. L., & Hagewood, J. H. (2011). Exploring negative emotion in women experiencing intimate partner violence: Shame, guilt, and PTSD. *Behavior Therapy, 42*(4), 740-750. https://doi.org/10.1016/j.beth.2011.04.001

Becker, L., & Rohleder, N. (2019). Time course of the physiological stress response to an acute stressor and its associations with the primacy and recency effect of the serial position curve. *PloS one, 14*(5), Article e0213883. https://doi.org/10.1371/journal.pone.0213883

Belleau, E. L., Chin, E. G., Wanklyn, S. G., Zambrano-Vazquez, L., Schumacher, J. A., & Coffey, S. F. (2017). Pre-treatment predictors of dropout from prolonged exposure therapy in patients with chronic posttraumatic stress disorder and comorbid substance use disorders. *Behaviour Research and Therapy, 91*, 43-50. https://doi.org/10.1016/j.brat.2017.01.011

Benish, S. G., Imel, Z. E., & Wampold, B. E. (2008). The relative efficacy of bona fide psychotherapies for treating post-traumatic stress disorder: A meta-analysis of direct comparisons. *Clinical Psychology Review, 28*(5), 746-758. https://doi.org/10.1016/j.cpr

Benson, H. (1997). *The relaxation response.* Avon.

Berceli, D. (2005). *Trauma releasing exercises: A revolutionary new method for stress/trauma recovery.* Create Space Publishers.

Berceli, D. (2007). *Evaluating the effects of stress reduction exercises* [Doctoral dissertation]. Arizona State University, Phoenix, AZ.

Berceli, D. (2009). *The revolutionary trauma release process: Transcend your toughest times.* Namaste.

Bergen-Cico, D., Possemato, K., & Pigeon, W. (2014). Reductions in cortisol associated with primary care brief mindfulness program for veterans with PTSD. *Medical Care, 52*, 25-31. https://doi.org/10.1097/MLR.0000000000000224

Bergstrom, K. J., & Hiscock, M. (1988). Factors influencing ocular motility during the performance of cognitive tasks. *Canadian Journal of Psychology, 42*, 1-23. https://doi.org/10.1037/h0084174

Berliner, L., Bisson, J., Cloitre, M., Forbes, D., Goldbeck, L., Jensen, T., Lewis, C., Monson, C., Olff, M., Pilling, S., Riggs, D., Roberts, N., & Shapiro, F. (2019). *ISTSS PTSD Prevention and Treatment Guidelines: Methodology and Recommendations.* International Society for Traumatic Stress Studies. https://istss.org/getattachment/Treating-Trauma/New-ISTSS-Prevention-and-Treatment-Guidelines/ISTSS_PreventionTreatmentGuidelines_FNL-March-19-2019.pdf.aspx

Bernardy, N. C., & Friedman, M. J. (2012). 2010 VA/DOD Clinical practice guideline for management of post-traumatic stress: How busy clinicians can best adopt updated recommendations. *Journal of Rehabilitation Research and Development, 49*(5), vii-viii. https://doi.org/10.1682/jrrd.2012.02.0036

Bezo, B., & Maggi, S. (2018). Intergenerational perceptions of mass trauma's impact on physical health and well-being. *Psychological Trauma: Theory, Research, Practice, and Policy, 10*(1), 87-94. https://doi.org/10.1037/tra0000284

Bisson, J. I., Ehlers, A., Matthews, R., Pilling, S., Richards, D., & Turner, S. (2007). Psychological treatments for chronic post-traumatic stress disorder: Systematic review and meta-analysis. *The British Journal of Psychiatry, 190*, 97-104. https://doi.org/10.1192/bjp.bp.106.021402

Black, S. W., Owen, J., Chapman, N., Lavin, K., Drinane, J. M., & Kuo, P. (2017). Feedback informed treatment: An empirically supported case study of psychodynamic treatment. *Journal of Clinical Psychology, 73*, 1499-1509. https://doi.org/10.1002/jclp.22529

Bloom, S. (2013). *Creating sanctuary. Toward the evolution of sane societies* (2nd ed.). Routledge.

Bonner, R., & Rich, A. (1988). Negative life stress, social problem-solving self-appraisal, and hopelessness: Implications for suicide research. *Cognitive Therapy and Research, 12*, 549-556. https://doi.org/10.1007/BF01205009

Bordoni, B., & Zanier, E. (2013). Anatomic connections of the diaphragm: Influence of respiration on the body system. *Journal of Multidisciplinary Healthcare, 6*, 281-291. https://doi.org/10.2147/JMDH.S45443

Borresen, K. (2018, February 2). Am I codependent? 10 signs you might be, according to experts. *Huffost.* https://www.huffpost.com/entry/signs-of-codependent-relationship_n_5a725f26e4b05253b27572ba

Bourne, E. J. (2010). *The anxiety and phobia workbook.* New Harbinger Publications.

Bremner, J. D. (2000). The neurobiology of post-traumatic stress disorder. In E. Fink (Ed.), *The encyclopedia of stress* (pp. 186-191). Academic Press.

Bremner, J. D., Narayan, M., Anderson, E. R., Staib, L. H., Miller, H. L., & Charney, D. S. (2000). Hippocampal volume reduction in major depression. *American Journal of Psychiatry, 157*(1), 115-118. https://doi.org/10.1176/ajp.157.1.115

Breslau, N., & Kessler, R. (2001). The stressor criterion in DSM-IV post-traumatic stress disorder: An empirical investigation. *Biological Psychiatry, 50*, 699-704. https://doi.org/10.1016/S0006-3223(01)01167-2

Briere, J., & Scott, C. (2012). *Principles of trauma therapy: A guide to symptoms, evaluation, and treatment* (2nd ed.). Sage Publications, Inc.

Burns, D. (1980). *Feeling good: The new mood therapy.* Morrow.

Cahill, S. P., Olasov Rothbaum, B., Resic, P. A., & Follette, V. M. (2009). Cognitive-behavioral therapy for adults. In E. B. Foa, T. M. Keane, M. J. Friedman, & J. A. Cohen (Eds.), *Effective treatments for PTSD: Practice guides from the International Society for Traumatic Stress Disorders* (2nd ed., pp. 617-639). The Guildford Press.

Carbonell, J. L., & Figley, C. R. (1996). When trauma hits home: Personal trauma and the family therapist. *Journal of Marital and Family Therapy, 22*(1), 53-58. https://doi.org/10.1111/j.1752-0606.1996.tb00186.x

Carbonell, J. L., & Figley, C. (1999). Promising PTSD treatment approaches a systematic clinical demonstration of promising PTSD treatment approaches. *Traumatology, 5*(1), 32-48. https://doi.org/10.1177/153476569900500106

Carlson, J., Kjos, D., & Miller, S. D. (Directors). (2000). *Client-directed interaction: Adjusting the therapy, not the person* [DVD]. Zeig, Tucker & Theisen, Inc. https://video-alexanderstreet-bc.orc.scoolaid.net/watch/client-directed-interaction-adjusting-the-therapy-not-the-person

Center for Substance Abuse Treatment. (2014). *Trauma-informed care in behavioral health services (Treatment Improvement Protocol (TIP) Series, No. 57).* Substance Abuse and Mental Health Services Administration (US). https://www.ncbi.nlm.nih.gov/books/NBK207201/

Chaby, L. E., Sheriff, M. J., Hirrlinger, A. M., & Braithwaite, V. A. (2015). Can we understand how developmental stress enhances performance under future threat with the Yerkes-Dodson law? *Communicative & Integrative Biology, 8*(3), e1029689. https://doi.org/10.1080/19420889.2015.1029689

Chadwell, M., Sikorski, J., Roberts, H., & Allen, K (2018). Process versus content in delivering ABA services: Does process matter when you have content that works? *Behavior Analysis: Research and Practice, 19*(1), 14–22. https://doi.org/10.1037/bar0000143

Charlton, B. G., & White, M. (1995). Living on the margin: A salutogenic model for socio-economic differentials in health. *Public Health, 109*(4), 235–243. https://doi.org/10.1016/s0033-3506(95)80200-2

Chow, D. L., Miller, S. D., Seidel, J. A., Kane, R. T., Thornton, J. A., & Andrews, W. P. (2015). The role of deliberate practice in the development of highly effective psychotherapists. *Psychotherapy, 52*(3), 337–345. https://doi.org/10.1037/pst0000015

Cloitre, M. (1998). Sexual revictimization: Risk factors and prevention. In V. M. Follette, J. I. Ruzek, & F. R. Abeug (Eds.), *Cognitive-behavioral therapies for trauma* (pp. 278–304). Guilford.

Cloitre, M., Courtois, C. A., Charuvastra, A., Carapezza, R. Stolbach, B. C., & Green, B. L. (2011). Treatment of complex PTSD: Results of the ISTSS Expert Clinician Survey on Best Practices. *Journal of Traumatic Stress, 24*, 615–627. https://doi.org/10.1002/jts.20697

Cloitre, M., Courtois, C. A., Ford, J. D., Green, B. L., Alexander, P., Briere, J., Herman, J. L., Lanius, R., Stolbach, B. C., Spinazzola, J., Van der Kolk, B. A., & Van der Hart, O. (2012). *The ISTSS expert consensus treatment guidelines for complex PTSD in adults.* https://psychotraumanet.org/en/istss-expert-consensus-guidelines-complex-ptsd-adults

Cocker, F., & Joss, N. (2016). Compassion fatigue among healthcare, emergency and community service workers: A systematic review. *International Journal of Environmental Research and Public Health, 13*, 618. https://doi.org/10.3390/ijerph13060618

Corrigan, F. M. (2002). Mindfulness, dissociation, EMDR and the anterior cingulate cortex: A hypothesis. *Contemporary Hypnosis, 19*(1), 8–17. https://doi.org/10.1002/ch.235

Covey, S. R. (1996). 7 keys to performance. *Executive Excellence, 13*(6), 8–9.

Covey, S. R., Merrill, A. R., & Merrill, R. R. (1997). *First things first every day: Daily reflections-because where you're headed is more important than how fast you get there.* Simon & Schuster.

Cox, C. L. (1992). Perceived threat as a cognitive component of state anxiety and confidence. *Perception and Motor Skills, 75*, 1092–1094. https://doi.org/10.2466/pms.1992.75.3f.1092

Craigie, M., Slatyer, S., Hegney, D., Osseiran-Moisson, R., Gentry, E., Davis, S., Dolan, T., & Rees, R. (2016). A pilot evaluation of a mindful self-care and resiliency (MSCR) intervention for nurses. *Mindfulness, 7*, 764–774. https://doi.org/10.1007/s12671-016-0516-x

Critchley, H. C., Melmed, R. N., Featherstone, E., Mathias, C. J., & Dolan, R. J. (2001). Brain activity during biofeedback relaxation. *Brain: A Journal of Neurology, 124*, 1003–1012. https://doi.org/10.1093/brain/124.5.1003

Crowder, J. A., Taylor, J. M., & Raskin, V. (2012, July). Autonomous creation and detection of procedural memory scripts. In *Proceedings of the 13th annual international conference on artificial intelligence, Las Vegas.*

Csikszentmihalyi, M. (1997). *Finding flow: The psychology of engagement with everyday life.* Basic Books.

De Champlain, J., Karas, M., Toal, C., Nadeau, R., & Larochelle, P. (1999). Effects of antihypertensive therapies on the sympathetic nervous system. *The Canadian Journal of Cardiology, 15*, 8A–14A.

DeFina, P. A., Fellus, J., Polito, M. Z., Thompson, J. W. G., Moser, R. S., & DeLuca, J. (2009). The new neuroscience frontier: Promoting neuroplasticity and brain repair in traumatic brain injury. *Clinical Neuropsychologist, 23*(8), 1391–1399. https://doi.org/10.1080/13854040903058978

Dennis, P. A., Kimbrel, N. A., Sherwood, A., Calhoun, P. S., Watkins, L. L., Dennis, M. F., & Beckham, J. C. (2017). Trauma and autonomic dysregulation: Episodic-versus systemic-negative affect underlying cardiovascular risk in posttraumatic stress disorder. *Psychosomatic Medicine, 79*(5), 496–505. https://doi.org/10.1097/PSY.0000000000000438

Diamond, D. M., Campbell, A. M., Park, C. R., Halonen, J., & Zoladz, P. R. (2007). The temporal dynamics model of emotional memory processing: A synthesis on the neurobiological basis of stress-induced amnesia, flashbulb and traumatic memories, and the Yerkes-Dodson law. *Neural plasticity, 2007*, 60803. https://doi.org/10.1155/2007/60803

Dietrich, A. M. (2000). A review of visual/kinesthetic disassociation in the treatment of posttraumatic disorders: Theory, efficacy and practice recommendations. *Traumatology, 6*(2), 85–107. https://doi.org/10.1177/153476560000600203

Doidge, N. (2007). *The brain that changes itself: Stories of personal triumph from the frontiers of brain science.* Penguin Group.

Dolan, Y. M. (1991). *Resolving sexual abuse: Solution-focused therapy and ericksonian hypnosis for adult survivors.* Norton.

Doublet, S. (2000). *The stress myth.* Science & Humanities Press.

Dovan, M. L. (2013). *Examining the effects of anxiety on running efficiency in a cognitive-motor dual-task.* [Unpublished doctoral dissertation]. Concordia University, Montreal, Canada.

Dudley, K. J., Li, X., Kobor, M. S., Kippin, T. E., & Bredy, T. W. (2011). Epigenetic mechanisms mediating vulnerability and resilience to psychiatric disorders. *Neuroscience and Biobehavioral Reviews, 35*(7), 1544–1551. https://doi.org/10.1016/j.neubiorev.2010.12.016

Dumovich, J., & Singh P. (2021, September 20). Physiology, trauma. In *StatPearls.* https://www.ncbi.nlm.nih.gov/books/NBK538478/

Duncan, B. L., Miller, S.D., & Sparks, J.A. (2004). *The heroic client: A revolutionary way to improve effectiveness through client-directed, outcome-informed herapy.* Jossey-Bass.

Duncan, B. L., Miller, S. D., Wampold, B. E., & Hubble, M. A. (Eds.). (2010). *The heart and soul of change: Delivering what works in therapy* (2nd ed.). American Psychological Association. https://doi.org/10.1037/12075-000

Dunkley, B. T., Wong, S. M., Jetly, R., Wong, J. K., & Taylor, M. J. (2018). Post-traumatic stress disorder and chronic hyperconnectivity in emotional processing. NeuroImage. *Clinical, 20*, 197–204. https://doi.org/10.1016/j.nicl.2018.07.007

Ehrenreich, J. H. (2001). *Coping with disaster: A guidebook to psychosocial intervention* (rev. ed.). https://www.hhri.org/wp-content/uploads/2021/01/Coping-With-Disaster.pdf

Ehrlichman, H., & Micic, D. (2012). Why do people move their eyes when they think? *Current Directions in Psychological Science, 21*(2), 96–100. https://doi.org/10.1177/0963721412436810

Ellis, A., & Harper, R. A. (1961). *A guide to rational living.* Prentice-Hall.

Erickson, M. H., & Rossi, E. L. (1989). *The February Man*. Brunner/Mazel.

Ericsson, K. A. (2006). The influence of experience and deliberate practice on the development of superior expert performance. In K. A. Ericsson, N. Charness, P. J. Feltovich, & R. R. Hoffman Eds.), *The Cambridge Handbook of Expertise and Expert Performance* (pp. 685–704). Cambridge University Press. https://doi.org/10.1017/CBO9780511816796

Eysenck, H. J. (1952). The effects of psychotherapy: An evaluation. *Journal of Consulting Psychology, 16*(5), 319–324. https://doi.org/10.1037/h0063633.

Falconer, E., Bryant, R., Felmingham, K. L., Kemp, A. H., Gordon, E., Peduto, A., & Williams, L. M. (2008). The neural networks of inhibitory control in Post-Traumatic Stress Disorder. *Journal of Psychiatry & Neuroscience, 33*(5), 413–422.

Felitti, V. J., Anda, R. F., Nordenberg, D., Williamson, D. F., Spitz, A. M., Edwards, V., & Koss, M. P. (1998). The relationship of adult health status to childhood abuse and household dysfunction. *American Journal of Preventive Medicine, 14*, 245–258. https://doi.org/10.1016/S0749-3797(98)00017-8

Fife, S. T, Whiting, J. B., Bradford, K., & Davis, S. (2014). The therapeutic pyramid: A common factors synthesis of techniques, alliance, and way of being. *Journal of Marital and Family Therapy, 40*(1), 20–33. https://doi.org/10.1111/jmft.12041

Figley, C. R., Bride, B. E., & Mazza, N. (Eds.). (1997). *Death and trauma: The traumatology of grieving*. Taylor & Francis.

Figley, C. R., Carbonell, J. L., Boscarino, J. A., & Chang, J. (1999). A clinical demonstration model for assessing the effectiveness of therapeutic interventions: an expanded clinical trials methodology. *International Journal of Emergency Mental Health, 1*(3), 155–164.

Firth, N., Saxon, D., Stiles, W. B., & Barkham, M. (2019). Therapist and clinic effects in psychotherapy: A three-level model of outcome variability. *Journal of Consulting and Clinical Psychology, 87*(4), 345–356. https://doi.org/10.1037/ccp0000388

Flarity, K., Gentry, J. E., Dietz, J. & Bebarta, V. S. (2021). Compassion fatigue resiliency. In R. Strauss & T. Mayer (Eds.), *Emergency department management* (Vol. 2; chapter 126). American College of Emergency Physicians.

Flarity, K., Gentry, J. E., & Mesnikoff, N. (2013). The Effectiveness of an educational program on preventing and treating compassion fatigue in emergency nurses. *Advanced Emergency Nursing Journal, 35*(3), 247–258. https://doi.org/10.1097/TME.0b013e31829b726f

Flarity, K., Holcomb, E., & Gentry, J. E. (2014). Promoting compassion fatigue resiliency among emergency department nurses. In B. A. Anderson, J. M. Knestrick, & R. Barroso (Eds.), *DNP capstone projects: Exemplars of excellence in practice* (pp. 67–78). Springer. https://doi.org/10.1891/9780826130266.0006

Flarity, K., Jones Rhodes, W. J. & Reckard, P. (2016). Intervening to improve compassion fatigue resiliency in nurse residents. *Journal of Nursing Education and Practice, 6*(12), 99–104. https://doi.org/10.5430/jnep.v6n12p99

Flarity, K., Moorer, A., & Rhodes Jones, W. (2018). Longitudinal study of a compassion fatigue resiliency intervention in nurse residents. *Journal of Nursing Education and Practice, 8*(9), 61–67. https://doi.org/10.5430/jnep.v8n9p61

Flarity, K., Nash, K., Jones, W., & Steinbruner, D. (2016). Intervening to improve compassion fatigue resiliency in forensic nurses. *Advanced Emergency Nursing Journal, 38*(2), 147–156. https://doi.org/10.1097/TME.0000000000000101

Flarity, K., Rhodes, W. J., & Reckard, P. (2016). Intervening to improve compassion fatigue resiliency in nurse residents. *Journal of Nursing Education and Practice, 6*(12), 99–104. https://doi.org/10.5430/jnep.v6n12p99

Foa, E. B., Davidson, J. R. T., & Frances, A. (1999). The expert consensus guideline series: Treatment of post-traumatic stress disorder. *The Journal of Clinical Psychiatry, 60*(Suppl. 16), 3–76.

Foa, E. B., Hembree, E., & Rothbaum, B. O. (2007). *Prolonged exposure therapy for PTSD: Emotional processing of traumatic experiences therapist guide*. Oxford University Press. https://doi.org/10.1093/med:psych/9780195308501.001.0001

Foa, E. B., Keane, T. M., & Friedman, M. J. (Eds.). (2000). *Effective treatments for PTSD*. Guilford.

Foa, E. B., Keane, T. M., Friedman, M. J., Cohen, J. A. (2009). *Effective treatments for PTSD: Practice guidelines from the International Society for Traumatic Stress Studies* (2nd ed.). Guilford.

Foa, E. B., & Kozak, M. J. (1998). Clinical applications of bioinformational theory: Understanding anxiety and its treatment. *Behavior Therapy, 29*(4), 675–690. https://doi.org/10.1016/S0005-7894(98)80025-7

Foa, E. B., & Meadows, E. A. (1997). Psychosocial treatments for post-traumatic stress disorder: A critical review. *Annual Review of Psychology, 48*, 449–480. https://doi.org/10.1146/annurev.psych.48.1.449

Follette, V. M., Ruzek, J. I., & Abueg, F. R. (1998). Cognitive behavioral therapies for trauma. In V. M. Follette, J. I. Ruzek, & F. R. Abueg (Eds.), *Cognitive-behavioral therapies for trauma*. Guilford.

Forbes, D., Creamer, M., Bisson, J. I., Cohen, J. A., Crow, B. E., Foa, E. B., Friedman, M. J., Keane, T. M., Kudler, H. S., & Ursano, R. J. (2010). A guide to guidelines for the treatment of PTSD and related conditions. *Journal of Traumatic Stress, 23*(5), 537–552. https://doi.org/10.1002/jts.20565

Ford, J. D. (2005). Treatment implications of altered affect regulation and information processing following child maltreatment. *Psychiatric Annals, 35*(5), 410. https://doi.org/10.3928/00485713-20050501-07

Ford, J. D., & Blaustein, M. E. (2013). Systemic self-regulation: A framework for trauma-informed services in residential juvenile justice programs. *Journal of Family Violence, 28*(7), 665–677. https://doi.org/10.1007/s10896-013-9538-5

Ford, J. D., & Russo, E. (2006). Trauma-focused, present-centered, emotional self-regulation approach to integrated treatment for post-traumatic stress and addiction: Trauma adaptive recovery group education and therapy. *American Journal of Psychotherapy, 60*(4) 335-355. https://doi.org/10.1176/appi.psychotherapy.2006.60.4.335

Frankl, V. E. (1963). *Man's search for meaning*. Washington Square Press, Simon and Schuster.

French, G. D., & Harris, C. (1998). *Traumatic incident reduction*. CRC Press.

Friedman, M. J. (1996). PTSD diagnosis and treatment for mental health clinicians. *Community Mental Health Journal, 32*, 173–189. https://doi.org/10.1007/BF02249755

Friedman, M. J., Cohen, J. A., Foa, E. B., & Keane, T. M. (2009). Integration and summary. In E. B. Foa, T. M. Keane, M. J. Friedman, & J. A. Cohen (Eds.), *Effective treatments for PTSD: Practice guides from the International Society for Traumatic Stress Disorders* (2nd ed., pp. 617–639). Guildford.

Friis, A. M., & Sollers, J. J. (2013). Yoga improves autonomic control in males a preliminary study into the heart of an ancient practice. *Journal of Evidence-Based Complementary & Alternative Medicine, 18*(3), 176–182. https://doi.org/10.1177/2156587212470454

Fuchs, E., & Flügge, G. (2014). Adult neuroplasticity: More than 40 years of research. *Neural Plasticity, 2014, Article 541870.* https://doi.org/10.1155/2014/541870

Gallegos, A. M., Lytle, M. C., Moynihan, J. A., & Talbot, N. L. (2015). Mindfulness-based stress reduction to enhance psychological functioning and improve inflammatory biomarkers in trauma-exposed women: A pilot study. *Psychological Trauma, 7*(6), 525–532. https://doi.org/10.1037/tra0000053

Gallo, F. P. (1996). Reflections on active ingredients in efficient treatments of PTSD, Part 2. *Traumatology, 2*(2), 9–14. https://doi.org/10.1177/153476569600200202

Gentry, J. E. (2002). Compassion fatigue: A crucible of transformation. *The Journal of Trauma Practice, 1*(3/4), 37–61. https://doi.org/10.1300/J189v01n03_03

Gentry, J. E. (2012). *Certified clinical trauma professional 2-day workshop manual.* PESI.

Gentry, J. E. (2016). *Forward-facing® trauma therapy: Healing the moral wound.* Compassion Unlimited Press.

Gentry, J. E. (2021). *Forward-facing® freedom: Healing the past, transforming the present: A future on purpose.* Outskirts Press.

Gentry, J. E., Baggerly, J., & Baranowsky, A. B. (2004). Training-as-treatment: The effectiveness of the Certified Compassion Fatigue Specialist Training. *International Journal of Emergency Mental Health, 6*(3), 147–155.

Gentry, J. E., & Baranowsky, A. B. (1998). *Treatment manual for the Accelerated Recovery Program: Set II.* Psych Ink Resources.

Gentry, J. E., Baranowsky, A. B., & Dunning, K. (2002). ARP: The Accelerated Recovery Program (ARP) for compassion fatigue. In C. R. Figley (Ed.), *Treating compassion fatigue* (pp. 123–137). Brunner-Routledge.

Gentry, J. E., Baranowsky, A. B., & Rhoton, R. (2017). Trauma competency: An active ingredients approach to treating posttraumatic stress disorder. *Journal of Counseling & Development, 95*(3), 279–287. https://doi.org/10.1002/jcad.12142

Gentry, J. E., & Dietz, J. D. (2020). *Forward-Facing® professional resilience: Prevention and resolution of burnout, toxic stress, and compassion fatigue.* Outskirts Press.

Gentry, J. E., & Schmidt, I. M. (1999). Safety reconnaissance for grieving trauma survivors. In C. R. Figley (Ed.), *Traumatology of grieving: Conceptual, theoretical, and treatment foundations* (pp. 201–216). Routledge.

George, M. S., Sackeim, H. A., Rush, A. J., Marangell, L. B., Nahas, Z., Husain, M. M., Lisanby, S., Burt, T., Goldman, J., & Ballenger, J. C. (2000). Vagus nerve stimulation: A new tool for brain research and therapy. *Biological Psychiatry, 47*, 287–295. https://doi.org/10.1016/S0006-3223(99)00308-X

Goldberg, E. (2001). *The executive brain: Frontal lobes and the civilized mind.* Oxford Press.

Goldstein D. S. (2010). Adrenal responses to stress. *Cellular and molecular neurobiology, 30*(8), 1433–1440. https://doi.org/10.1007/s10571-010-9606-9

Gray, R. (2011). NLP and PTSD: The visual-kinesthetic dissociation protocol. *Current Research in NLP, 2*(1), 33–42.

Grinder, J., & Bandler, R. (1981). *Trance-formations: Neuro-linguistic programming and the structure of hypnosis.* Real People Press.

Hamarat, E., Thompson, D., Zabrucky, K. M., Steele, D., Matheny, K. B., & Aysan, F. (2001). Perceived stress and coping resource availability as predictors of life satisfaction in young, middle-aged, and older adults. *Experimental Aging Research, 27*, 181–196. https://doi.org/10.1080/036107301750074051

Hanh, T. N. (1990). *The path of mindfulness in everyday life.* Bantam.

Hanson, R. (2013). *Hardwiring happiness: The new brain science of contentment, calm, and confidence.* Harmony.

Havens, J., Hughes, J. H., McMaster, F., & Kingerlee, R. (2019). Planned dream interventions: A pragmatic randomized control trial to evaluate a psychological treatment for traumatic nightmares in UK military veterans. *Military Behavioral Health, 7*(4), 401–413. https://doi.org/10.1080/21635781.2018.1526148

Heim, C., Ehlert, U., Hanker, J. P., & Hellhammer, D. H. (1998). Abuse-related post-traumatic stress disorder and alterations of the hypothalamic-pituitary-adrenal axis in women with chronic pelvic pain. *Psychosomatic Medicine, 60*, 309–331. https://doi.org/10.1097/00006842-199805000-00017

Heinzelmann, M., & Gill, J. (2013). Epigenetic mechanisms shape the biological response to trauma and risk for PTSD: A critical review. *Nursing Research and Practice, 2013*, Article 417010. https://doi.org/10.1155/2013/417010

Herman, J. L. (1981). *Father-daughter incest.* Harvard University Press. https://doi.org/10.1037/0735-7028.12.1.76

Herman, J. L. (1992). *Trauma and recovery.* Basic Books.

Hersen, M., & Gross, A. M. (Eds.). (2008). *Handbook of clinical psychology, children and adolescents* (Vol. 2). John Wiley & Sons, Inc.

Hoffman, J. W., Benson, H., Arns, P. A., Stainbrook, G. L., Landsberg, G. L., Young, J. B., & Gill, A. (1982). Reduced sympathetic nervous system responsivity associated with the relaxation response. *Science, 215*(4529), 190–192. https://doi.org/10.1126/science.7031901

Holbrook, T. L., Hoyt, D. B., Stein, M. B., & Sieber, W. J. (2001). Perceived threat to life predicts post-traumatic stress disorder after major trauma: Risk factors and functional outcome. *The Journal of Trauma: Injury, Infection, and Critical Care, 51*, 287–293. https://doi.org/10.1097/00005373-200108000-00010

Holland, J. C., Morrow, G. R., Schmale, J., Derogatis, L., Stefanek, M., Berenson, S., Carpenter, P. J., Breitbart, W., & Feldstein, M. (1991). A randomized clinical trial of alprazolam versus progressive muscle relaxation in cancer patients with anxiety and depressive symptoms. *Journal of Clinical Oncology, 9*, 1004–1011. https://doi.org/10.1016/0163-8343(91)90082-8

Honore, C. (2004). *In praise of slowness: How a worldwide movement is challenging the cult of speed.* HarperSanFrancisco.

Hubble, M. A., Duncan, B. L., & Miller, S. D. (1999). *The heart and soul of change: What works in therapy.* American Psychological Association. https://doi.org/10.1037/11132-000

Huttenlocher, P. R. (2002). *Neural plasticity: The effects of environment on the development of the cerebral cortex.* Harvard University Press. https://doi.org/10.4159/9780674038936

International Society for Traumatic Stress Studies, ISTSS. (n.d.). *Resources for the public.* https://istss.org/public-resources

Ironson, G., Freund, B., Strauss, J. L., & Williams, J. (2002). Comparison of two treatments for traumatic stress: A community-based study of EMDR and prolonged exposure. *Journal of Clinical Psychology, 58*(1), 113-128. https://doi.org/10.1002/jclp.1132

Jackson, S., Baity, M. R., Bobb, K., Swick, D., & Giorgio, J. (2019). Stress inoculation training outcomes among veterans with PTSD and TBI. *Psychological trauma: Theory, research, practice, and policy, 11*(8), 842-850. https://doi.org/10.1037/tra0000432

Jacobson, E. (1938). *Progressive relaxation.* University of Chicago Press. https://doi.org/10.1097/00000441-193811000-00037

James, K., & MacKinnon, L. (2012). Integrating a trauma lens into a family therapy framework: Ten principles for family therapists. *Australian & New Zealand Journal of Family Therapy, 33*(3), 189-209. https://doi.org/10.1017/aft.2012.25

Jamison, J. (1999). Stress: The chiropractic patients' self-perceptions. *Journal of Manipulative and Physiological therapeutics, 22*(6), 395-398. https://doi.org/10.1016/S0161-4754(99)70085-0

Jamison, R. N. (1996). *Mastering chronic pain: A professional's guide to behavioral treatment.* Professional Resource Exchange.

Jonas, D. E., Cusack, K., Forneris, C. A., Wilkins, T. M., Sonis, J., Middleton, J. C., Feltner, C., Meredith, D., Cavanaugh, J., Brownley, K. A., Olmsted, K. R., Greenblatt, A., Weil, A., & Gaynes, B. N. (2013). *Psychological and pharmacological treatments for adults with posttraumatic stress disorder (PTSD).* Agency for Healthcare Research and Quality.

Kabat-Zinn, J. (1990). *Full catastrophe living: Using the wisdom of your body and mind to face stress, pain, and illness.* Delta.

Kabat-Zinn, J., & Hanh, T. N. (2009). *Full catastrophe living: Using the wisdom of your body and mind to face stress, pain, and illness.* Random House LLC.

Kar, N. (2011). Cognitive behavioral therapy for the treatment of post-traumatic stress disorder: A review. *Neuropsychiatric Disease and Treatment, 7,* 167-181. https://doi.org/10.2147/NDT.S10389

Karver, M. S., Handelsman, J. B., Fields, S., & Bickman, L. (2006). Meta-analysis of therapeutic relationship variables in youth and family therapy: The evidence for different relationship variables in the child and adolescent treatment outcome literature. *Clinical Psychology Review, 26*(1), 50-65. https://doi.org/10.1016/j.cpr.2005.09.001

Kashani, F., Kashani, P., Moghimian, M., & Shakour, M. (2015). Effect of stress inoculation training on the levels of stress, anxiety, and depression in cancer patients. *Iranian Journal of Nursing and Midwifery Research, 20*(3), 359-364.

Katz, C. L., & Yehuda, R. (2006). Neurobiology of trauma. In L. A. Schein, H. I. Spitz, G. M. Burlingame, & P. R. Muskin (Eds.), *Psychological effects of catastrophic disasters: Group approaches to treatment* (pp. 61-81). Haworth Press.

Kays, J. L., Hurley, R. A., & Taber, K. H. (2012). The dynamic brain: Neuroplasticity and mental health. *The Journal of Neuropsychiatry and Clinical Neurosciences, 24*(2), 118-124. http://search.proquest.com/docview/1315542057?accountid=14771 https://doi.org/10.1176/appi.neuropsych.12050109

Keating, L., Muller, R. T., & Wyers, C. (2021). LGBTQ+ people's experiences of barriers and welcoming factors when accessing and attending intervention for psychological trauma. *Journal of LGBTQ Issues in Counseling, 15*(1), 77-92. https://doi.org/10.1080/15538605.2021.1868376

Kegel, A. H. (1951). Physiologic therapy for urinary stress incontinence. *Journal of the American Medical Association, 146,* 915-917. https://doi.org/10.1001/jama.1951.03670100035008

Kim, S. H., Schneider, S. M., Bevans, M., Kravitz, L., Mermier, C., Qualls, C., & Burge, M. (2013). PTSD symptom reduction with mindfulness-based stretching and deep breathing exercise: Randomized controlled clinical trial of efficacy. *Journal of Clinical Endocrinology and Metabolism, 98,* 2984-2992. https://doi.org/10.1210/jc.2012-3742

Kinsella, S. M., & Tuckey, J. P. (2001). Perioperative bradycardia and asystole: relationship to vasovagal syncope and the Bezold-Jarisch reflex. *British Journal of Anaesthesia, 86,* 859-868. https://doi.org/10.1093/bja/86.6.859

Kirmayer, L. J., Lemelson, R., & Barad, M. (2007). *Understanding trauma: Integrating biological, clinical, and cultural perspectives* (pp. 27-40). Cambridge University Press. https://doi.org/10.1017/CBO9780511500008

Knerr, M., Bartle-Haring, S., McDowell, T., Adkins, K., Delaney, R. O., Gangamma, R., Glebova, T., Grafsky, E., & Meyer, K. (2011). The impact of initial factors on therapeutic alliance in individual and couple's therapy. *Journal of Marital and Family Therapy, 37*(2), 182-199. https://doi.org/10.1111/j.1752-0606.2009.00176.x

Krishnamurthy, K., Laskowitz, D. T. (2016). Cellular and molecular mechanisms of secondary neuronal injury following traumatic brain injury. In D. Laskowitz, G. Grant (Eds.), *Translational research in traumatic brain injury* (chapter 5). CRC Press/Taylor and Francis Group. https://www.ncbi.nlm.nih.gov/books/NBK326718

Kyeong, S., Kim, J., Kim, D. J., Kim, H. E., & Kim, J. J. (2017). Effects of gratitude meditation on neural network functional connectivity and brain-heart coupling. *Scientific Reports, 7*(1), 5058. https://doi.org/10.1038/s41598-017-05520-9

Lambert, M. J. (1992). Psychotherapy outcome research: Implications for integrative and eclectic therapists. In J. C. Norcross & M. R. Goldfried (Eds.), *Handbook of psychotherapy integration* (pp. 92-129). Basic Books.

Lancaster, C. L., Teeters, J. B., Gros, D. F., & Back, S. E. (2016). Posttraumatic stress disorder: Overview of evidence-based assessment and treatment. *Journal of Clinical Medicine, 5*(11), Article 105. https://doi.org/10.3390/jcm5110105

Lanius, U. F. (2014). Attachment, neuropeptides, and autonomic regulation: A vagal shift hypothesis. In U. F. Lanius, S. L. Paulsen, & F. M. Corrigan (Eds.), *Neurobiology and treatment of traumatic dissociation: Towards an embodied self* (pp. 105-129). Springer. https://doi.org/10.1891/9780826106322

LeDoux, J. E. (2015). *Anxious: Using the brain to understand and treat fear and anxiety.* Penguin.

LeDoux, J. E., & Pine, D. S. (2016). Using neuroscience to help understand fear and anxiety: A two-system framework. *The American Journal of Psychiatry, 173*(11), 1083-1093. https://doi.org/10.1176/appi.ajp.2016.16030353

LePera, N. (2021). *How to do the work: Recognize your patterns, heal from your past, and create your self.* Harper Wave.

Lewis, C., Roberts, N. P., Gibson, S., & Bisson, J. I. (2020). Dropout from psychological therapies for post-traumatic stress disorder (PTSD) in adults: systematic review and meta-analysis. *European Journal of Psychotraumatology, 11*(1), Article 1709709. https://doi.org/10.1080/20008198.2019.1709709

Levine, P. A. (2010). *In an unspoken voice: How the body releases trauma and restores goodness.* North Atlantic Books.

Levine, P. A., & Frederick, A. (1997). *Waking the tiger: Healing trauma.* North Atlantic Books.

Lim, S. H., Anantharaman, V., Goh, P. P., & Tan, A. T. (1998). Comparison of treatment of supraventricular tachycardia by Valsalva maneuver and carotid sinus massage. *Annals of Emergency Medicine, 31,* 30–35. https://doi.org/10.1016/S0196-0644(98)70277-X

Llewelyn, S., Macdonald, J., & Aafjes-van Doorn, K. (2016). Process-outcome studies. In J. C. Norcross, G. R. VandenBos, D. K. Freedheim, & B. O. Olatunji (Eds.), *APA handbook of clinical psychology: Theory and research* (p. 451–463). American Psychological Association. https://doi.org/10.1037/14773-020

Lohrasbe, R. M. S. (2012). *Resourcing: The experience of children attending individualized tri-phasic trauma therapy* [Unpublished doctoral dissertation]. University of Victoria, Canada.

Luecken, L., Dausch, B., Gulla, V., Hong, R., & Compas, B. (2004). Alterations in morning cortisol associated with PTSD in women with breast cancer. *Journal of Psychosomatic Research, 56,* 13–15. https://doi.org/10.1016/S0022-3999(03)00561-0

Lutz, W., Leon, S. C., Martinovich, Z., Lyons, J. S., & Stiles, W. B. (2007). Therapist effects in outpatient psychotherapy: A three-level growth curve approach. *Journal of Counseling Psychology, 54*(1), 32–39. https://doi.org/10.1037/0022-0167.54.1.32

Maeng, L. Y., & Milad, M. R. (2017). Post-traumatic stress disorder: The relationship between the fear response and chronic stress. *Chronic Stress, 1,* 1–13. https://doi.org/10.1177/2470547017713297

Magee, J. C., Harden, K. P., & Teachman, B. A. (2012). Psychopathology and thought suppression: A quantitative review. *Clinical Psychology Review, 32*(3), 189–201. https://doi.org/10.1016/j.cpr.2012.01.001

Management of Post-Traumatic Stress Working Group. (2010). *VA/DoD clinical practice guideline for management of post-traumatic stress* (Version 2.0). Department of Veterans Affairs & Department of Defense. https://www.rehab.research.va.gov/jour/2012/495/pdf/VADODclinicalguidlines495.pdf

Management of Posttraumatic Stress Disorder Work Group. (2017). *VA/DoD clinical practice guideline for the management of post-traumatic stress* (Version 3.0). Department of Veterans Affairs & Department of Defense. https://www.healthquality.va.gov/guidelines/MH/ptsd/VADoDPTSDCPGFinal.pdf

Mandle, C. L., Jacobs, S. C., Acari, P. M., & Domar, A. D. (1998). The efficacy of relaxation response interventions with adult patients: A review of the literature. In C. E. Guzzetta (Ed.), *Essential readings in holistic nursing* (pp. 243–263). Aspen.

Mariotti, A. (2015). The effects of chronic stress on health: New insights into the molecular mechanisms of brain–body communication. *Future Science OA, 1*(3), Article FSO23. https://doi.org/10.4155/fso.15.21

Marmar, C. R. (1990). Psychotherapy process research: Progress, dilemmas, and future directions. *Journal of Consulting and Clinical Psychology, 58*(3), 265–272. https://doi.org/10.1037/0022-006X.58.3.265

McCann, I. L., & Pearlman, L. A. (1990). Vicarious traumatization: A framework for understanding the psychological effects of working with victims. *Journal of Traumatic Stress, 3,* 131–149. https://doi.org/10.1007/BF00975140

McClelland, M., Geldhof, J., Morrison, F., Gestsdóttir, S., Cameron, C., Bowers, E., Duckworth, A., Little, T., Grammar, J. (2018). Self-regulation. In N. Halfon, C. B. Forrest, R. M. Lerner, & E. M. Faustman (Eds.), *Handbook of life course health development* (pp. 275–298). Springer. https://doi.org/10.1007/978-3-319-47143-3_12

McNaughton, N. (1997). Cognitive dysfunction resulting from hippocampal hyperactivity: A possible cause of anxiety disorder? *Pharmacology Biochemistry and Behavior, 56,* 603–611. https://doi.org/10.1016/S0091-3057(96)00419-4

Meichenbaum, D. (1994). *A clinical handbook/practical therapist manual: For assessing and treating adults with post-traumatic stress disorder (PTSD).* Institute Press.

Meichenbaum, D. (2012). *Roadmap to resilience: A guide for military, trauma victims and their families.* Institute Press.

Miller, S., Bargmann, S., Chow, D., Seidel, J., & Maeschalck, C. (2016). Feedback-informed treatment (FIT): Improving the outcome of psychotherapy one person at a time. In W. O'Donohue & A. Maragakis (Eds.), *Quality improvement in behavioral health* (pp. 247–262). Springer International Publishing. https://doi.org/10.1007/978-3-319-26209-3_16

Miller, S. D., Hubble, M. A., & Chow, D. (2020). *Better results: Using deliberate practice to improve therapeutic effectiveness.* American Psychological Association. https://doi.org/10.1037/0000191-000

Miller, S. D., Hubble, M. A., Chow, D. L., & Seidel, J. A. (2013). The outcome of psychotherapy: Yesterday, today, and tomorrow. *Psychotherapy, 50*(1), 88–89. https://doi.org/10.1037/a0031097

Miller, S. D., Hubble, M. A., Chow, D., & Seidel, J. (2015). Beyond measures and monitoring: Realizing the potential of feedback-informed treatment. *Psychotherapy, 52*(4), 449–457. https://doi.org/10.1037/pst0000031

Montirosso, R., Borgatti, R., & Tronick, E. (2010). Lateral asymmetries in infant's regulatory and communicative gestures. In R. A. Lanius, E. Vermetten, & C. Pain (Eds.), *Impact of early life trauma on health and disease: The hidden epidemic.* Cambridge University Press. https://doi.org/10.1017/CBO9780511777042.013

Mower, O. H. (1960). *Learning theory and behavior.* Wiley. https://doi.org/10.1037/10802-000

Murray, L. K., Dorsey, S., Haroz, E., Lee, C., Alsiary, M. M., Haydary, A., Weiss, W. M., & Bolton, P. (2014). A common elements treatment approach for adult mental health problems in low-and middle-income countries. *Cognitive and Behavioral Practice, 21*(2), 111–123. https://doi.org/10.1016/j.cbpra.2013.06.005

Najmi, S, & Wegner, D.M. (2009). Hidden complications of thought suppression. *International Journal of Cognitive Therapy, 2*(3), 210–223. https://doi.org/10.1521/ijct.2009.2.3.210

Neff, K. (2011). *Self-compassion: The proven power of being kind to yourself.* HarperCollins Publishers.

Nestler, E. J. (2012). Stress makes its molecular mark: Trauma affects people differently. Epigenetics may be partly to blame. *Nature, 490*(7419), 171–172.

Neumeister, A., Henry, S., & Krystal, J. H. (2007). Neurocircuitry and neuroplasticity in PTSD. In M. J. Friedman, T. M. Keane, & P. A. Resick (Eds.), *Handbook of PTSD: Science and practice* (pp. 151–165). Guilford Press.

Nixon, R., Best, T., Wilksch, S., Angelakis, S., Beatty, L., & Weber, N. (2016). Cognitive processing therapy for the treatment of acute stress disorder following sexual assault: A randomised effectiveness study. *Behaviour Change, 33*(4), 232–250. https://doi.org/10.1017/bec.2017.2

Norcross, J. C., & Lambert, M. J. (2018). Psychotherapy relationships that work III. *Psychotherapy, 55*(4), 303–315. https://doi.org/10.1037/pst0000193

Norsworthy, C., Thelwell, R., Weston, N., Jackson, S. A. (2018). Flow training, flow states, and performance in elite athletes. *International Journal of Sport Psychology, 49*(2), 134–152. https://doi.org/10.7352/IJSP.2018.49.134

Ogden, P., & Minton, K. (2000). Sensorimotor psychotherapy: One method for processing traumatic memory. *Traumatology, 6*(3), 149–173. https://doi.org/10.1177/153476560000600302

Ogden, P., Minton, K., & Pain, C. (2006). *Trauma and the body: A sensorimotor approach to psychotherapy.* WW Norton & Company.

Pavlov, I. P. (1902). *The work of the digestive glands.* Griffin. (Original published in 1897)

Pavlov, I. P. (2015). *Conditioned reflexes: An investigation of the physiological activity of the cerebral cortex* (G. V. Anrep, Trans. & Ed.). Oxford University Press. (Original published 1927).

Pennebaker, J. W. (1997). Writing about emotional experiences as a therapeutic process. *Psychological Science, 8*(3), 162–166. https://doi.org/10.1111/j.1467-9280.1997.tb00403.x

Perry, B. D. (2007). Keep the cool in school: Self-regulation – The second core strength. *Scholastic: Early Childhood Today.* Retrieved from https://www.scholastic.com/teachers/articles/teaching-content/keep-cool-school-self-regulation-second-core-strength/

Perry, B. D., & Szalavitz, M. (2007). *The boy who was raised as a dog: And other stories from a child psychiatrist's notebook – What traumatized children can teach us about loss, love and healing.* Basic Books.

PESI Mental Health. (2016, November 4). *Bessel Van Der Kolk on effective trauma treatment with EMDR.* YouTube. www.youtube.com/watch?v=EgCDzYro2I8

Pickersgill, M., Martin, P., & Cunningham-Burley, S. (2015). The changing brain: Neuroscience and the enduring import of everyday experience. *Public Understanding of Science, 24*(7), 878–892. https://doi.org/10.1177/0963662514521550

Porges, S. W. (1973). Heart rate variability: An autonomic correlate of reaction time performance. *Bulletin of the Psychonomic Society, 1*(4), 270–272. https://doi.org/10.3758/BF03333367

Porges, S. W. (1985, September 27–30). The vagal tone monitor: Application in sleep research. In J. C. Lin & B. N. Frainberg, *Proceedings of the 7th Annual Conference of the IEEE Engineering in Medicine and Biology Society* (pp. 868–869). IEEE Service Center.

Porges, S. W. (1992). Vagal tone: A physiologic marker of stress vulnerability. *Pediatrics, 90,* 498–504. https://doi.org/10.1542/peds.90.3.498

Porges, S. W. (1995). Orienting in a defensive world: Mammalian modifications of our evolutionary heritage. A polyvagal theory. *Psychophysiology, 32*(4), 301–318. https://doi.org/10.1111/j.1469-8986.1995.tb01213.x

Porges, S. W. (1999). Emotion: An evolutionary by-product of the neural regulation of the autonomic nervous system. In C. S. Carter, I. I. Lederhendler, & B. Kirpatrick (Eds.), *The integrative biology of affiliation.* MIT Press.

Porges, S. W. (2002). Polyvagal theory: Three neural circuits regulate behavioral reactivity. *Psychological Science Agenda, 15,* 9–11.

Porges, S. W. (2007). The polyvagal perspective. *Biological psychology, 74*(2), 116–143. https://doi.org/10.1016/j.biopsycho.2006.06.009

Porges, S. W. (2009). Reciprocal influences between body and brain in the perception and expression of affect: A polyvagal perspective. In D. Fosha, D. J. Siegel, & M. F. Solomon, *The healing power of emotion: Affective neuroscience, development & clinical practice* (pp. 27–54). Norton.

Porges, S. W. (2011a). *Clinical applications of polyvagal theory* [DVD]. PESI Incorporated.

Porges, S. W. (2011b). *The polyvagal theory: Neurophysiological foundations of emotions, attachment, communication, and self-regulation.* Norton.

Porges, S. W. (2015). *Clinical insights from the polyvagal theory.* Norton.

Porges, S. W. (2018, April 23). *Dr. Stephen Porges: What is the Polyvagal Theory* [Video]. YouTube. https://www.youtube.com/watch?v=ec3AUMDjtKQ

Porges, S. W. (2018, November 3). *Trauma and intimacy through the lens of the polyvagal theory: Understanding the transformative power of feeling safe* [Presenation]. United States Association for Body Psychotherapy Conference Pioneer Award Lecture conducted at the USABP National Conference, Santa Barbara, CA.

Porges, S. W. (2021). Polyvagal theory: A biobehavioral journey to sociality. *Comprehensive Psychoneuroendocrinology, 7, Article 100069.* https://doi.org/10.1016/j.cpnec.2021.100069

Porges. S. W., & Dana, D. (2018). *Clinical applications of the polyvagal theory: The emergence of polyvagal-informed therapies.* WW Norton.

Porges, S. W., & Furman, S. A. (2011). The early development of the autonomic nervous system provides a neural platform for social behavior: A polyvagal perspective. *Infant and Child Development, 20,* 106–118. https://doi.org/10.1002/icd.688

Potter, P., Berger, J. A., Olsen, S., & Chen, L. (2013, March). Evaluation of a compassion fatigue resiliency program for oncology nurses. *Oncology Nursing Forum, 40*(2), 180–187. https://doi.org/10.1188/13.ONF.180-187

Potter, P., Deshields, T., Divanbeigi, J., Berger, J. A., Cipriano, D., Norris, L., & Olsen, S. (2010). Compassion fatigue and burnout. *Clinical Journal of Oncology Nursing, 14*(5), E56–E62. https://doi.org/10.1188/10.CJON.E56-E62

Potter, P., Deshields, T., & Rodriguez, S. (2013). Developing a systemic program for compassion fatigue. *Nursing Administration Quarterly, 37*(4), 326–332. https://doi.org/10.1097/NAQ.0b013e3182a2f9dd

Potter, P., Pion, S., & Gentry, J. E. (2015). Compassion fatigue resiliency training: the experience of facilitators. *Journal of Continuing Education in Nursing, 46*(2), 83–88. https://doi.org/10.3928/00220124-20151217-03

Powers, M. B., Halpern, J. M., Ferenschak, M. P., Gillihan, S. J., & Foa, E. B. (2010). A meta-analytic review of prolonged exposure for posttraumatic stress disorder. *Clinical Psychology Review, 30*(6), 635–641. https://doi.org/10.1016/j.cpr.2010.04.007

Prescott, D. S., Maeschalck, C. L., & Miller, S. D. (Eds.). (2017). *Feedback-informed treatment in clinical practice: Reaching for excellence.* American Psychological Association. https://doi.org/10.1037/0000039-000

Radley, J. J., Kabbaj, M., Jacobson, L., Heydendael, W., Yehuda, R., & Herman, J. P. (2011). Stress risk factors and stress-related pathology. Neuroplasticity, epigenetics and endophenotypes. *Stress, 14*(5), 481–497. https://doi.org/10.3109/10253890.2011.604751

Rank, M. G., Zapparanick, T. L., & Gentry, J. E. (2009). Nonhuman-animal care compassion fatigue: Training as treatment. *Best Practices in Mental Health: An International Journal, 5*(2), 40-61.

Rauch, S. A., Eftekhari, A., & Ruzek, J. I. (2012). Review of exposure therapy: A gold standard for PTSD treatment. *Journal of Rehabilitation Research and Development, 49*(5), 679-688. https://doi.org/10.1682/JRRD.2011.08.0152

Resick, P. A., Monson, C. M., & Chard, K. M. (2006). Cognitive processing therapy: Veteran/military version. *Clinical Psychology, 74*, 898-907.

Resick, P. A., & Schnicke, M. K. (1992). Cognitive processing therapy for sexual assault victims. *Journal of Consulting and Clinical Psychology, 60*, 748-756. https://doi.org/10.1037/0022-006X.60.5.748

Resick, P. A., & Schnicke, M. K. (1993). *Cognitive processing therapy for rape victims: A treatment manual.* Sage.

Rhoton, P. R. (2012). *Understanding symptoms related to traumagenesis* [Conference address]. Touchstone Behavioral Health Conference on Child Trauma, Phoenix, AZ.

Rhoton, R., & Gentry, J. E. (2021). *Trauma competency for the 21st Century: A salutogenic "active ingredients" approach.* Outskirts Press.

Rogers, C. R. (1966). Client-centered therapy. In A. Silvano (Ed.), *American handbook of psychiatry* (pp. 183-200). Basic Books.

Rollnick, S., & Miller, W. R. (1995). What is motivational interviewing? *Behavioural and Cognitive Psychotherapy, 23*, 325-334. https://doi.org/10.1017/S135246580001643X

Romano, L. A. (2020). *The codependency manifesto: Clearing the way out of the codependent mind.* Outskirts Press, Inc.

Rothbaum, B., Foa, E., & Hembree, E. (2007). *Reclaiming your life from a traumatic experience: A prolonged exposure treatment program workbook.* Oxford University Press.

Rothbaum, B. O., Meadows, E. A., Resick, P., & Foy, D. W. (2000). Cognitive-behavioral therapy. In E. B. Foa, T. M. Keane, & M. J. Friedman (Eds.), *Effective treatments for PTSD* (pp. 60-83). Guilford.

Rothschild, B. (2000). *The body remembers: The psychophysiology of trauma and trauma treatment.* Norton.

Rousmaniere, T. (2016). *Deliberate practice for psychotherapists: A guide to improving clinical effectiveness.* Routledge. https://doi.org/10.4324/9781315472256

Roy, M. J., Costanzo, M. E., Blair, J. R., & Rizzo, A. A. (2014). Compelling evidence that exposure therapy for PTSD normalizes brain function. *Studies in Health Technology and Informatics, 199*, 6-65.

Sadigh, M. R., & Montero, R. P. (2013). *Autogenic training: A mind-body approach to the treatment of fibromyalgia and chronic pain syndrome.* Taylor Francis - CRC Press.

Sapolsky, R. M. (1996). Why stress is bad for your brain. *Science, 273*(5276), 749-750. https://doi.org/10.1126/science.273.5276.749

Sapolsky, R. M. (2004). *Why zebras don't get ulcers: The acclaimed guide to stress, stress-related diseases, and coping.* Holt paperbacks.

Sapolsky, R. M. (2017). *Behave: The biology of humans at our best and worst.* Penguin.

Sato, W., Kochiyama, T., Uono, S., Yoshikawa, S., & Toichi, M. (2016). Direction of amygdala–neocortex interaction during dynamic Facial expression processing. *Cerebral Cortex, 27*(3), 1878-1890. https://doi.org/10.1093/cercor/bhw036.

Sayers, W. M., & Sayette, M. A. (2013). Suppression on your own terms: Internally generated displays of craving suppression predict rebound effects. *Psychological Science, 24*(9), 1740-1746. https://doi.org/10.1177/0956797613479977

Scaer, R. C. (2001). *The body bears the burden: Trauma, dissociation, and disease.* Hawthorne.

Scaer, R. C. (2005). *The trauma spectrum: Hidden wounds and human resiliency.* WW Norton & Co.

Scaer, R. C. (2006). *The trauma spectrum: Hidden wounds, human resiliency.* Basic Books.

Scaer, R. C. (2014). *The body bears the burden: Trauma, dissociation, and disease* (3rd ed.). Routledge.

Scarlet, J., Lang, A. J., & Walser, R. D. (2016). Acceptance and commitment therapy for posttraumatic stress disorder. In D. M. Benedek & G. H. Wynn (Eds.), *Complementary and alternative medicine for PTSD* (pp. 35-57). Oxford University Press. https://doi.org/10.1093/med/9780190205959.003.0003

Schnarch, D. M. (1997). *Passionate marriage: Love, sex, and intimacy in emotionally committed relationships.* WW Norton & Company.

Schnurr, P. P., Lunney, C. A., & Sengupta, A. (2004). Risk factors for the development versus maintenance of post-traumatic stress disorder. *Journal of Trauma Stress, 17*, 85-95. https://doi.org/10.1023/B:JOTS.0000022614.21794.f4

Scotland-Coogan, D., & Davis, E. (2016). Relaxation techniques for trauma. *Journal of Evidence-Informed Social Work, 13*(5), 434-441. https://doi.org/10.1080/23761407.2016.1166845

Schnyder, U., Ehlers, A., Elbert, T., Foa, E. B., Gersons, B. P. R., Resick, P. A., Shapiro, F., & Cloitre, M. (2015). Psychotherapies for PTSD: What do they have in common? *European Journal of Psychotraumatology, 6*(1), Article 28186. https://doi.org/10.3402/ejpt.v6.28186

Schultz, D. F. (2004). *A language of the heart: Therapy stories that heal.* Rainbow Books.

Schultz, D. F. (2016). *A language of the heart: Therapy stories that heal* (2nd ed.). Peppertree Press.

Schultz, D. F. (2005). *A language of the heart workbook.* Rainbow Books.

Schumann, C. M., Bauman, M. D., & Amaral, D. G. (2011). Abnormal structure or function of the amygdala is a common component of neurodevelopmental disorders. *Neuropsychologia, 49*(4), 745-759. https://doi.org/10.1016/j.neuropsychologia.2010.09.028

Sealy, M. (2014, December 16). *Guided body scan meditation for mind & body healing* [video]. YouTube. https://youtu.be/i7xGF8F28zo

Seidel, J. A. (2012). Using feedback-informed therapy (FIT) to build a premium-service, private-pay practice. In C. E. Stout (Ed.), *Getting better at private practice* (pp. 279-291). Wiley. https://doi.org/10.1002/9781118089972.ch18

Seligman, M. (2002). *Authentic happiness.* Free Press.

Shaffer J. (2016). Neuroplasticity and clinical practice: Building brain power for health. *Frontiers in Psychology, 7*, Article 1118. https://doi.org/10.3389/fpsyg.2016.01118

Shah, L. B., Klainin-Yobas, P., Torres, S., & Kannusamy, P. (2014). Efficacy of psychoeducation and relaxation interventions on stress-related variables in people with mental disorders: A literature review. *Archives of psychiatric nursing, 28*(2), 94-101. https://doi.org/10.1016/j.apnu.2013.11.004

Shalev, A., Bonne, O., & Eth, S. (1996). Treatment of post-traumatic stress disorder: A review. *Psychosomatic Medicine, 58*, 165-182. https://doi.org/10.1097/00006842-199603000-00012

Shapiro, F. (1989). Efficacy of the eye movement desensitization procedure: A new treatment for post-traumatic stress disorder.

*Journal of Traumatic Stress, 2,* 199-223. https://doi.org/10.1002/jts.2490020207

Shapiro, F. (1995). *Eye movement desensitization and reprocessing: Basic principles, protocols and procedures.* Guilford.

Shapiro, F., & Solomon, R. (1995). Eye movement desensitization and reprocessing: Neurocognitive information processing. In G. Everley (Ed.), *Innovations in disaster and trauma psychology* (Vol. 1, pp. 216-237). Chevron Publishing.

Sherin, J. E., & Nemeroff, C. B. (2011). Post-traumatic stress disorder: The neurobiological impact of psychological trauma. *Dialogues in Clinical Neuroscience, 13*(3), 263-278. https://doi.org/10.31887/DCNS.2011.13.2/jsherin

Shubina, I. (2015). Cognitive-behavioral therapy of patients with PTSD: Literature review. *Procedia - Social and Behavioral Sciences, 165,* 208-216. https://doi.org/10.1016/j.sbspro.2014.12.624

Shusterman, V., & Barnea, O. (2005). Sympathetic nervous system activity in stress and biofeedback relaxation. *Engineering in Medicine and Biology Magazine, IEEE, 24,* 52-57. https://doi.org/10.1109/MEMB.2005.1411349

Siegel, D. J. (2010). *Mindsight: The new science of personal transformation.* Random House.

Sikirov, B. A. (1990). Cardio-vascular events at defecation: Are they unavoidable? *Medical Hypothesis, 32,* 231-233. https://doi.org/10.1016/0306-9877(90)90128-2

Sinha, S. (2016). Trauma-induced insomnia: A novel model for trauma and sleep research. *Sleep Medicine Reviews, 25,* 74-83. https://www.sciencedirect.com/science/article/abs/pii/S1087079215000209?via%3Dihub https://doi.org/10.1016/j.smrv.2015.01.008

Skinner, B. F. (1938). *The behavior of organisms: An experimental analysis.* Appleton-Century-Crofts.

Solomon, Z., & Horesh, D. (2007). Changes in diagnostic criteria for PTSD: Implications from two prospective longitudinal studies. *American Journal of Orthopsychiatry, 77*(2), 182-188. https://doi.org/10.1037/0002-9432.77.2.182

Spilsbury, J. C., Belliston, L., Drotar, D., Drinkard, A., Kretschmar, J., Creeden, R., Flannery, D. J., & Friedman, S. (2007). Clinically significant trauma symptoms and behavioral problems in a community-based sample of children exposed to domestic violence. *Journal of Family Violence, 22,* 487-499. https://doi.org/10.1007/s10896-007-9113-z

Staugaard-Jones, J. A. (2012). *The vital psoas muscle: Connecting physical, emotional, and spiritual well-being.* North Atlantic Books.

Stop Breathe Think. (2017, September 28). *Body scan meditation: Tame anxiety* [video]. YouTube. https://youtu.be/QS2yDmWk0vs

Stoppelbein, L. A., Greening, L., & Elkin, T. D. (2006). Risk of posttraumatic stress symptoms: A comparison of child survivors of pediatric cancer and parental bereavement. *Journal of Pediatric Psychology, 31,* 367-376. https://doi.org/10.1093/jpepsy/jsj055

Tabibnia, G., & Radecki, D. (2018). Resilience training that can change the brain. *Consulting Psychology Journal: Practice and Research, 70*(1), 59-88. https://doi.org/10.1037/cpb0000110

Takahashi, T., Ikeda, K., Ishikawa, M., Kitamura, N., Tsukasaki, T., Nakama, D., & Kameda, T. (2005). Anxiety, reactivity, and social stress-induced cortisol elevation in humans. *Neuroendocrinology Letters, 4,* 351-354.

Taub, E. (2000). Constraint-induced movement therapy and massed practice. *Stroke, 1*(4), 986-988. https://doi.org/10.1161/01.STR.31.4.983-c

Taylor, A. H. (2012). *Assessing the effects of stress resilience training on visual discrimination skills: Implications for perceptual resilience in US warfighters* [Doctoral dissertation]. Virginia Commonwealth University Richmond, Virginia.

Tedeschi, R., & Calhoun, L. (1996). The posttraumatic growth inventory: Measuring the positive legacy of trauma. *Journal of Traumatic Stress, 9*(3), 455-471. https://doi.org/10.1002/jts.2490090305

Tindle, J., & Tadi, P. (2020). Neuroanatomy, parasympathetic nervous system. In *StatPearls.* StatPearls Publishing. https://www.ncbi.nlm.nih.gov/books/NBK553141/

Tinnin, L. (1994). *Time-limited trauma therapy: A treatment manual.* Gargoyle.

Trott, S. (1995). *The holy man.* Thorndike Press.

Tull, M. (2020, December 12). Imagery rehearsal therapy to treat nightmares with PTSD. *Very Well Mind.* https://www.verywellmind.com/imagery-rehearsal-therapy-2797304

US Department of Veterans Affairs & Department of Defense. (2017). *VA/DoD clinical practice guideline for the management of posttraumatic stess disorder and acute stress disorder: Clinician summary (Version 3.0).* https://www.healthquality.va.gov/guidelines/MH/ptsd/VADoDPTSDCPGClinicianSummaryFinal.pdf

Valiente-Gómez, A., Moreno-Alcázar, A., Treen, D., Cedrón, C., Colom, F., Pérez, V., & Amann, B. L. (2017). EMDR beyond PTSD: A systematic literature review. *Frontiers in Psychology, 8,* Article 1668. https://doi.org/10.3389/fpsyg.2017.01668

Van der Hart, O., & Brown, P. (1992). Abreaction re-evaluated. *Dissociation, 5*(3), 127-140.

Van der Kolk, B. A. (1986). *Psychological trauma.* American Psychiatric Publishing.

Van der Kolk, B. A. (1996a). The complexity of adaptation to trauma: Self-regulation, stimulus discrimination, and characterological development. In B. A. van der Kolk, A. C. McFarlane, & L. Weisaeth (Eds.), *Traumatic stress: The effects of overwhelming experience on mind, body, and society* (pp. 182-213). Guilford.

Van der Kolk, B. A. (1996b). The black hole of trauma. In B. A. van der Kolk, A. C. McFarlane, & L. Weisaeth (Eds.). *Traumatic stress: The effects of overwhelming experience on mind, body, and society* (pp. 3-23). Guilford.

Van der Kolk, B. A. (2015). *The body keeps the score: Brain, mind, and body in the healing of trauma.* Viking.

Van der Kolk, B. A., McFarlane, A. C., & Weisaeth, L. (Eds.). (1996). *Traumatic stress: The effects of overwhelming experience on mind, body, and society.* Guilford.

Wampold, B. E. (2005). Establishing specificity in psychotherapy scientifically: Design and evidence issues. *Clinical Psychology: Science and Practice, 12*(2), 194-197. https://doi.org/10.1093/clipsy.bpi025

Wampold, B. E., & Imel, Z. E. (2015). *The great psychotherapy debate: The evidence for what makes psychotherapy work.* Routledge. https://doi.org/10.4324/9780203582015

Wampold, B. E., Imel, Z. E., Laska, K. M., Benish, S., Miller, S. D., Flückiger, C., Del Re, A. C., Baardseth, T. P., & Budge, S. (2010).

Determining what works in the treatment of PTSD. *Clinical Psychology Review, 30*(8), 923–933. https://doi.org/10.1016/j.cpr.2010.06.005

Watkins, L. E., Sprang, K. R., & Rothbaum, B. O. (2018). Treating PTSD: A review of evidence-based psychotherapy interventions. *Frontiers in Behavioral Neuroscience, 12*, Article 258. https://doi.org/10.3389/fnbeh.2018.00258

Waxman, M. B., Wald, R. W., Finley, J. P., Bonet, J. F., Downar, E., & Sharma, A. D. (1980). Valsalva termination of ventricular tachycardia. *Circulation, 62*, 843–851. https://doi.org/10.1161/01.CIR.62.4.843

Webb, J. (2017). *Running on empty no more: Transform your relationships with your partner, your parents and your children.* Morgan James Publishing.

Wenzel, A. (2012). Modification of core beliefs in cognitive therapy. In I. Reis de Oliviera (Ed.), *Standard and innovative strategies in cognitive behavior therapy.* InTechOpen. https://www.intechopen.com/chapters/31822 https://doi.org/10.5772/30119

Winders, S. J., Murphy, O., Looney, K., & O'Reilly, G. (2020). Self-compassion, trauma, and posttraumatic stress disorder: A systematic review. *Clinical Psychology & Psychotherapy, 27*(3), 300–329. https://doi.org/10.1002/cpp.2429

Winkeljohn Black, S., Owen, J., Chapman, N., Lavin, K., Drinane, J. M., & Kuo, P. (2017). Feedback informed treatment: An empirically supported case study of psychodynamic treatment. *Journal of Clinical Psychology, 73*(11), 1499–1509. https://doi.org/10.1002/jclp.22529

Wolpe, J. (1954). Reciprocal inhibition as the main basis of psychotherapeutic effects. *AMA Archives of Neurology & Psychiatry, 72*(2), 205–226. https://doi.org/10.1001/archneurpsyc.1954.02330020073007

Wolpe, J. (1958). *Psychotherapy by reciprocal inhibition.* Stanford University Press.

Wolpe, J. (1968). Psychotherapy by reciprocal inhibition. *Conditional Reflex: A Pavlovian Journal of Research & Therapy, 3*(4), 234–240. https://doi.org/10.1007/BF03000093

Wolpe, J. (1969). *The practice of behavioral therapy.* Pergamon.

Wolynn, M. (2016). *It didn't start with you: How inherited family trauma shapes who we are and how to end the cycle.* Viking.

World Health Organization. (2007). *The World Health Report 2007 – A safer future: Global public health security in the 21st century.* https://www.who.int/publications/i/item/9789241563444

Yaribeygi, H., Panahi, Y., Sahraei, H., Johnston, T. P., & Sahebkar, A. (2017). The impact of stress on body function: A review. *EXCLI Journal, 16*, 1057–1072. https://doi.org/10.17179/excli2017-480

Yartz, A. R., & Hawk, L. W. (2001). Psychophysiological assessment of anxiety: Tales from the heart. In M. Antony, S. Orsillo, & L. Roemer (Eds.), *Practitioner's guide to empirically based measures of anxiety* (pp. 25–30). Springer.

Yahuda, R. (2016). *GCPH lecture 5: How the effects of traumatic stress are transmitted to the next generation* [Video]. https://edshare.ecs.soton.ac.uk/id/eprint/1265/

Yehuda, R. (2001). Biology of post-traumatic stress disorder. *Journal of Clinical Psychiatry, 62*, 41–46.

Yehuda, R., & Lehrner, A. (2018). Intergenerational transmission of trauma effects: putative role of epigenetic mechanisms. *World Psychiatry, 17*(3), 243–257. https://doi.org/10.1002/wps.20568

Yeomans, P. D., Forman, E. M., Herbert, J. D., & Yuen, E. (2010). A randomized trial of a reconciliation workshop with and without PTSD psychoeducation in Burundian sample. *Journal of Traumatic Stress, 23*(3), 305–312. https://doi.org/10.1002/jts.20531

Yerkes, R. M., & Dodson, J. D. (1908). The relation of strength of stimulus to rapidity of habit-formation. *Journal of Comparative Neurology and Psychology, 18*, 459–482. https://doi.org/10.1002/cne.920180503

Youssef, N. A., Lockwood, L., Su, S., Hao, G., & Rutten, B. (2018). The effects of trauma, with or without PTSD, on the transgenerational DNA methylation alterations in human offsprings. *Brain Sciences, 8*(5), Article 83. https://doi.org/10.3390/brainsci8050083

# Appendices

# Appendix 1
# Self-Regulation

## Transformation: Shift From Sympathetic to Parasympathetic Nervous System

Brain imaging research has shown that anxiety is a brain killer – the more anxiety a person experiences, the less effectively our brains operate. It is clear that professional and personal effectiveness require self-regulation skills. By relaxing the muscles of the pelvic region (i.e., kegels, sphincter, and psoas), we are able to affect profound systemic muscle relaxation. This relaxation facilitates a shift in the autonomous nervous system (ANS) from the *sympathetic* system (i.e., fight-or-flight reflex utilized during periods of perceived threat) to the *parasympathetic* system (i.e., relaxation and optimal functioning utilized during period of safety). By maintaining this pelvic relaxation, we are able to thwart the ANS from shifting to sympathetic dominance each time we perceive even the mildest threats (e.g., criticism).

By practicing the release and relaxation of these muscles, we can gradually shift from sympathetic to parasympathetic dominance. The rewards of this transformation include comfort in our bodies, maximal motor and cognitive functioning, ability to tolerate intimacy, self-regulation, internal vs. external locus of control, ability to remain mission/principle driven, increased tolerance, increased effectiveness, and increased health of our body's systems.

## What Happens When My Sympathetic Nervous System Is Dominant?

When you perceive a threat, your body responds to either neutralize or move away from this perceived threat. This is true for all species of living things and is known as the fight-or-flight reflex. If we are truly in danger of losing our lives, then this reflex is arguably useful. However, we are rarely confronted with threats and circumstances that are this dire in our daily lives. Instead, we perceive some mild threat, our sympathetic nervous system (SNS) activates, and we find ourselves trying to either kill or run away from our boss, coworker, or spouse. This overactive and very sensitive threat identification and early warning system is the cause of all stress.

When our SNS is activated and dominant, we are preparing for battle or flight. Our circulation becomes constricted, our heart rate increases, and our muscles become tense and ready to act. Inside our brains, the neocortex becomes less functional while the brain stem, basal ganglia, and thalamus become more active. This is because the perceived need to survive has superseded all other brain functioning. As we become more stressed, and the longer we are in this state of sympathetic dominance, the more likely we are to compromise the functioning of higher-order brain systems such as language, speech, motor activity, filtering, and compassion. This loss of functioning may partially account for why people have trouble thinking logically during stressful times, or why they have trouble being kind when they perceive threat, or even why they have trouble with peak physical performance (e.g., sports) when they are "nervous." By simply relaxing and keeping relaxed our pelvic muscles we can reverse this process of sympathetic dominance and return to parasympathetic systems. This return to parasympathetic dominance will allow the individual to regain optimal functioning of speech, language (remember, intentional thought is simply talking to ourselves – something for which we need to be able to create language and speech), motor coordination, filtering, and compassion. Once an individual is able to successfully transition from sympathetic to parasympathetic dominance, without external agents (i.e., drugs) and without regard for the external events (i.e., crises) the individual has become self-regulatory. A person who becomes skilled in making this transition has developed an internal locus of control and is no longer a victim of circumstances.

## Where Are the Pelvic Muscles? How Do I Find Them?

While conducting seminars students often ask us this question. We cannot help but feel a twinge of sadness when this question is asked. The sadness comes from the awareness that the person asking this question has learned to be unaware of these muscles. People who are not aware of the muscles in their midbody are not aware for good reason – it has been a coping strategy since childhood. Children who grew up in anxious and dangerous environments learned to keep their bodies tight in anticipation of danger. With no skills for self-regulating, these children often learn to numb and dissociate their awareness away from the pain in their bodies. These children grow into adults that have difficulty being "in" their bodies – they have difficultly monitoring and regulating muscle tension and, ultimately, anxiety.

### Exercise

1. While sitting, put your hands under your butt.
2. Feel the two pointed bones upon which you are sitting.
3. Now, touch the two bony points on your right and left side just below the waist.
4. You have made a touch memory for four distinct points. Connect those four points to make a square.
5. Now, allow your breath to get to the area in the middle of the square. Also, allow the square to expand.
6. Release and relax all muscles that traverse the area of the square so that there are *no clenched muscles* in the square.

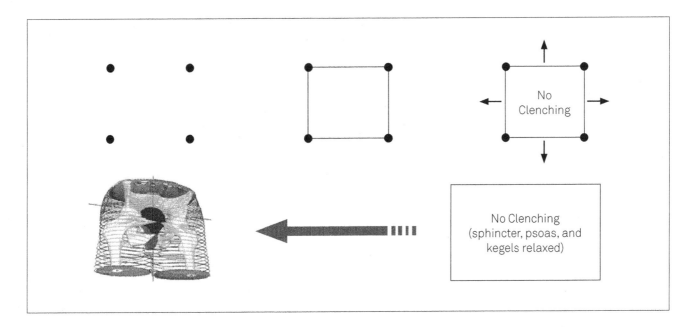

## What Now That My Pelvic Muscles Are Relaxed?

Keep them that way. If you are able to keep your pelvic muscles released and relaxed for 20–30 seconds, then you will begin to notice the clear differences in yourself as you transition from sympathetic to parasympathetic dominance. You will first notice comfort in your body. As you release the tension and stress that you have been generating you will become aware that your body is comfortable – no matter what is going on around you. Your thoughts may still be racing and producing warning messages. If this is happening, *do nothing*; just concentrate on keeping your pelvic muscles relaxed. This will be difficult for many people because, since childhood, we have taken action when we experience this alarm. However, if we are able to keep our pelvic muscles relaxed then we will be rewarded with a lessening of stress and the restoration of optimal functioning in our thinking and actions. With this self-regulation, we will be able to comfortably seek creative solutions to problems and situations that used to leave us baffled, exhausted, and frustrated.

By developing and practicing the skills of self-regulation we will find ourselves able to maintain fidelity to our intention – our mission. We will find that we no longer need to react to every little crisis as though it is a life-or-death situation. We will become free from our pasts to live for ourselves the lives that we create without having to be perpetually "on guard" for the next danger. We will be able to function at peak effectiveness anytime we choose – a transformation indeed.

Sympathetic = Reactive = Stress = Diminished Functioning= No Choice

Parasympathetic = Intentional = Comfort = Optimal Functioning = Choice

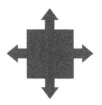

You Choose

# Appendix 2
# Training Opportunities

For up-to-date information on training opportunities and to arrange for training at your location, contact:
Dr. Anna B. Baranowsky, CEO
Traumatology Institute (Canada) Training & Development, Inc.
4789 Yonge Street, Suite 703
Toronto, ON M2N 0G3
Canada
https://psychink.com and https://whatisptsd.com

For organizations or teaching institutions that would like more information about the full Traumatology Institute Training Curriculum (TITC), please contact the Traumatology Institute (Canada). The TITC is a comprehensive set of training programs for developing specialization in the area of posttraumatic response and recovery. The TITC is internationally recognized by the American Academy of Experts in Traumatic Stress and the Academy of Traumatology – Commission on Certification and Accreditation.

We would be happy to discuss options to become a fully recognized provider of the Traumatology Institute Training Curriculum.

The full TITC is available for qualifying organizations or institutions who would like to establish recognized site licenses through the Traumatology Institute.

J. Eric Gentry, PhD, LMHC, FAAETS
President
Forward-Facing® Institute, LLC
PO Box 937
Phoenix, AZ 85001
USA
www.forward-facing.com

More information about Forward-Facing® services including Forward-Facing® Trauma Therapy and Forward-Facing® Professional Resilience training can be found at https://forward-facing.com/training/

# Notes on Supplementary Materials

**DOWNLOAD**

The following materials for your book can be downloaded free of charge once you register on our website:

## Using the Tools

USING THE TOOLS 1: Trigger-List Exercise (Multiple Events)

USING THE TOOLS 2: Trigger-List Exercise (One Event – Multiple Hot Points)

USING THE TOOLS 3: Autogenic Relaxation (R)

USING THE TOOLS 4: 3-6 Breathing (R)

USING THE TOOLS 5: Anchoring Part II: Safety I

USING THE TOOLS 6: Ten Errors of Thinking

USING THE TOOLS 7: CHANGES – Positive Challenges to Errors in Thinking

USING THE TOOLS 8: Reflection Sheet #1 & Reflection Sheet #2

USING THE TOOLS 9: Flashback Journal

USING THE TOOLS 10: Rituals

USING THE TOOLS 11: Contract for Safety and Self-Care

USING THE TOOLS 12: Safety Net Plan

USING THE TOOLS 13: Safe Place Imagery: My Committee of Comfort and Support

USING THE TOOLS 14: Make Peace With Your Sleep

USING THE TOOLS 15: Layering (Baranowsky, 1997)

USING THE TOOLS 16: Cognitive Continuum

USING THE TOOLS 17: Looped Tape Scripting – Installing the Positive

USING THE TOOLS 18: Cognitive Processing Therapy

USING THE TOOLS 19: Corrective Messages from Old Storylines

USING THE TOOLS 20: SIT Phase Oriented – Task Checklist

USING THE TOOLS 21: SIT Book Developer

USING THE TOOLS 22: IATP NET Checklist, Graphic Timeline, Written Narrative, & Pictorial Narrative

USING THE TOOLS 23: Sadness Script

USING THE TOOLS 24: Thematic Map and Release

USING THE TOOLS 25: Exploring Your Cognitive Map

USING THE TOOLS 26: Self-Compassion Reflections

USING THE TOOLS 27: Your Heart's Desire

USING THE TOOLS 28: Picture Positive

USING THE TOOLS 29: Memorials

USING THE TOOLS 30: Connections with Others

USING THE TOOLS 31: Algorithm for Forward-Facing® Trauma Therapy

USING THE TOOLS 32: Vision Statement Exercise

USING THE TOOLS 33: Covenant/Mission Exercise

USING THE TOOLS 34: My Code of Honor

USING THE TOOLS 35: Reactive to Intentional Worksheet

USING THE TOOLS 36: Individualized Compassion Fatigue Resiliency Plan

# Video Material

**TP_Videos_Phase_0_1-4.zip**

TP_Video_1_Recovery-Now-TRAUMA

TP_Video_2_The-Emotional-Brain-Landmine

TP_Video_3_Inherited-Family-Trauma-w-Mark-Wolynn

TP_Video_4_Learn-about-Adrenaline&Cortisol

**TP_Videos_Phase_I_5-10.zip**

TP_Video_5_Relaxation-Autogenics

TP_Video_6_Diaphragmatic-Breathing

TP_Video_7_3-6-Breathing

TP_Video_8_Breath-Training-3-6-Breathing

TP_Video_9_Grounding-&-Containment

TP_Video_10_Simple-Grounding-Containment-Exercise

**TP_Videos_Phase_I_11-13.zip**

TP_Video_11_NLP-Anchoring

TP_Video_12_Manage-Stress-&-Anxiety-w-Your-Breath

TP_Video_13_Guided-Body-Scan-Exercise

**TP_Videos_Phase_I_14-15.zip**

TP_Video_14_Deep-Relaxation-w-Safe-Place

TP_Video_15_Circle-of-Support

**TP_Videos_Phase_I_16-19.zip**

TP_Video_16_How-to-Create-a-Containment-Vessel

TP_Video_17_Embrace-Positivity-With-a-Hope-Box

TP_Video_18_Day-17_Making-Peace-With-Your-Sleep

TP_Video_19_Make-Peace-With-Your-Sleep

**TP_Videos_Phase_I_20-21.zip**

TP_Video_20_Improve-Sleep,-Relax-Deeply,-&-Embed

TP_Video_21_Day-7_Relaxed-Breathing-Guided

**TP_Videos_Phase_II_22-26.zip**

TP_Video_22_Layering

TP_Video_23_Comfort-on-Palms-of-Hand

TP_Video_24_Hands-over-Heart-Space-Exercise

TP_Video_25_Paced-Breathing

TP_Video_26_Traumagram-and-Epigenetics

**TP_Video_Phase_II_27.zip**

TP_Video_27_Thematic-Map-&-Release-Full-Session

**TP_Videos_Phase_II_28-29.zip**

TP_Video_28_Thematic-Map-&-Release-Short-Version

TP_Video_29_Grounding-Light-Stream-Exercise!

**TP_Videos_Phase_III_30-32.zip**

TP_Video_30_How-to-Overcome-Emotional-Neglect

TP_Video_31_Emotional-Neglect-&-Loneliness

TP_Video_32_Recover-Childhood-Emotional-Neglect

**TP_Video_Phase_III_33.zip**

TP_Video_33_Healing-Relationships-After-Neglect

**TP_Videos_Phase_III_34-35.zip**

TP_Video_34_Tame-and-Decode-Bad-Dreams

TP_Video_35_Go-Slow-to-Heal-After-Trauma

**TP_Videos_Phase_III_36-37.zip**

TP_Video_36_Shake-to-Release-Stress-Exercise

TP_Video_37_From-Fear-to-Shake-&-Laughter

**TP_Videos_Phase_III_38-41.zip**

TP_Video_38_Day31-Self-Compassion-Reflection

TP_Video_39_Reflection-on-Self-Compassion

TP_Video_40_Create-a-Wellness-Mind-Map

TP_Video_41_The-Importance-of-Community

## How to proceed:

### 1. Create a user account (or, if you have already one, please log in)

For customers from the USA and Canada:

hgf.io/login-us

For customers from the rest of the world:

hgf.io/login-eu

### 2. Download your supplementary materials

Go to My supplementary materials in your account dashboard and enter the code below. You will automatically be redirected to the download area, where you can access and download the supplementary materials.

**Code: B-P268YS**

To make sure you have permanent direct access to all the materials, we recommend that you download them and save them on your computer.